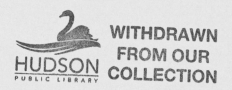

HOMEGROWN HERBS

A Complete Guide to Growing, Using, and Enjoying More than **100 Herbs**

Tammi Hartung

Photography by Saxon Holt

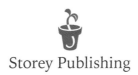

Storey Publishing

Dedicated to Chris and M'lissa, with love

The mission of Storey Publishing is to serve our customers by publishing practical information that encourages personal independence in harmony with the environment.

Edited by Carleen Madigan and Anne Halpin White
Art direction and book design by Jessica Armstrong

Photography by © Saxon Holt except for © CuboImages/Alamy 227 right; © GAP Photos, Ltd./BBC Magazines, Ltd. 215 right; © Bob Gibbons/Alamy 188; © Storey Publishing 56 & 96; Mars Vilaubi 111
Garden plan illustrations by Alison Kolesar
Insect illustrations by Brigita Fuhrmann and Kurt Musfeldt

Indexed by Christine R. Lindemer, Boston Road Communications

© 2011 by Tammi Hartung
An earlier version of this book was published under the title *Growing 101 Herbs That Heal* (Storey Publishing, 2000)

Storey books are available for special premium and promotional uses and for customized editions. For further information, please call 1-800-793-9396.

Storey Publishing
210 MASS MoCA Way
North Adams, MA 01247
www.storey.com

Printed in China by Toppan Leefung Printing Ltd.
10 9 8 7 6 5 4 3 2 1

Library of Congress Cataloging-in-Publication Data

Hartung, Tammi, 1961–
  Homegrown herbs / Tammi Hartung ; photography by Saxon Holt.
    p. cm.
  Includes index.
  ISBN 978-1-60342-703-6 (pbk. : alk. paper)
  ISBN 978-1-60342-705-0 (hardcover : alk. paper)
  1. Herbs. 2. Herb gardening. 3. Herbs—Utilization. 4. Herbs—Therapeutic use.
  5. Cooking (Herbs) I. Holt, Saxon. II. Title.
SB351.H5H3236 2011
635'.7—dc22
                                                    2010043055

CONTENTS

ACKNOWLEDGMENTS

MY DANCE WITH THE PLANTS began a long time ago, over 30 years now. My journey to understand how to grow and use them will be ongoing for all the rest of the days that I walk on this earth. Many people have played a role in my understanding of and inspiration for working with herbs.

I offer my gratitude and appreciation to my elders, within my family and my community, and to the teachers who have helped me learn about plants.

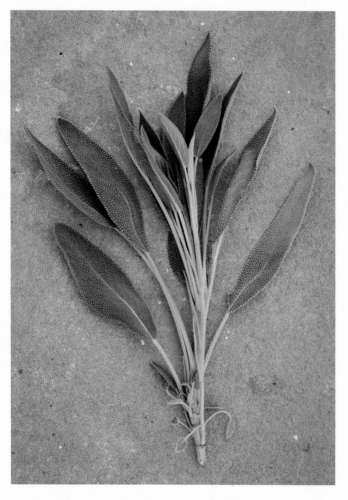

My love and deepest thanks to my husband, Chris, my daughter, M'lissa, and my wonderful parents, Alvin and Carroll. They nurture and love me in every way and have given me so much support in the writing of this book.

Thank you to Rosemary Gladstar, who came into my life as my teacher, who has enriched my life as one of my most treasured friends. She has done me the great honor of writing the foreword for this book. Much love to you, Rosemary.

I offer my thanks to Saxon Holt, the photographer. He made the photo shoots easy and fun, for which I am very grateful. He is a joyful man with great talent.

I am deeply indebted to Carleen, my editor at Storey, who has been a constant source of guidance, kind and inspiring words, and good editorial advice. Thank you, Carleen. I appreciate you! To the rest of the Storey staff, thank you for being so helpful in every way.

This book reflects all the positive energy I've been gifted with by many individuals during the course of my life and my work with plants. I hold every one of you in my heart with honor and respect. You are each a piece of the reason that I embrace this passion for plants and have chosen this lifestyle.

Foreword by Rosemary Gladstar

FOR THE PAST 40 YEARS I HAVE SPENT MUCH OF MY TIME IN A GARDEN — watering, tending, weeding, planting, and mostly enjoying. I've had the great good fortune to have planted two gardens that became public gardens, sanctuaries for plants that many others came to enjoy. And I've had the pleasure of visiting hundreds of other gardens and the lucky people who tended them. One of the most amazing and most prolific of gardeners is Tammi Hartung, the astute authoress of this amazing book you hold in your hands. I've known Tammi for so many years now, I can't even recall the first time I met her. But for as long as I've known her, she's been a gardener extraordinaire and a brilliant plantsperson, deeply engrossed in the secret life of plants, and versed in with their inner teachings.

Tammi is a master gardener with all plants and can coax anything to grow, but first and foremost she loves herbs — those magic healing plants that were used so aptly by our ancestors for health, healing, spiritual, and culinary purposes. Though a renowned gardener, Tammi is also an accomplished medical herbalist and educator, and is often asked to speak at conferences and events around the country. But there's nowhere she's more at home than in her gardens at Desert Canyon Farm, and nothing that she'd rather talk about than gardening and her beloved herbs.

Tammi and her husband, Chris, settled on their farm over a decade ago. Located at the base of a mountain in the high desert of southern Colorado, one would hardly call the land that they settled on a gardener's haven. With too little water, too much sun, and very cold winters, those first few years were challenging; but with hard work and ingenuity, they transformed this high desert property into a gardener's paradise. Even more than a garden, Desert Canyon Farm became a sanctuary, a pleasant refuge for flocks of birds, butterflies and other beneficial insects, wild animals, and people who are hungry to learn about the green world. Here, in the gardens, Tammi holds a variety of popular community events, and hosts programs specially geared toward schoolchildren. Much of her work centers on the healing property of herbs.

When Tammi talks about the healing power of plants, her message is of much broader scale than using them only as medicine for humans. She understands and appreciates the plants also as medicines of and for the earth, within the garden and the larger landscape that surrounds our garden plots. As Stephen Buhner, herbalist and author, states in the foreward to *Plant Spirit Healing* by Pam Montgomery,

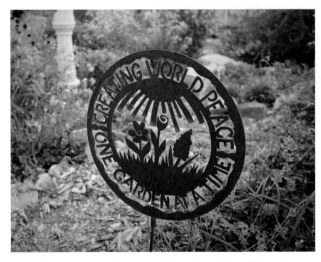

When everyone has good food on their table and herbal remedies for health and well-being in their cupboard, the world will indeed be a more peaceful and sustainable place.

"That plant medicines are used throughout ecosystems by insects, birds, reptiles, mammals, and other plants is something long overlooked by reductionist researchers. Overlooked as well is that plants can, and will, determine just what particular chemical an ill member of an ecosystem needs, and further, they will then begin making it for them." Tammi applies these principles — using the herbs' own inherent healing properties to help balance and heal the garden's ecosystem — to problem-solve the issues that

This entire book teaches us to "think like a plant" when we garden.

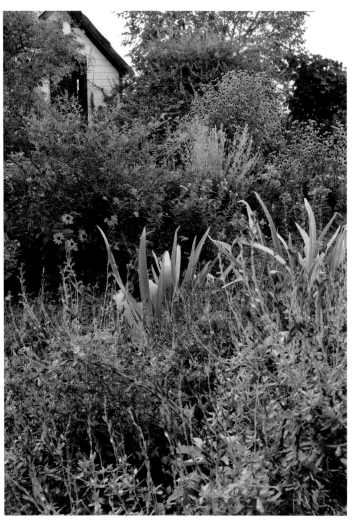

Gardens should be beautiful, as well as practical. They can nourish our bodies while also lifting our spirits with their rich colors and intoxicating fragrances!

arise in a garden. And it's in her gardens — walking among the diverse beds of flowers, herbs, vegetables, and wild plants, with hummingbirds darting about, bird feeders full of songbirds, and an occasional rabbit or even a deer strolling at the outskirts of the garden — that one sees this healing power and rich biodiversity at its best.

It is here at Desert Canyon Farm that Tammi perfected her skills and expanded her view of gardening beyond the normal realms of what belongs and what doesn't belong in a garden. *The rules change here.* That's one of the things I find so intriguing about this book. Tammi is, without doubt, eminently practical, and her advice in growing plants is always simple and direct. But there's also an interconnectedness woven into everything she does, so that what appears as simple is in fact profound, as in this "simple" piece of advice she offers us: "If you are new to growing herbs, then remember the only rule is that there *are* no rules." She then goes on to tell us, "Many of the herbs — especially those closest to their wild roots — seem to hate rules, and they are very good at breaking them." Oh, I love that! Or how about "Set aside technology for a moment and begin to think like the plant you want to grow." This entire book teaches us to "think like a plant" when we garden.

Thinking like a plant isn't all that difficult, thanks to Tammi's wonderfully clear instructions. Her approach is mostly about common sense and awareness. It's also about reevaluating our current notions about garden weeds, wild animals, and soil, and envisioning our gardens as part of the greater ecosystem. She says, "Everything in a growing environment is interwoven: soil, water, temperature, insect populations, and pollinators." How to welcome, enhance, and encourage them is part of our goal as gardeners.

Few people can take such broad concepts, weave them into simple doable steps, and manifest a garden. That's the brilliance of Tammi's teachings. She herself is eminently practical: What's going to make my garden thrive, make the plants stronger, the soil richer, my body healthier, and my community happier? She's thinking of the whole interconnected weave of life as she weeds and hoes, and considers which herbs to plant next to one another, who and what to chase out of the garden, and who to invite in. It's a philosophy that begins with the best choice of seed, where best to plant them, what to feed the soil, what method of watering is best, which insects to encourage, how to attract beneficial pollinators, and what's really the best way to manage the deer "problem" and those carrot-loving rabbits.

Tammi's ideas are refreshing, and they work. Even though I've gardened for a long time, I still find this book to be rich with earthly wisdom and enthralling ideas that continuously encourage me to review my gardening methods. Isn't that the best book of all, one that teaches us quietly, doesn't scream too loudly, and encourages us to review our methods and belief systems? Who says that deer, after all, are always a threat to a garden? And perhaps there are solutions to our deer problems other than deer fencing and/or shooting them? There *are* other solutions offered herein. . . .

Tammi gardens, too, because she's dedicated to medicinal plant conservation and knows that one of the best ways to help conserve wild plant populations is by growing high-quality organic herbs for market. Poor logging practices, urban sprawl, poor harvesting techniques, and the rapidly growing herbal market have caused a dearth of some of our most popular and effective native herbal medicines, some of them found growing nowhere else in the world other than North America. In 1994, a group of herbalists and plant lovers came together to form a small grassroots organization, United Plant Savers (UpS), that is dedicated solely to the preservation and cultivation of native medicine plants. From the beginning, Tammi was active in the organization and served as a dedicated advisory board member for many years. Her gardens are a reflection of her conservation work with medicinal plants, and Desert Canyon Farm is a designated UpS Botanical Sanctuary, providing a safe haven for many of the plants that are at risk in the wild. We grow herbs to use them and we also grow them to protect them from extinction.

* * *

This book is meant to make us think like a plant and like a gardener of plants. It also gives readers every skill they need to create a successful, bountiful garden. From soil to seed to harvest, there is nothing missing here. If I were just a novice, I could

pick up my hoe (that special kind she tells me about in the pages of her book that makes my job of hoeing so much easier), order my seeds, and start turning the soil, knowing that I have the knowledge needed to begin the sacred act of creating a garden, a sanctuary for all living beings. Even for me, an experienced gardener, there's so much in these pages that stimulate me and encourage me to try new ideas and methods.

How wonderful to see gardening becoming popular again as people reinvest in their food sources as a direct route to better health, and as they yearn, out of dire need born in their souls, to reconnect to the earth again. Nothing connects us more than digging in the rich, moist soil teeming with microbial activity, planting those seeds, and watching them grow. It is life manifest! People have been doing gardening for millennia, knowing it not only produces the best food possible but that it also fosters a deep sense of belonging.

And what better accomplishment to not only have a garden and grow your own food, but also be able to make your own medicine from your garden plants. Tammi, an accomplished herbalist as well as a gardener, has been making herbal medicine and teaching herb classes for many years. I don't think she could write a book about growing herbs without including a wonderful array of her favorite herbal recipes and remedies for home health care. Growing plants and making one's own kitchen remedies has been such a long tradition of human beings. Our ancestors all over the planet have been doing the same things for eons — caretaking, planting, growing, making food and medicine.

In the simple act of sharing the bounty from her garden (both through her harvest and through her teachings), Tammi is ensuring that this ancient tradition survives.

As she writes in the preface of her first book, "This is my work, play, rest and spirituality." Dig deeply. Delve into these pages. You'll find not only practical advice and endless tips on growing herbs, but a wise, deep, friendly voice, poetic and kind, guiding you on.

Preface

THIS BOOK REFLECTS A CONTINUATION OF MY LIFE STORY. It offers a peek into the lifestyle my husband, Chris, and I follow, as well as the work we do here at Desert Canyon Farm. Both our lifestyle and our work are interwoven with plants and people. The farm is our home and sits at the base of the mountains in the high desert of southern Colorado. Chris and I decided in 1996, after many years of working for others, that it was time to stop managing arboretums, working at herbal manufacturing facilities, and propagating plants for other people, and to do something on our own. That first spring, we planted 34 different medicinal plants in our field, and the following fall we put up a greenhouse. We started an herb school with a few public workshops and a two-year herbal apprenticeship program. We were in business.

Much has changed through the years, as this is the nature of farming. Our strategy is to remain diversified in our products, but to keep the focus on herbs, heirloom and ethnic food plants, and open-pollinated seed crops, all grown with earth-friendly, organic methods. Our business and our personal life revolve around the plants. Our field production has moved away from medicinal herbs and we now produce perennial flower and grass seed crops instead. That first greenhouse has grown to seven. They hold our field starts and provide us with our primary income-producing wholesale potted herbs, heirloom vegetables, and the miniature plants used in fairy gardens.

Today's society is fast-paced, and all about accomplishing more than is reasonable in each day's time. Our society has become consumed with "stuff," and we often can be so intent on accumulating more that we forget to enjoy the very things and events we want to be the building blocks of our lifestyle. This book is about acknowledging what is important and nurturing in your life. It will offer you guidance, skills, and inspiration to grow and use herbs in every aspect of your lifestyle. It is about honoring what is simple, beautiful, and empowering. I want to share here in these pages, from the many lessons of my own life, how to choose ways to enrich your lifestyle by allowing herbs to play an important role.

A few years ago we made the decision to close our herb school and my private practice, and to stop doing consulting work. This allows us the time, beyond the growing of plants, to focus on hosting groups of schoolchildren at the farm, as well as time for me to write about all the things related to an earth-friendly lifestyle. Seldom does a day pass when the farm isn't as busy as a beehive.

When we arrived, no one knew what to think of us, those crazy herb growers up on the hill. One gentleman, who works in the prison industry here, reminded us as he was introducing himself that a neighbor of ours was "busted for having pot in his barn." Chris smiled and said, "Well, the only thing you'll find in our barn is catnip." Since that wary neighbor's introduction, much has changed, and the community has become very much a part of the farm. Spring brings our annual series of public open-farm dates and workshops, plus a huge farm plant sale. Neighbors constantly drop in for visits and to seek a bit of plant advice for their gardens. We have become very much a part of our community, and it feels great!

Chris and I maintain our tradition of finding time to sit on the porch and enjoy the chiminea (a Southwestern outdoor fireplace) in the evening or take in a soak at the local hot springs. Chris is a jazz musician and a dedicated bike rider and lap swimmer, while I do my needlework, bake sourdough breads, and take my morning walks along the Arkansas River. Our daughter, M'lissa, has long since flown the nest, but she visits often, and helps out occasionally with farm projects while studying for her master's degree in archaeology.

For us, our work affords us this lifestyle, which we feel is nurturing and important and allows us to live in a beautiful geographic location. We're not likely ever to get close to a high income bracket, and it is doubtful that retirement will be part of our future. Those are the trade-offs. We have everything we need and much of what we want in a place where the pace of life is a bit gentler. Life is rich in abundance.

I hope this book will help you to embrace your relationship with the place you call home and the plants that live in that space. Design and plant gardens that are practical and bring beauty into your home. Take advantage of the gifts plants offer you, and trust in your intuition and creativity. Use herbs to prepare delicious meals, support your good health and well-being, and make your home a comfortable, sacred place. As you bring herbs into every part of your life, offer your gratitude to the plants and the gifts they offer you. Take care of your gardens in a way that is earth-friendly and supports our great planet. Teach your children what you know and what you are still learning, for they are the caretakers of the future.

The fields at Desert Canyon Farm are more beautiful than ever, the gardens have grown to gorgeous maturity, and our ponds are alive with the earth's creatures. Chris and I often reflect on the fact that we have come a long way from when we arrived in Cañon City as just a couple of "crazy herb farmers," and we are in a place of gratitude.

I hope my passion for herbs and an earth-friendly philosophy will infuse the pages of this book in

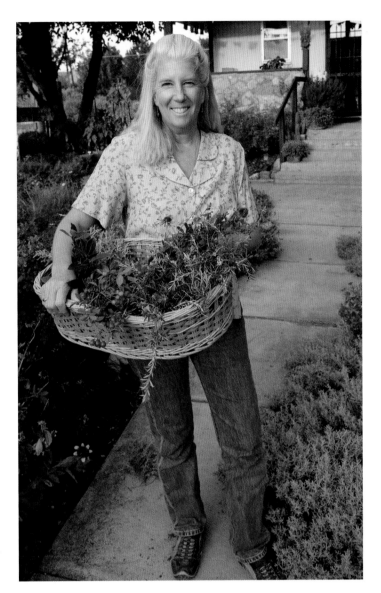

such a way that I am a good and humble voice for the plants. I hope that the gifts and lessons that Chris and I have learned through the years will offer helpful insights as you grow your gardens and use the herbs to enrich your lifestyle. That passion is what I'm all about, and my wish is that it will inspire you.

With green thoughts,

Tammi Hartung

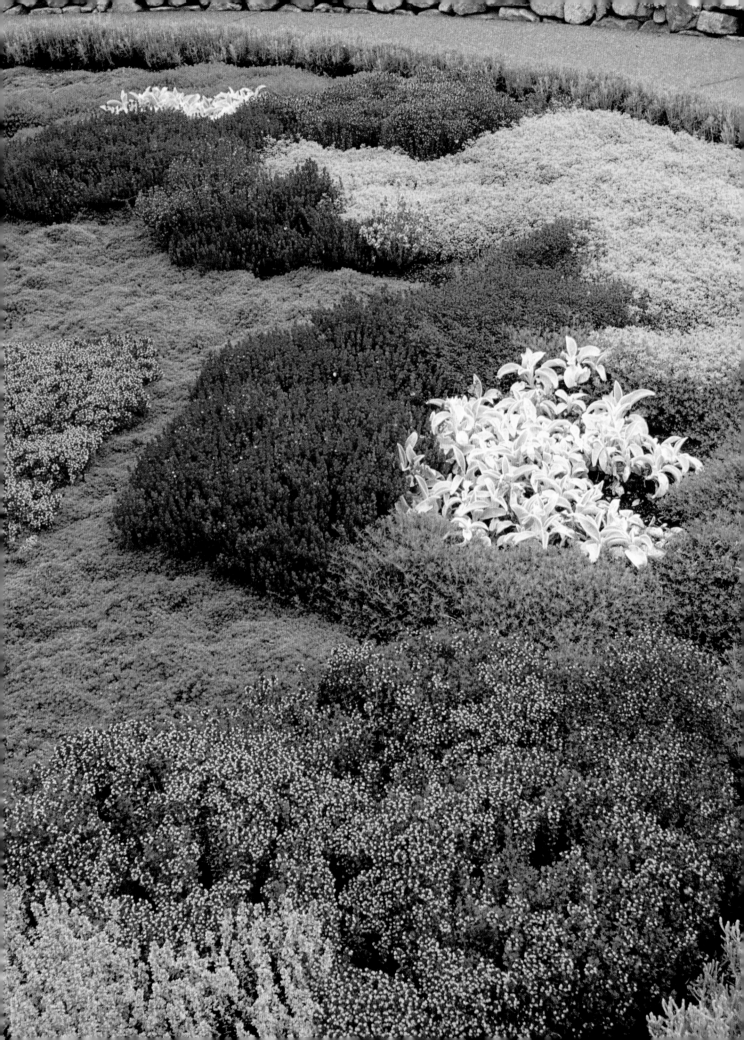

CHAPTER ONE

An Introduction to Growing and Using Herbal Plants

Since the beginning of human history, we have needed plants for our very survival. And from the earliest days, humankind has learned that cultivating plants was often easier and more reliable than harvesting wild plants. Our knowledge and skills have developed through the years, so that we choose plants for our gardens that are not only useful, but also beautiful. Although we still need plants for survival, we also count on them to help us enhance our lifestyles. Indeed, the history of our relationship with the garden is constantly evolving. Its roots are very long — and still growing.

Remembering Our Roots

Through time, we have learned how to use plants for food and medicine, to make them into textiles and structures, and for our personal needs. Through the centuries, gardens have maintained their usefulness, but they have also become places that stimulate our sense of beauty and well-being. Growing a garden brings pleasure, the prospect of improving one's health, and the abundance of harvest. A garden can also contribute to the health of the earth, when it's grown in a sustainable, earth-friendly way. I ask you to explore the richness of herb gardening as a lifestyle and as a way to do your part to improve the well-being of our glorious planet.

The tradition of cultivating plants for a specific need has always been an integral part of human history. Early on we used plants to survive; in our more recent history, we've come to use plants also for the pleasure of improving our lifestyle. As time continues, we begin to understand that we humans are not the only living beings depending on these plants, and we are beginning to develop the wisdom to be good caretakers, in order to ensure that plant populations thrive. This brings to the forefront of our consciousness an important concept: It is not our intended purpose to control the world, but rather to exist in partnership with all other living creatures. My question to you is simply this: Have you thought about the positive impact you can have on the earth by simply growing an herb garden?

SAVING WILD PLANTS

By encouraging conservation, herb gardeners can have an important, positive impact on the well-being of wild plant populations. Unfortunately, many wild herbs are under stress from habitat destruction, overharvesting by commercial product manufacturers, and climate change (to name just a few reasons). United Plant Savers is a nonprofit organization that strives to save wild medicinal plants through education, research, and encouraging organic cultivation. See Resources, page 245, for contact information.

Let me share a story, one you will most likely recognize.

In the beginning of humankind, we honored our relationship with the green nation. We used plants for food and medicine, to make clothing and practical utensils, and as an integral part of our spiritual traditions. We carefully gathered and thanked each plant in anticipation of how we would use it. Later, we learned to cultivate some of the plants, primarily those we used for food. Other plants, such as those with medicinal properties, we still gathered from the wild. As time passed, the larger percentage of the plants we used were cultivated.

Now well into the twenty-first century, I look around and see more and more people returning to their roots. That sense of improving one's lifestyle through individual empowerment continues to grow in popularity. People of all ages are holding on to the desire to take more control over the foods they eat, their health care, the clothing and household linens they want to use . . . the list goes on and on.

We are all concerned about the quality of the things we use in our daily lives. We want to make sure we have plenty of options that reflect our preferences. Each of us seems to be seeking personalized ways to enrich the day-to-day tasks of living, whether that be cooking, bathing, taking care of our health, or simply making life fun for our family and even our pets.

People everywhere are more conscious of how their lifestyle choices affect the greater reality of life on this earth. We are becoming acutely aware that our decisions as consumers have very serious impacts on the sustainability of our planet, our personal quality of life, and the quality of life of all the other members of the human society in this complicated world we call home.

More and more of us are also thinking about all the ways we can improve how we live. We are taking greater responsibility for the richness of our seniors' lives, the completeness of our adult lives, and the future quality of our children's and grandchildren's lives. As crazy as it may sound, growing and using herbs fits perfectly into a responsible and sustainable way of living healthy lives and protecting the future.

Let's Start in the Garden

Everything begins in the simplest (yet also most complicated) place, one of pure magic and positive energy: the garden.

The decision to plant an herb garden of some kind — be it a formal knot garden, a patio container garden, a few pots of herbs on a windowsill or a countertop, or herbs tucked into an existing garden — is a huge step toward enriching your lifestyle.

Growing herbs is a practical idea. It means you will have on hand the fresh herbs you need for cooking. Perhaps you want to find natural ways to support your health and would like to have a ready supply of medicinal herbs for the medicine chest. If you drink herbal teas, your goal may be to ensure that your teas are of the highest quality. And for those of us who are concerned about our budgets, growing herbs gives us the abundance of harvest at very little expense.

Although practicality is important to me, I also choose to grow herbs for their simple beauty and for the richness they add to my life through their colors and textures and fragrance. I love how they look in my gathering spaces, on the back porch and in my kitchen sitting area. They impart a sense of welcome, comfort, and good energy!

Nourishing Our Bodies and Our Earth

As we plant our gardens, we must cultivate them in a nurturing and honoring way. We must learn to grow these plants organically, without synthetic chemicals. This means using great discrimination in what types of fertilizers we choose, as well as finding the most effective and least harmful ways to control pests, diseases, and weed problems. We must learn how to nurture the soil, use water in a conservative way, and take advantage of companion/complementary planting. It is equally important to honor the wild creatures that give us a helping hand with our gardening: the honeybees and bats pollinating our sage flowers, the wild birds eating caterpillars off our comfrey leaves, the microbes aerating our soil.

As we create garden schemes and designs, we must learn to think a bit more like a plant and a little less like a person. I challenge you to think about where each plant grows in nature, the ideal place

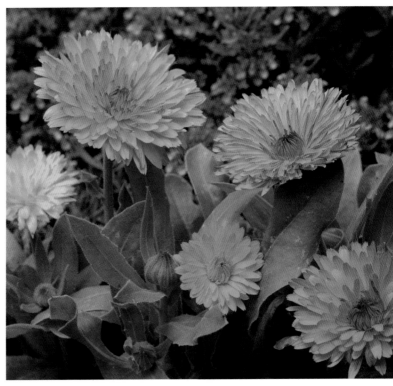

A popular herb, calendula can be used in a variety of ways. This cheerful flower might act as a coloring agent for your cake frosting, or be an important ingredient in your sunburn relief spray.

THE IMPORTANCE OF ORGANIC GARDENING

If I'm going to use a plant herbally, I want to know that it's not going to be full of chemicals that not only do nothing to promote health but also, and worse, may actually harm my body. I also must know that the earth has not been compromised or contaminated. Gardening organically — that is, without using harmful substances that poison the earth and our bodies — is essential.

of its own choosing. Would a plant choose a shady place near a stream or would it find a sunny, gravelly slope more to its liking? What will a seed need in order to sprout? Maybe it requires a harsh winter, or perhaps it must land in a dark place, like under a fallen leaf, before it finds the right circumstances to germinate. If we learn the personality of each plant, we can then decide how best to incorporate it into our gardens.

Gardening for the Soul

Whether you garden for pure pleasure or for practicality, growing herbs is important and enjoyable. It may be a way for you to improve your health by taking advantage of the medicinal benefits of the plants, or to offer healing remedies to your family and friends. And the act of gardening itself is therapeutic and healing.

Organic gardening most certainly will be an opportunity for you to nurture the piece of the earth where you live. It is a chance for you to make a grassroots statement about how important it is to have organically grown herbs in your foods, teas, and medicines (and anything else you use them for). It is a way for you to immediately affect the earth's environment, simply by growing your own herbs instead of buying herbs imported from distant places that require a huge carbon input to get them from where they grow to your table. This type of social responsibility is easy and painless, and produces positive results on many levels.

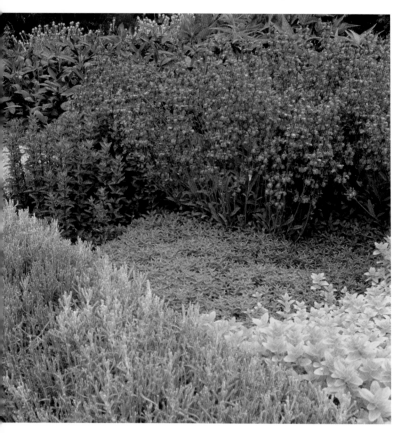

The beauty of the garden space heals the spirit and soul, just as the plants offer healing to the body. The design can be as simple as a set of containers or as elaborate as a formal knot garden.

Encouraging an Herbal Lifestyle

Growing herbs is only one piece of the pie. As you use herbs to enrich your own lifestyle, you will also be leading by example. Every meal you prepare with herbs and serve to company may inspire someone else to expand his culinary creativity. Every herbal foot soak you give to someone else is a wonderful gift, and because she enjoyed it so much, she may just turn around and gift someone else with a foot soak. Each time you encourage a child to grow an herb and then make it into a necklace for dress-up, you give her life skills as a gardener and nourish her imagination . . . both wonderful! As you intentionally bring herbs into your own life, just think how many other people you will be teaching through your own living example.

Picking and Choosing

I'm often asked how I decide which herbs to grow. There are many factors involved. You might want to plant a garden based on personal health issues. You may like to cook a specific type of cuisine and want to have appropriate herbs for those dishes. Always begin with plants for which you have a personal liking, plants you think you will use the most.

In selecting the plants for this book, I wanted to share those for which I have a special fondness, but also plants that are broadly useful and fun to grow. I like a lot of variety in my life and hence I love having lots of herbs to choose from. I'm hoping that my enthusiasm for variety will be contagious. Be prepared: As you read and use this book, you will probably fall in love with many of these plants. Keep in mind, however, that this is just the tip of the iceberg. There are thousands of herbs you could consider growing as you travel on your gardening journey.

I also give consideration to plants for which it isn't always easy to find growing information. My experience has often been one of frustration as I struggled to discover how to design an herb garden, and to propagate and organically grow and maintain herbal plants. But I have learned to turn my frustration into an adventure. Now I want to save you some of that frustration and encourage you to become adventurous in your herb gardening experiences.

Enjoy the journey!

A GUIDE TO USING THIS BOOK

THIS BOOK HAS BEEN ARRANGED to make it easy and fun to read. You will find information that speaks of my own experiences. The step-by-step adventure begins with planning and designing your garden (chapter 2). An in-depth look at maintaining healthy soils (chapter 3) follows. Then you'll discover how to propagate different herbs (chapter 4), and to incorporate them into your garden.

Of course, no gardening book would be complete without instructions for maintaining healthy plants, so you'll find that information in chapter 5. Be sure to read chapter 6 carefully for general insight into organic insect and disease management, as well as how to make your garden more wildlife-friendly in ways that you and nature can both live with.

I want to inspire you to harvest your plants, so I've provided a detailed harvesting guide in chapter 7. You'll find information on cooking with herbs and using them throughout your home in chapters 8 and 9, which include delectable recipes and fun projects (even directions for making your own herbal cat toys). I provide easy-to-follow directions for the kitchen "pharmacy" (chapter 9), where you will prepare your own medicinal remedies. So you can get to know many different herbs up close and personal, I have profiled each

one of them in chapter 10, Herb Personalities. Come back to this section whenever you want to understand or experiment with a specific herb and need to know a lot about it individually. In addition, I've included many detailed charts that will be great quick reference points when you need a bit of information fast. Finally, a note about the botanical Latin names in the book. You will notice that whenever a genus name for a plant is listed several times together, only the first letter will be given as an abbreviation of the genus, followed by the species and variety names.

If you need some guidance on where to buy seeds or other gardening supplies, or if you're looking for further information on a particular subject, simply turn to page 246. There you'll find a reading list of my favorite plant books, so you can explore individual subjects further. There is also information on resources such as gardening supply companies and professional organizations.

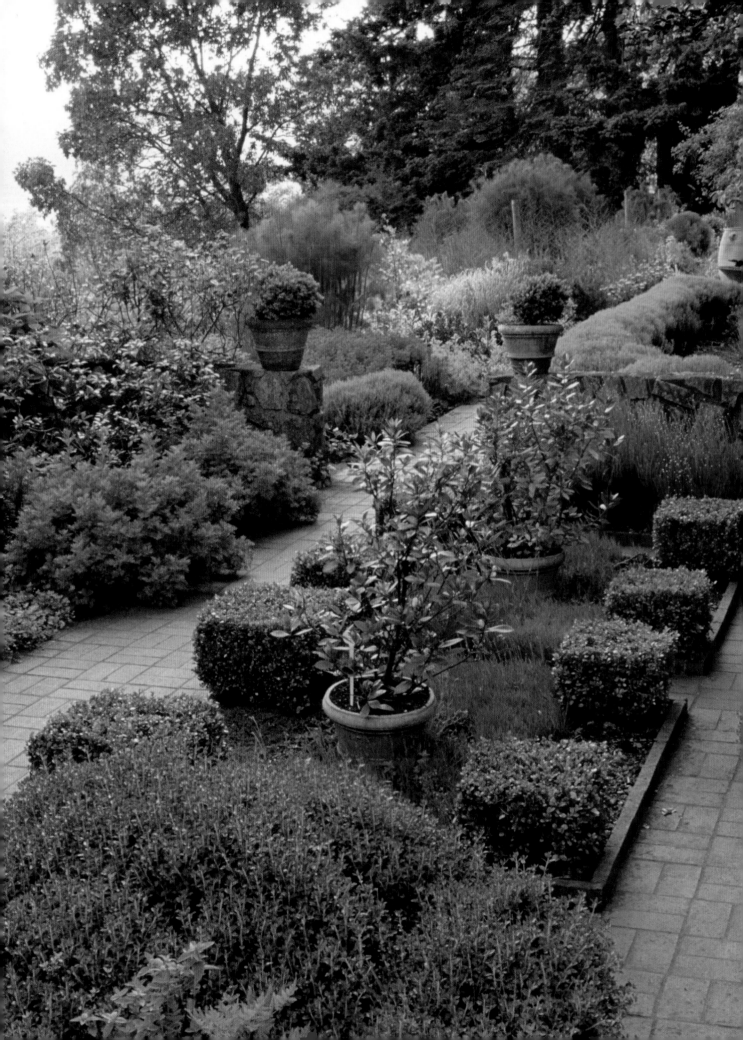

CHAPTER TWO

Selecting Plants and Designing Your Garden

As every gardener — seasoned and beginner — knows, the next best thing to actually planting the garden is designing and planning it. This is certainly one of my favorite parts of the process. There are many things to ponder, like how big it will be, whether it will be located in the sun or shade, what kinds of colors it will display. So many possibilities! Still, as creative as designing and planning are, there are some guidelines to consider that will make a project come together smoothly. And so you begin...

Discovering Your Garden Personality

The first question you must answer is a personal one. What type of garden personality are you? Do you like a very formal garden? Maybe you're a practical-garden personality, or perhaps you're a wild-garden type.

It is also possible that the garden space itself has some personality traits that need to be considered. Do you want this garden to be easily accessible from the kitchen? You might want to plant a scented medicinal garden beneath a bathroom or bedroom window. Perhaps you would prefer to grow herbs in containers on a deck or balcony.

> The garden you plant today
> may be very different from the one
> you plant five years from now.

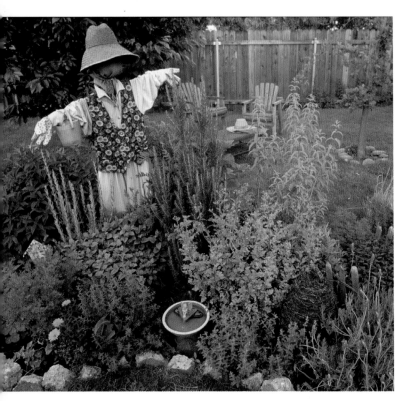

The colorful and fun addition of a scarecrow in this herb garden reflects the whimsical personality of the gardener.

Usually the more formal the garden is, the more time will be required to care for it. I always recommend a bit of soul-searching before designing a garden. It will bring you little pleasure if you design a garden for yourself that fits another's garden personality. (If you are asked to design a garden for someone else, keep your own personality to yourself and be sensitive to the other person's preferences.) This is also the most appropriate time to do a reality check with yourself. Ask yourself these crucial but sometimes difficult questions: "How much time do I plan to spend caring for this garden? Is that a reasonable expectation for the type of garden I hope to plant and for the lifestyle I'm currently leading?" The answers to these questions will be different at various times in your life. The garden you plant today may be very different from the one you plant five years from now.

For example, when my daughter was young, I grew many herbs that could be used for children's illnesses, like lemon balm for symptom relief of common viruses and spearmint for tummyaches. I also offered a corner of the garden space to M'lissa, for her to plant her own herbs. She grew chamomile for tea, violas to snack on (they are delicious, you know), and woolly lamb's ears for soothing skinned knees.

Now that I no longer have a small child at home, my garden has taken on a different face. My garden today features red clover for supporting my bone health as I get older and plantain to soothe an angry bee sting. Because I love to cook, I grow lots of culinary herbs. And still there are all colors of violas, because they are delicious and beautiful after all! I am passionate about growing my own food gardens and through the years the gardens have become an intermingled blend of herbs growing alongside strawberries, radicchio, and climbing beans of all sorts. Ten years from now, I'm sure my garden will take on a different character yet again, perhaps with more containers or planter boxes as I become less inclined to crawl around on my knees to weed in my elder years. Gardens are, and should be, flexible to change as our lifestyles shift.

Siting the Garden

In order to design your garden, you must first determine where in your yard it will be. Sit quietly for a moment and observe the potential areas. Consider these questions:

- What existing features are in the area? Are there buildings or fences, trees and shrubs, or maybe a stream?

- What will border the garden space — a patio, lawn, woodland?

- What type of light does each area get? Is it in full shade, in sun, a bit of both?

- Do you plan to plant in beds, in rows, or in containers?

- Is the existing soil decent or will you need to prepare it more extensively?

- Is the location visually pleasing, or is it most important that it just be a practical space?

I find it's always wise to answer these questions as best I can while I'm sitting *in* the proposed garden space, where I can see and feel the situation. I take detailed notes about all I observe. These are very helpful to me during the design process.

Planning for Easy Access

Whether you are establishing a brand-new garden or integrating herbs into an existing bed, easy access is key. Several factors should be considered at this point. First and foremost, is the garden in a place where you can work in it easily and harvest from it on a whim? Many times I've listened to the same story: that a garden was planted and it turned out to be quite lovely, "but I never seem to use any of the herbs. They're just not handy." Being able to pop into the garden to pick some basil or heartsease flowers enables you to use fresh basil in your spaghetti sauce and to serve a salad dressed with beautiful edible flowers. Ease of harvesting herbs is important. Often in our busy lives we spend only short bits of time working in the garden; if the garden is located conveniently, then all is well. If not,

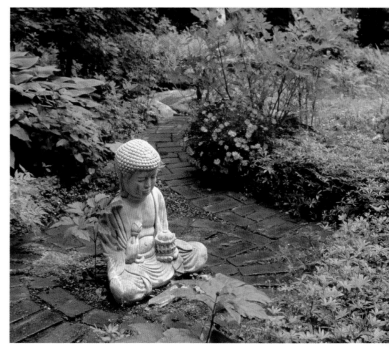

An herb garden holds useful plants, but at the same time it can be a restful, sacred, and beautiful place to relax.

the weeds tend to gain the upper hand and the mint begins to ramble beyond its allocated space.

Considering the logistics of access before the garden is planted will make your life much easier. Discovering *after* the garden is planted that a key factor doesn't work very well is one of my most frustrating gardening experiences. As an example, imagine that you planted a glorious garden only to discover that there isn't easy access to a hose for watering. Or perhaps you put the garden in your dog's favorite running location and he isn't willing to "give way" to your garden. These are frustrations that usually happen to all gardeners at some time in their gardening career, but taking a bit of time ahead of the actual planting to problem-solve will mean far fewer of these kinds of gardening difficulties.

If you think about these challenges after the garden is in place, you'll find yourself grumbling as you drag heavy hoses around the yard. And you certainly don't want to be pushing a rototiller all over the place, trying to figure out how to access a new garden area without causing damage to trees and fences, for example. Just imagine how entertaining that would be for onlookers, and how disastrous it would be for your garden preparation!

Determining Size

Once you know where the garden will be, measure the space with a tape measure. Be reasonable in determining the size of your garden. All of us have eyes that are bigger than our abilities or our budget when it comes to planning a beautiful garden. It's no great pleasure to prepare a huge garden space and discover that it's too much to care for, or that it will be too expensive to plant the entire area.

Start with a reasonable amount of space that will match the level of commitment you can make to gardening it. You might feel you're being overcautious, but remember that garden additions are as much fun as the originals. Once you've decided on the size, write down those measurements for later reference.

Staking out the dimensions is a good approach to sizing, especially if you have trouble visualizing the actual size of an area. To do this, measure the length and width of the garden. Pound a stake into each of the four corners, and then run string between the parallel posts. This will give you a more accurate idea of the garden size you have chosen.

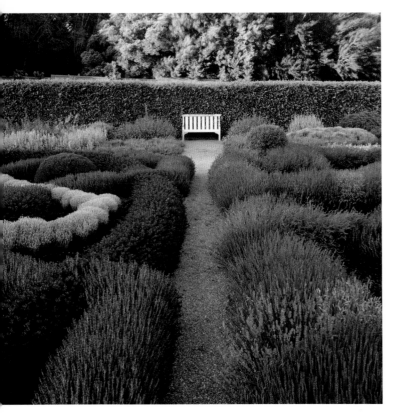

A large, labor-intensive knot garden can quickly become overwhelming.

START SMALL

For a new gardener, it's wise to begin with a small garden space and add to it as you feel comfortable. Start with a space that is 6 to 8 feet (1.8–2.4 m) square or round; use the guidelines in this chapter to help you. When you feel ready to expand, enlarge the perimeter by 2 to 6 feet (0.6–1.8 m) and then plant. You may decide to create a different shape for the garden as you're expanding. This is easily accomplished by creating a shape outside of the existing garden and then joining it to the garden as an extension.

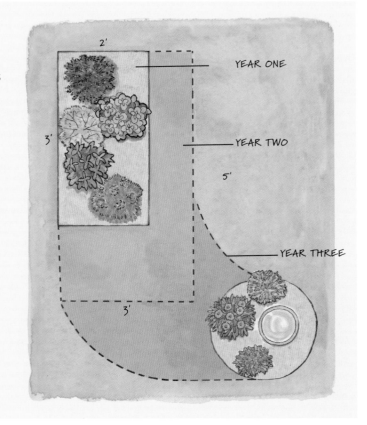

Drafting a Design

I like to work with a piece of graph paper when I'm designing a garden space. Pencil in the perimeters of the garden, using whatever scale you prefer. I usually make each square equal to ½ foot (15 cm), so that four graph squares equal one square foot (0.09 m²).

Add the Hardscaping

The next step is to draw in the hardgoods of the garden. These are the pathways, rocks, benches, focal points, and other structural elements. Be sure to include any existing features of the space, such as a patio, a fence, and buildings. Make decisions about what types of pathways or stepping-stones you would like to use — flagstones, grass, gravel, and even bark mulch are all very nice choices. Pathways and stepping-stones are among the most important components of garden design — they give access to maintain and harvest the garden without stepping on, and thus compacting, the soil around the plants.

Will you welcome birds (beneficial for controlling insect pests) or other wildlife into your garden? If so, be sure to include a bird feeder or birdbath or other watering spot. We also have a pond for the deer, turtles, and Canada geese to enjoy. If you want to entice honeybees and bumblebees to improve pollination, incorporate a water source for them, also — shallow pottery dishes work well — somewhere in the design.

Will your garden be a place to go and sit for a spell? There are many wonderful choices for a peaceful retreat. You might decide you'd like an elegant iron bench, or perhaps a willow chair would be more to your taste. Even a glorious old stump or flat boulder can make a lovely seat. I often combine a bench with an arbor to create a shaded place to sit and read or sketch. Arbors and trellises can also be important elements in the garden if you plan to grow climbing plants like hops and passionflower.

Focal Points

Every garden design benefits from having a focal point from which the rest of the garden flows. Sometimes there's more than one focal point, especially if a garden is large. You certainly could use one of your hardgoods — such as a bench, a trellis, a statue, or a fountain — as a focal point. The focal point may be a special plant, like a specimen tree or a rosebush. It's also nice to create the focus of the garden around a cluster of plants, such as three or four mullein plants or hollyhocks. Both mullein and hollyhocks are quite tall and their flowers add a splash of color along the spires, making them eye-catching as focal points.

> Will your garden
> be a place to go and
> sit for a spell?

If the garden is also a children's space, it might be fun to create a sunflower and morning glory playhouse as the focal point for the rest of the garden. Simply train the morning glories to climb up the stalks of the sunflowers, thus filling in the spaces to create "walls." Be sure to provide an entry to the playhouse.

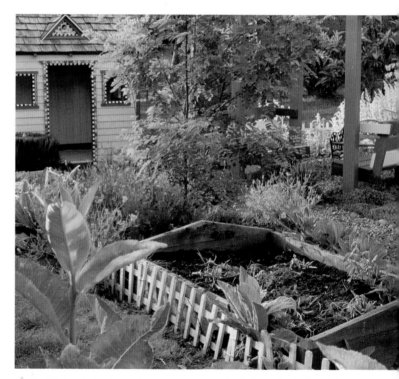

A children's herb garden can be a magical place that stimulates imagination and fun for even very young children. At the same time, it's a place to learn about gardening, harvesting, and using herbs.

Which Plant Where?

As you are drawing all of your ideas on graph paper, consider some basic points. Spacing requirements are a common concern. Plant height and flower color are always good to consider, too. I really appreciate knowing if a plant will grow in a clump or if it has a spreading nature. You will find specifics on spacing and flower color and other helpful details about the individual plants in the Plant Characteristics and Requirements chart on page 24.

Spacing Requirements

First of all, how much space should you give each plant. The answer will vary a bit depending on the individual plant you're working with, but as a general guideline, allow 10 to 12 inches (25–30 cm) for most plants. Of course there will be some that can be spaced much more closely than that, and certainly some will need more room to mature.

> Planning ahead goes a long way toward making a garden a great success.

WHICH PLANT WHEN?

As you prepare to plant your garden, you'll want to know if the time is right to put out a specific herb. Has all danger of frost passed yet? Many herbs are very tender, especially when they are young. They cannot stand up to freezing temperatures, so make sure you plant these tender ones in the garden late enough in spring to avoid frost.

Other herbs are quite durable and actually may prefer to be planted out earlier in the spring. It's helpful to know which ones may be started early from seed indoors and then transplanted out in late spring. Many plants do well if they are divided or transplanted in the fall. With the help of your local Cooperative Extension Service, determine approximate last frost dates for your area and plant accordingly. See chapter 4 for more details about the best times and methods of seeding and/or transplanting each herb.

Don't be deceived in the spring when you're putting out young plants. Most people forget to allow enough room between the plants and they end up with a garden that looks unpleasantly crowded as the plants come into maturity. The May garden will be much different from the July or August garden, and a second-year perennial garden will look a lot less sparse than it did during its first growing season. If you do plant too closely, you can dig up some plants and move them around a bit to provide more growing space; crowded conditions are not usually the end of the world. They do, however, create extra work. As you plan which plants to grow, check the spacing requirements and draw them into your design accordingly.

Light Exposure

As you are deciding the plan for your garden, spend some time watching how the sun travels across the space you are considering. Will the garden be located in full sun, partial shade, or full shade? Perhaps the garden will contain areas of many types of light exposure. This is important when you begin to select the plants you will grow.

Soil Type

What type of soil will you have available? Is it sandy, rich loam, clay, or gravel? You may have areas that are a combination of soil types. There are very few instances in which the soil is so poor that a good variety of herbs cannot be grown in it. However, defining the soil type before you plant will help you choose the most appropriate herbs to grow. Growing black cohosh in a gravelly soil is not the best idea. Penstemons, on the other hand, will thrive in it. Planning ahead goes a long way toward making a garden a great success.

Plant Height

The next important detail to know is approximately how tall a plant will be at maturity. You don't want to place short plants behind tall ones. If you set in herbs as front-of-the-border plants and later discover that they grow to 3 feet (0.9 m) tall and everything planted behind them is only 1 to 2 feet (30–60 cm) tall, your border becomes a living wall that will screen all that is behind it.

The Color Palette

Designing a garden is like painting a picture. Colors are what make the difference between a complex-looking garden and one that is simply planted with no attention to detail.

WHITE FLOWERS AND SILVERY OR GRAY FOLIAGE will play a critical role in how lively your garden looks throughout the growing season. I like to make sure I have 30 to 40 percent of my flower and foliage color in the white/gray/silver range. This allows the garden to look spunky during the late part of the season when even the best of gardens begin to look weary and faded.

PURPLES AND BLUES in foliage and flower color are beautiful, but planting from only that palette will produce a bluish hue in the garden when viewed even from nearby, because those colors lose their definition with distance. Try planting bright yellow, orange, red, or pink flowers throughout a blue or purple color scheme. This will visually separate the individual blue and purple flowers, so that you will see them all specifically, even from a distance.

RED AND ORANGE flowers and foliage look great together, but take care when planting a lot of these colors. This is a fiery and spicy combination; it can be a lot of fun, but it can just as easily look harsh.

PINKS are always pretty, but they sometimes clash with other colors. When using a lot of pinks, I like to utilize white and silver along with blue and purple foliage and flowers to create a watercolor effect.

As you contemplate the flower color, don't forget to use foliage textures, colors, and shapes to make your garden design more interesting. Foliage is always there, even after blooming has finished. In some cases, the foliage distinctions may be what really liven up a garden all year long, as many plants will remain green even through the winter months.

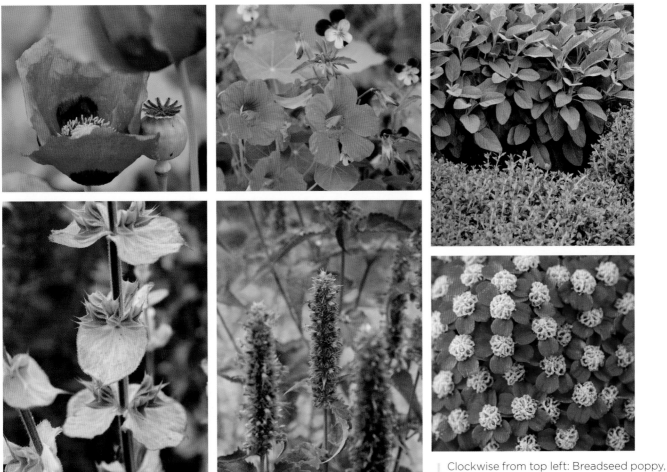

Clockwise from top left: Breadseed poppy, nasturtium, garden sage and santolina, yarrow, anise hyssop, and clary sage.

PLANT CHARACTERISTICS & REQUIREMENTS

THIS CHART PROVIDES THE BASIC INFORMATION you need to know about each herb in order to be able to incorporate it into a garden plan. Unlike the Plant Habitat Preferences chart (page 38), which gives a plant's first choices, the growing guidelines here are based on my experience. Although some information may not seem typical for a specific plant, I have learned that plants are often more flexible than we think. Over time you will learn each plant's limits and won't ask it to grow in a situation that is too far beyond its natural choices.

COMMON NAME (*LATIN NAME*)	CYCLE	GROWING NATURE	LIGHT REQUIREMENTS	HEIGHT
Agastache (*Agastache* species)	Perennial	Clumps	Full sun	15–18 inches (38–45 cm)
Angelica (*Angelica archangelica*)	Biennial	Clumps	Full sun, partial shade, shade	4–6 feet (1.2–1.8 m)
Anise hyssop (*Agastache foeniculum*)	Perennial	Clumps	Full sun, partial shade	2–3 feet (0.6–0.9 m)
Astragalus, Chinese (*Astragalus membranaceus*)	Perennial	Clumps	Full sun, partial shade	3–4 feet (0.9–1.2 m)
Basil (*Ocimum* species)	Annual	Clumps	Full sun	15 inches (38 cm)
Borage (*Borago officinalis*)	Annual	Clumps	Full sun, partial shade	3 feet (0.9 m)
Breadseed poppy (*Papaver somniferum*)	Annual	Clumps	Full sun	2 feet (0.6 m)
Calendula (*Calendula officinalis*)	Annual	Clumps	Full sun	12–15 inches (30–38 cm)
California poppy (*Eschscholzia californica*)	Annual	Clumps	Full sun, partial shade	12 inches (30 cm)
Catmint (*Nepeta × faassenii*)	Perennial	Clumps	Full sun, partial shade	15 inches (38 cm)
Catnip (*Nepeta cataria*)	Perennial	Clumps	Full sun, partial shade, shade	15–24 inches (38–60 cm)
Cayenne (*Capsicum* species)	Annual	Clumps	Full sun	to 24 inches (60 cm)
Chamomile, German (*Matricaria recutita*)	Annual	Clumps	Full sun, partial shade	24 inches (60 cm)
Chamomile, Roman (*Chamaemelum nobile*)	Perennial	Spreads	Full sun, partial shade	8–10 inches (20–25 cm)
Chasteberry (*Vitex agnus-castus*)	Perennial	Clumps	Full sun, partial shade	2–10 feet (0.6–3.0 m)
Chives (*Allium schoenoprasum*)	Perennial	Clumps	Full sun, shade	10–12 inches (25–30 cm)
Cilantro, Coriander (*Coriandrum sativum*)	Annual	Clumps	Full sun, partial shade, shade	10–12 inches (25–30 cm)
Clary sage (*Salvia sclarea*)	Biennial	Clumps	Full sun	3 feet (0.9 m)
Comfrey (*Symphytum × uplandicum*)	Perennial	Clumps	Full sun, partial shade	3–4 feet (0.9–1.2 m)
Costmary (*Tanacetum balsamita*)	Perennial	Clumps	Full sun, partial shade	18 inches (45 cm)

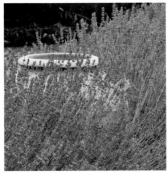

Lavender, see page 202

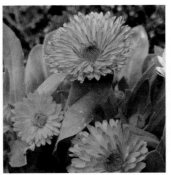

Calendula, see page 179

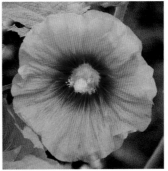

Hollyhock, see page 198

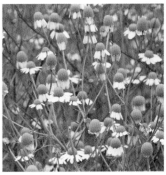

German chamomile, see page 183

SPACING	BLOOM COLOR	WATER REQUIREMENTS	SOIL PREFERENCES
12 inches (30 cm)	Salmon to hot pink	Low to moderate	Dry, gravelly, sandy, well-drained
15 inches (38 cm)	Yellowish green	Moderate to high	Rich loam
15 inches (38 cm)	Purple	Low to moderate	Dry, gravelly, or sandy
15 inches (38 cm)	Yellow	Moderate	Dry, sandy, well drained, slightly alkaline
12 inches (30 cm)	White, purple, pink	Low to moderate	Well drained
15 inches (38 cm)	Blue	Moderate	No special needs
12 inches (30 cm)	White, pink, purple	Moderate	No special needs
10 inches (25 cm)	Yellow, orange	Low to moderate	No special needs
10–12 inches (25–30 cm)	Orange	Low to moderate	No special needs
12–15 inches (30–38 cm)	Blue	Low	Well drained
12 inches (30 cm)	White	Low to moderate	No special needs
12 inches (30 cm)	White, red fruit	Low	Fertile, slightly acid
10 inches (25 cm)	White	Low	No special needs
8 inches (20 cm)	White	Moderate	Well drained
12–24 inches (30–60 cm)	Lavender	Moderate	Well drained
8 inches (20 cm)	Pink	Moderate	No special needs
8–10 inches (20–25 cm)	White	Moderate to high	No special needs
24 inches (60 cm)	Lavender, pink, white	Moderate	Well drained
24 inches (60 cm)	Purple	Moderate	Loam or sandy
24 inches (60 cm)	White	Moderate	No special needs

COMMON NAME (*LATIN NAME*)	CYCLE	GROWING NATURE	LIGHT REQUIREMENTS	HEIGHT
Coyote mint (*Monardella odoratissima*)	Perennial	Spreads	Full sun	10-12 inches (25-30 cm)
Cutting celery (*Apium graveolens*)	Biennial	Clumps	Partial shade	12 inches (30 cm)
Dill (*Anethum graveolens*)	Annual	Clumps	Full sun	3-5 feet (0.9-1.5 m)
Echinacea (*Echinacea* species)	Perennial	Clumps	Full sun	2-4 feet (0.6-1.2 m)
Epazote (*Chenopodium ambrosioides*)	Annual	Clumps	Full sun	12-15 inches (30-38 cm)
Eucalyptus (*Eucalyptus* species)	Tender perennial	Clumps	Full sun, partial shade	4 feet plus (1.2 m plus)
Fennel (*Foeniculum vulgare*)	Perennial	Clumps	Full sun	4-5 feet (1.2-1.5 m)
Feverfew (*Tanacetum parthenium*)	Perennial	Clumps	Full sun, partial shade	24 inches (60 cm)
Garlic (*Allium sativum*)	Perennial, but treated as an annual	Clump	Full sun, partial shade	15 inches (38 cm)
Garlic chives (*Allium tuberosum*)	Perennial	Clump	Full sun, partial shade	12 inches (30 cm)
Ginger (*Zingiber officinale*)	Perennial	Clumps	Shade, partial shade	3-4 feet (0.9-1.2 m)
Goldenrod (*Solidago* species)	Perennial	Clumps	Full sun	2-4 feet (0.6-1.2 m)
Goldenseal (*Hydrastis canadensis*)	Perennial	Clumps	Shade, partial shade	10-15 inches (25-38 cm)
Gotu kola (*Centella asiatica*)	Tender perennial	Spreads	Shade, partial shade	6-8 inches (15-20 cm)
Heartsease (*Viola tricolor, V. cornuta*)	Perennial, short-lived	Clumps	Full sun, shade	6 inches (15 cm)
Hollyhock (*Alcea* species)	Perennial	Clumps	Full sun, partial shade	6-8 feet (1.8-2.4 m)
Hops (*Humulus lupulus*)	Perennial	Spreads	Full sun, partial shade	8 feet (2.4 m) and taller
Horehound (*Marrubium vulgare*)	Perennial	Clumps	Full sun	12-24 inches (30-60 cm)
Horseradish (*Armoracia rusticana*)	Perennial	Clumps	Full sun, partial shade	24 inches (60 cm)
Hyssop (*Hyssopus officinalis*)	Perennial	Clumps	Full sun, partial shade	12-24 inches (30-60 cm)
Lady's mantle (*Alchemilla vulgaris*)	Perennial	Clumps	Partial to full shade	12-15 inches (30-38 cm)
Lavender (*Lavandula* species)	Perennial	Clumps	Full sun	24 inches (60 cm)
Lemon balm (*Melissa officinalis*)	Perennial	Clumps	Full sun, partial shade	24 inches (60 cm)
Lemongrass, East Indian, West Indian (*Cymbopogon flexuosus, C. citratus*)	Tender perennial	Clumps	Full sun, partial shade, shade	3-4 feet (0.9-1.2 m)
Lemon verbena (*Aloysia triphylla*)	Tender perennial	Clumps	Full sun, partial shade	3-4 feet (0.9-1.2 m)
Licorice (*Glycyrrhiza glabra*)	Perennial	Clumps	Full sun, partial shade	4-5 feet (1.2-1.5 m)

SPACING	BLOOM COLOR	WATER REQUIREMENTS	SOIL PREFERENCES
12–15 inches (30–38 cm)	Lavender	Low	Nutrient-poor
12 inches (30 cm)	White	Moderate	Well worked, high in organic matter
10–12 inches (25–30 cm)	Yellow	Moderate	Well drained, slightly acid
12 inches (30 cm)	Pink, yellow	Low	Nutrient-poor to high in organic matter, depending on species
10–12 inches (25–30 cm)	Green	Low	No special needs
3 feet (0.9 m)	White	Moderate	No special needs
12–15 inches (30–38 cm)	Yellow	Low to moderate	Well worked and well drained
12 inches (30 cm)	White	Moderate	Rich loam
10 inches (25 cm)	Greenish white	Moderate	Well drained
10 inches (25 cm)	White	Low to moderate	No special needs
15 inches (38 cm)	Yellowish green	High	Rich loam
12 inches (30 cm)	Yellow	Low to moderate	No special needs
8–10 inches (20–25 cm)	Greenish white	Moderate	Humus
10 inches (25 cm)	Greenish	High	Rich loam
6 inches (15 cm)	Multicolored	Moderate	No special needs
15 inches (38 cm)	Varies	Moderate	No special needs
6–8 feet (1.8–2.4 m)	Green	Moderate to high	Rich loam
12 inches (30 cm)	White	Low	Nutrient-poor
3 feet (0.9 m)	White	Moderate	Well drained
12 inches (30 cm)	Purple	Low to moderate	Well drained, sandy
12 inches (30 cm)	Chartreuse	Moderate to high	High in organic matter
12–15 inches (30–38 cm)	Purple	Low	Well drained, sandy
12 inches (30 cm)	White	Moderate	Well drained
12–15 inches (30–38 cm)	None	Moderate to high	Rich loam or sandy
12–15 inches (30–38 cm)	White	Moderate to high	Rich loam
24 inches (60 cm)	Lavender	Moderate	Well drained or sandy

COMMON NAME (*LATIN NAME*)	CYCLE	GROWING NATURE	LIGHT REQUIREMENTS	HEIGHT
Lovage (*Levisticum officinale*)	Perennial	Clumps	Full sun, partial shade, shade	2–3 feet (0.6–0.9 m)
Marjoram (*Origanum majorana, O. syriaca*)	Tender perennial	Clumps	Full sun, partial shade	10–12 inches (25–30 cm)
Marsh mallow (*Althaea officinalis*)	Perennial	Clumps	Full sun, partial shade, shade	3–4 feet (0.9–1.2 m)
Melaleuca, Tea tree (*Melaleuca alternifolia*)	Tender perennial	Clumps	Full sun, partial shade	4 feet plus (1.2 m plus)
Mexican oregano (*Lippia graveolens*)	Tender perennial	Clumps	Full sun	24 inches (60 cm)
Monarda (*Monarda* species)	Perennial	Clumps	Full sun, partial shade	2–3 feet (0.6–0.9 m)
Motherwort (*Leonurus cardiaca*)	Perennial	Clumps	Full sun, partial shade, shade	2–4 feet (0.6–1.2 m)
Mugwort (*Artemisia vulgaris*)	Perennial	Clumps	Full sun, partial shade	4–5 feet (1.2–1.5 m)
Mullein (*Verbascum thapsus*)	Biennial	Clumps	Full sun	5–6 feet (1.5–1.8 m)
Nasturtium (*Tropaeolum majus*)	Annual	Vining or trailing	Partial to full shade	4 foot plus (1.2 m plus)
Nettle (*Urtica dioica*)	Perennial	Spreads	Full sun, partial shade, shade	2–4 feet (0.6–1.2 m)
Oats (*Avena sativa*)	Annual	Clumps	Full sun	4–5 feet (1.2–1.5 m)
Oregano (*Origanum* species)	Perennial	Spreads	Full sun, partial shade	to 24 inches (60 cm)
Parsley (*Petroselinum crispum*)	Biennial	Clumps	Sun, partial shade	12–20 inches (30–50 cm)
Passionflower (*Passiflora incarnata, P. edulis*)	Tender perennial	Spreads	Shade, partial shade	8 feet (2.4 m) and much taller
Pennyroyal (*Mentha pulegium*)	Perennial	Spreads	Full sun, partial shade, shade	10–12 inches (25–30 cm)
Peppermint (*Mentha piperita*)	Perennial	Spreads	Full sun, partial shade, shade	24 inches (60 cm)
Potentilla (*Potentilla* species)	Perennial	Clumps, spreads	Full sun, partial shade, shade	6–20 inches (15–50 cm)
Prickly pear (*Opuntia* species)	Perennial	Clumps, spreads	Full sun	10–15 inches (25–38 cm)
Red clover (*Trifolium pratense*)	Perennial	Clumps	Full sun, partial shade	12–15 inches (30–38 cm)
Rosemary (*Rosmarinus* species)	Tender perennial	Clumps	Full sun	12–36 inches (30–90 cm) and taller
Rue (*Ruta graveolens*)	Perennial	Clumps	Full sun	12–15 inches (30–38 cm)
Sage (*Salvia officinalis*)	Perennial	Clumps	Full sun	24 inches (60 cm)
Salad burnet (*Sanguisorba minor*)	Annual	Clumps	Partial shade	12–15 inches (30–38 cm)
Santolina (*Santolina* species)	Perennial	Clumps	Full sun	12–24 inches (30–60 cm)

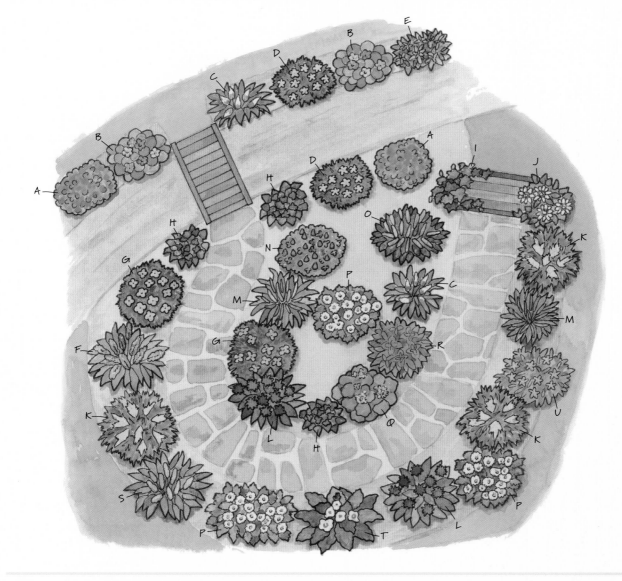

AN ECOSYSTEM GARDEN

A: Watercress

B: Nasturtium

C: Self-heal

D: Potentilla

E: Nettle

F: Wood betony

G: California poppy

H: Violet

I: Hops

J: Passionflower

K: Goldenrod

L: Monarda

M: Blue vervain

N: Red clover

O: Agastache

P: Feverfew

Q: Lady's mantle

R: Mint

S: Anise hyssop

T: Marsh mallow

U: St.-John's-wort

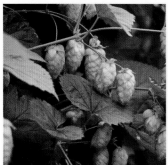

Hops, see page 198

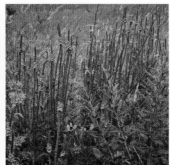

Blue vervain, see page 234

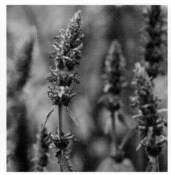

Wood betony, see page 238

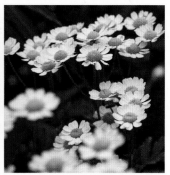

Feverfew, see page 192

than many of the surrounding areas, and plants growing there will have full sun or dappled shade, whereas mountain plants grow in partial to full shade.

DESERT/MEDITERRANEAN: A desert habitat is hotter and drier than are other habitats. It may offer sun or shade. Water may be abundant for a short time in spring and monsoon seasons, but usually not the remaining part of the year. Temperatures will be hot as a rule, but winter nights can get extremely cold. The Mediterranean habitat, found in southern Europe and surrounding regions, also offers hot and dry climates, with soil that is not always nutrient-rich. Night temperatures do not usually go below the mid 30°F range; plants from this region will not be hardy in colder climates.

RIVER/STREAM/LAKE/POND: This habitat is rich in moisture. Plants growing in any of these areas will require extra moisture and may grow in sun, shade, or partial shade. Often the soil is richer in this type of habitat.

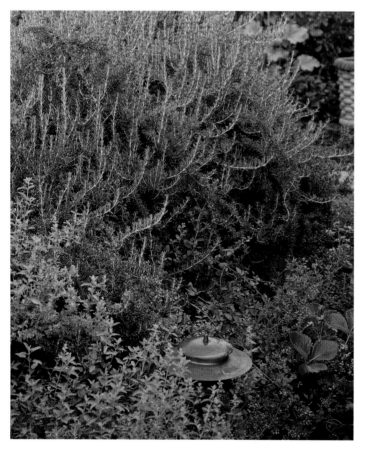

A wild garden creates the illusion of nature untouched by the human hand. Rosemary and other dryland herbs evoke a wild Mediterranean feel.

DISTURBED AREA: Water, sun, and shade may have altered the soil in this habitat. Disturbed areas often reflect overuse by humans or animals (for development, recreation, or livestock grazing, for example) and the native habitat is seriously compromised or no longer present. Many plants thrive in these places.

GARDENS ONLY: There are some plants that no longer exist outside of a garden environment. Because of circumstances like habitat destruction or lack of pollinators, they have become dependent upon humans for their existence. However, they do tend to be very specific in their preferences for garden habitats. For example, some will require a desert garden habitat, while others may prefer a mountain or meadow garden habitat.

TEMPERATE: In temperate climates, the temperatures never go into the ranges of extreme cold or extreme hot. Temperate climatic zones exist all over the world, between tropic climatic zones and the polar circle zones.

SUBTROPICAL: This is the climatic region between the tropics and the temperate zones. Temperatures are generally warmer than those in temperate zones, with more natural moisture, but cold spells and droughts can easily influence these habitats.

TROPICAL: This climate is very hot and humid. Plants in this habitat often grow very lush. They are not cold-hardy or drought-tolerant, so care must be taken to provide adequate moisture and warm temperatures.

The Wild Garden

Some people really enjoy a garden that is designed to look as if Mother Nature herself planted it. These types of gardens have many of the basic hardgoods in place, as well as a main focal point, but can be quite different from a traditional border garden. Imagine how it would feel to walk through a wild meadow; wild gardens impart the same feel.

These gardens are not planted with as much organizational detail as other types are — or at least that's how they appear. A little planned chaos works wonders. For instance, it's fine if a taller plant sits slightly in front of a smaller one or if the chamomile seeds itself into the pathways. It's a little bit wild and wonderfully enchanting!

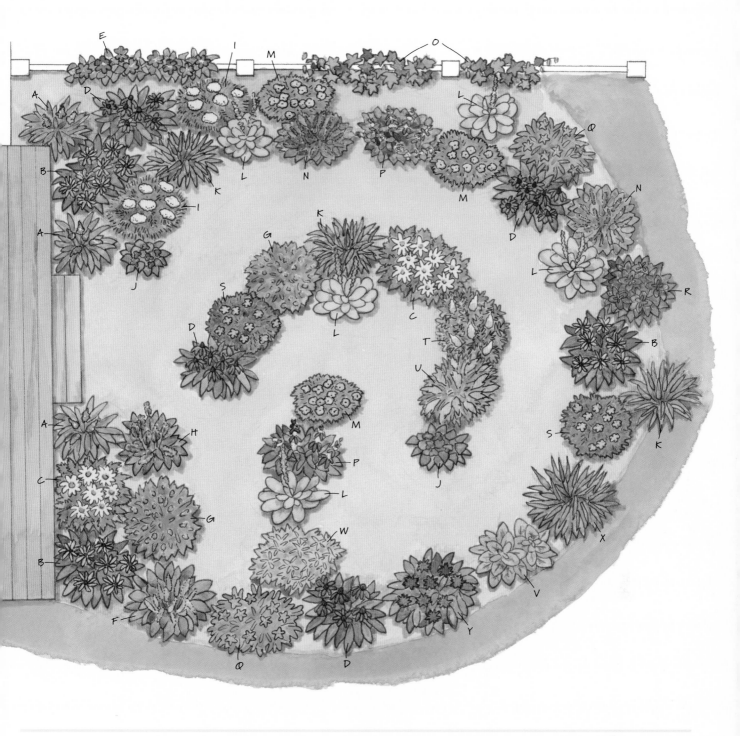

THE WILD GARDEN

A: Self-heal

B: Black-eyed Susan

C: Ox-eye daisy

D: Echinacea

E: Passionflower

F. Agastache
    (sunset hyssop)

G: Skullcap

H: Wood betony

I: Yarrow

J: Violet

K: Blue vervain

L: Mullein

M: California poppy

N: Catmint

O: Hops

P: Horehound

Q: St.-John's-wort

R: Nettle

S: Potentilla

T: Licorice

U: Goldenrod

V: Red-veined sorrel

W: White sage

X: Chasteberry

Y: Monarda

Raised-Bed Gardens

Raised beds have become very popular in the last couple of decades, although it was the monks of the European monasteries who originally brought this method into common practice. They created garden beds that were approximately 4 feet (1.2 m) wide and whatever length was desired. Raised beds are easy to reach into for maintenance or harvesting without stepping on the soil and compacting it.

Make raised beds simply by raking the soil into bed formations, leaving pathway access on all sides.

You can also create the beds using stones or landscaping timbers if you would like to make a more permanent or formalized look. Anything will work! I've used scrap lumber and old bricks; even cinderblocks are great. *Note:* It is extremely difficult to find untreated landscaping timbers; if you prefer not to use chemically treated lumber, you will most likely have to use a wood such as redwood or cedar. If you're very ambitious, install metal landscaping edging, which will outlast other materials and will help keep aggressive plants under control.

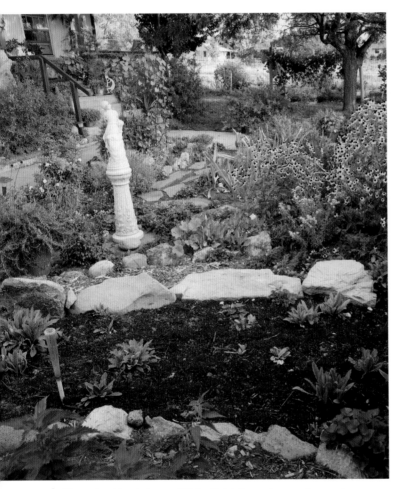

The raised beds in my White Rabbit garden are formed by stones collected from our farm. Mulch pathways travel throughout the garden, helping to manage weeds and conserve the soil moisture.

SPACE-SAVING GARDENS

If you have limited space or you would like to grow a small garden near a door or patio, consider creating a wagon-wheel or ladder garden. Simply lay a straight wooden ladder or old wagon wheel on the soil where you want the garden to be. Fill the space between the ladder rungs or wheel spokes with good soil, mix this soil with the top 3 to 4 inches (7.5–10 cm) of existing soil, and you're ready to plant. Do not place this type of garden over a patch of grass; the grass will grow right up through the soil and into the garden.

Another space-saving garden is the checkerboard. First create a checkerboard pattern using 12-inch-square (30 cm) garden stones or patio blocks. Once the pattern is in place, fill the areas between the stones with soil and plant one type of herb in each soil space. This is a fantastic way to get children involved in gardening, because they can plant something different in each block. Seniors who would like to decrease the size of a garden area for ease of maintenance may find this approach appealing.

A great benefit of the checkerboard garden is the easy access to every part of it via the stones. The extra heat that is collected and given off by the stones may also enable you to grow plants that would not normally be hardy in your climate.

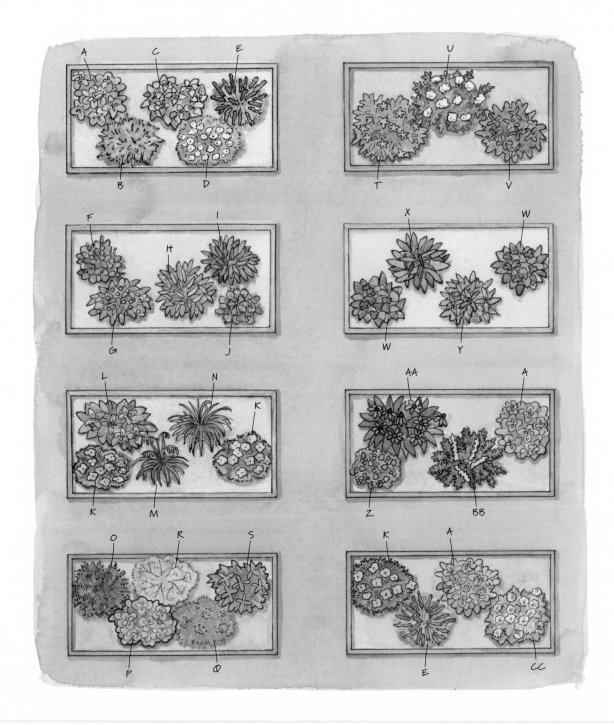

A RAISED-BED GARDEN

A: Lemon balm
B: Summer savory
C: Catnip
D: Chamomile
E: Lavender
F: Pennyroyal
G: Spilanthes
H: Chasteberry

I: Skullcap
J: Shiso
K: California poppy
L: Nettle
M: Oats
N: Garlic chives
O: Rosemary
P: Basil

Q: Dill
R: Fennel
S: Peppermint
T: St.-John's-wort
U: Valerian
V: Spearmint
W: Violet
X: Cayenne

Y: Epazote
Z: Red clover
AA: Echinacea
BB: Chinese astragalus
CC: Feverfew

PLANT HABITAT PREFERENCES

This is a general habitat guide to give you an idea of what type of environment these plants prefer and grow best in. Please remember that these are general guidelines only and that every plant will have some degree of tolerance for other circumstances. Look in chapter 10 for more specific growing guidelines.

COMMON NAME (*LATIN NAME*)	PREFERRED LOCATION	PREFERRED GROWING CLIMATE
Agastache (*Agastache* species)	Prairie/grassland, mountain/meadow	Temperate
Angelica (*Angelica archangelica*)	River/stream/lake/pond	Temperate
Anise hyssop (*Agastache foeniculum*)	Mountain/meadow	Temperate
Astragalus, Chinese (*Astragalus membranaceus*)	Prairie/grassland	Temperate, subtropical
Basil (*Ocimum* species)	Cultivated gardens only	Temperate, subtropical, tropical
Borage (*Borago officinalis*)	Desert/Mediterranean	Temperate
Breadseed poppy (*Papaver somniferum*)	Mountain/meadow	Temperate
Calendula (*Calendula officinalis*)	Cultivated gardens only	Temperate, subtropical
California poppy (*Eschscholzia californica*)	Prairie/grassland, disturbed area	Temperate
Catmint (*Nepeta × faassenii*)	Prairie/grassland, desert/Mediterranean	Temperate
Catnip (*Nepeta cataria*)	Prairie/grassland, river/stream/lake/pond, disturbed area	Temperate, subtropical
Cayenne (*Capsicum* species)	Desert/Mediterranean types of gardens	Temperate, subtropical, tropical
Chamomile (*Matricaria recutita, Chamaemelum nobile*)	Prairie/grassland	Temperate
Chasteberry (*Vitex agnus-castus*)	Desert/Mediterranean	Temperate
Chives (*Allium schoenoprasum*)	Mountain/meadow types of gardens	Temperate
Cilantro, Coriander (*Coriandrum sativum*)	Cultivated gardens only	Temperate, subtropical, tropical
Clary sage (*Salvia sclarea*)	Desert/Mediterranean	Temperate
Comfrey (*Symphytum × uplandicum*)	River/stream/lake/pond	Temperate
Costmary (*Tanacetum balsamita*)	River/stream/lake/pond, desert/Mediterranean	Temperate
Coyote mint (*Monardella odoratissima*)	Mountain/meadow, desert/Mediterranean	Temperate
Cutting celery (*Apium graveolens*)	Gardens only	Temperate, subtropical
Dill (*Anethum graveolens*)	Cultivated and desert/Mediterranean types of gardens	Temperate
Echinacea (*Echinacea* species)	Prairie/grassland	Temperate
Epazote (*Chenopodium ambrosioides*)	Desert/Mediterranean	Temperate
Eucalyptus (*Eucalyptus* species)	Woodland/forest	Temperate, subtropical
Fennel (*Foeniculum vulgare*)	Desert/Mediterranean, disturbed areas	Temperate

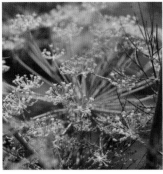
Dill, see page 189

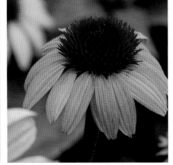
Echinacea, see page 190

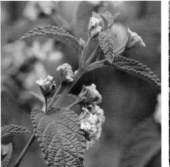
Mexican oregano, see page 208

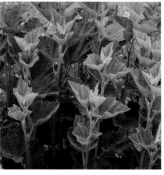
Marsh mallow, see page 207

COMMON NAME (LATIN NAME)	PREFERRED LOCATION	PREFERRED GROWING CLIMATE
Feverfew (Tanacetum parthenium)	Cultivated and desert/Mediterranean	Temperate
Garlic (Allium sativum)	Cultivated gardens only	Temperate, subtropical
Garlic chives (Allium tuberosum)	Mountain/meadow types of gardens	Temperate, subtropical
Ginger (Zingiber officinale)	Cultivated gardens only	Tropical
Goldenrod (Solidago species)	Prairie/grassland, mountain/meadow, river/stream/lake/pond	Temperate
Goldenseal (Hydrastis canadensis)	Woodland/forest	Temperate
Gotu kola (Centella asiatica)	River/stream/lake/pond, disturbed area	Tropical
Heartsease (Viola tricolor, V. cornuta)	Disturbed area, river/stream/lake/pond, mountain/meadow, woodland/forest	Temperate
Hollyhock (Alcea species)	Cultivated gardens only	Temperate
Hops (Humulus lupulus)	Woodland/forest, prairie/grassland, mountain/meadow, river/stream/lake/pond	Temperate
Horehound (Marrubium vulgare)	Prairie/grassland, desert/Mediterranean, disturbed area	Temperate
Horseradish (Armoracia rusticana)	Disturbed areas and cultivated gardens	Temperate
Hyssop (Hyssopus officinalis)	Desert/Mediterranean	Temperate
Lady's mantle (Alchemilla vulgaris)	River/stream/lake/pond, mountain/meadow	Temperate
Lavender (Lavandula species)	Desert/Mediterranean	Temperate
Lemon balm (Melissa officinalis)	Desert/Mediterranean	Temperate
Lemongrass, East Indian, West Indian (Cymbopogon flexuosus, C. citratus)	Cultivated gardens only	Tropical
Lemon verbena (Aloysia triphylla)	Cultivated gardens only	Tropical
Licorice (Glycyrrhiza glabra)	Desert/Mediterranean	Temperate
Lovage (Levisticum officinale)	Desert/Mediterranean, mountain meadow	Temperate
Marjoram (Origanum majorana, O. syriaca, O. vulgare)	Desert/Mediterranean types of gardens	Temperate
Marsh mallow (Althaea officinalis)	Mountain/meadow, river/stream/lake/pond	Temperate
Melaleuca, Tea tree (Melaleuca alternifolia)	Woodland/forest	Temperate, subtropical
Mexican oregano (Lippia graveolens)	Desert/Mediterranean	Temperate
Monarda (Monarda species)	Mountain/meadow, river/stream/lake/pond	Temperate

COMMON NAME (*LATIN NAME*)	PREFERRED LOCATION	PREFERRED GROWING CLIMATE
Motherwort (*Leonurus cardiaca*)	Disturbed area	Temperate
Mugwort (*Artemisia vulgaris*)	Mountain/meadow, desert/Mediterranean, disturbed area	Temperate
Mullein (*Verbascum thapsus*)	Prairie/grassland, mountain/meadow, desert/Mediterranean, river/stream/lake/pond, disturbed area	Temperate
Nasturtium (*Tropaeolum majus*)	Cultivated gardens	Temperate, subtropical, tropical
Nettle (*Urtica dioica*)	Mountain/meadow, river/stream/lake/pond, disturbed area	Temperate, subtropical
Oats (*Avena sativa*)	Prairie/grassland, mountain/meadow	Temperate
Oregano (*Origanum* species)	Desert/Mediterranean	Temperate
Parsley (*Petroselinum crispum*)	Desert/Mediterranean	Temperate
Passionflower (*Passiflora incarnata, P. edulis*)	Woodland/forest, mountain/meadow	Subtropical, tropical
Pennyroyal (*Mentha pulegium*)	Mountain/meadow, desert/Mediterranean	Temperate
Peppermint (*Mentha piperita*)	River/steam/lake/pond, disturbed area	Temperate
Potentilla (*Potentilla* species)	Mountain/meadow, river/stream/lake/pond	Temperate
Prickly pear (*Opuntia* species)	Desert/Mediterranean	Subtropical, temperate
Red clover (*Trifolium pratense*)	Mountain/meadow, disturbed area	Temperate
Rosemary (*Rosmarinus* species)	Desert/Mediterranean	Temperate
Rue (*Ruta graveolens*)	Desert/Mediterranean, disturbed area	Temperate, tropical
Sage (*Salvia officinalis*)	Desert/Mediterranean	Temperate
Salad burnet (*Sanguisorba minor*)	Cultivated gardens and disturbed areas	Temperate
Santolina (*Santolina* species)	Desert/Mediterranean	Temperate
Savory, summer (*Satureja hortensis*)	Desert/Mediterranean	Temperate
Savory, winter (*Satureja montana*)	Desert/Mediterranean	Temperate
Self-heal (*Prunella vulgaris, P. grandiflora* subsp. *pyrenaica*)	Woodland/forest, mountain/meadow, river/stream/lake/pond	Temperate
Shiso (*Perilla frutescens*)	Mountain/meadow types of gardens	Tropical
Skullcap (*Scutellaria lateriflora*)	Mountain/meadow, river/stream/lake/pond	Temperate
Sorrel, French, Red-veined (*Rumex acetosa, R. sanguineus*)	River/stream/lake/pond, mountain/meadow	Temperate
Southernwood (*Artemisia abrotanum*)	Prairie/grassland, desert/Mediterranean	Temperate
Spearmint (*Mentha spicata*)	River/stream/lake/pond, disturbed area	Temperate
Spilanthes (*Spilanthes oleracea*)	River/stream/lake/pond	Tropical
St.-John's-wort (*Hypericum perforatum*)	Mountain/meadow, disturbed area	Temperate
Stevia (*Stevia rebaudiana*)	River/stream/lake/pond	Tropical
Sunflower (*Helianthus annuus*)	Prairie/grassland, mountain/meadow, desert/Mediterranean, disturbed area	Temperate, subtropical, tropical

COMMON NAME (*LATIN NAME*)	PREFERRED LOCATION	PREFERRED GROWING CLIMATE
Sweetgrass (*Hierochloe odorata*)	Prairie/grassland	Temperate
Sweet woodruff (*Galium odoratum*)	Desert/Mediterranean	Tropical
Thyme (*Thymus* species)	Desert/Mediterranean	Temperate
Turmeric (*Curcuma longa*)	Woodland/forest and cultivated gardens	Tropical
Valerian (*Valeriana officinalis*)	Woodland/forest, river/stream/lake/pond	Temperate
Vervain, Blue vervain (*Verbena* species)	Prairie/grassland, mountain/meadow, desert/Mediterranean, disturbed area	Temperate
Vietnamese coriander (*Polygonum odorata*)	Cultivated gardens	Subtropical, tropical
Violet (*Viola* species)	Woodland/forest, mountain/meadow, river/stream/lake/pond	Temperate
Watercress (*Nasturtium officinale*)	River/stream/lake/pond	Temperate, subtropical
White sage (*Salvia apiana*)	Prairie/grassland, desert/Mediterranean	Temperate
Wood betony (*Stachys officinalis*)	Woodland/forest	Temperate
Yarrow (*Achillea* species)	Prairie/grassland, mountain/meadow, desert/Mediterranean, disturbed areas	Temperate
Yerba mansa (*Anemopsis californica*)	Desert/Mediterranean, river/stream/lake/pond	Temperate
Yucca (*Yucca* species)	Mountain/meadow, desert/Mediterranean	Temperate

Herbs Grown in Food Gardens

One of my favorite types of garden combines food plants with herbs and edible flowers. Indeed, I have several of these gardens here at our farm. Fresh food is as important to me as fresh herbs, and I like to have plenty of both always available for my use, especially in cooking.

Growing herbs intermixed with fruit and vegetable plants is very easy to accomplish and is quite lovely. This is an excellent approach for gardeners who want beauty from their garden, at the same time insisting that the garden be a practical and productive space. I've noticed many such gardens these days, as the need and desire for locally and personally grown food is ever increasing. The same gardeners who want to grow their own food are likely to be interested in growing herbs to use in any number of ways, thus increasing their empowerment over their own lives. Growing our own food and herbs goes hand in hand with the desire to be as sustainable as possible in providing for our family's needs.

Some folks turn their entire yards into gardens filled with herbs and food plants. I visited a very small garden a few years ago where the yard was filled with herbs, veggies, and edible flowers. It was about 50 feet long and maybe 30 feet wide, and contained a large patio space and flagstone walking paths. It also had a small garden shed in the back to store tools, pots, and other supplies. The garden had borders of lettuce and parsley all along the pathways. There were trellises up the sides of the shed and the house with passionflowers, beans, and cucumbers climbing up. The 6-foot-high wooden fence was covered with nasturtiums, morning glories, and scarlet runner beans. An arbor over the patio had grapes growing on it, and underneath were hanging baskets filled with strawberries, creeping rosemary, and gotu kola. The back fence, along the alley, was of chain link and was festooned with sunflowers, providing much-needed privacy in the garden space and food for wild birds and squirrels. They also looked incredibly cheerful!

Incorporating herbs into food gardens is easy. Simply plant some thyme next to the carrots. Grow a row of cilantro in partial shade alongside the lettuces and spinach. Basil intermixed with tomatoes and peppers will give those vegetables a stronger and more delicious flavor. Echinacea and hyssop are really lovely growing with beans and cucumbers. I like to plant nasturtiums with tomatillos. Beets, onions, or garlic woven among my rosemary plants is really lovely. The strawberries complement lady's mantle and dill in the partial shade of the garden. I also grow strawberries in a narrow bed around the perimeter of one of our farm buildings. This is a permanent planting, but each spring I interplant the strawberries with trellis beans, peas, and epazote. The planting is pretty thick, which helps keep down the amount of weeds in this bed, so it is quite low-maintenance.

Consider how you can combine your own food and herb gardens. Let your imagination soar!

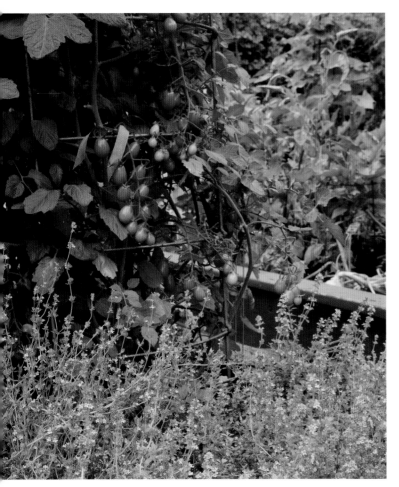

When herbs are included in a vegetable garden, harvesting ingredients in preparation for a meal is a snap! Many kinds of herbs also help deter insect pests.

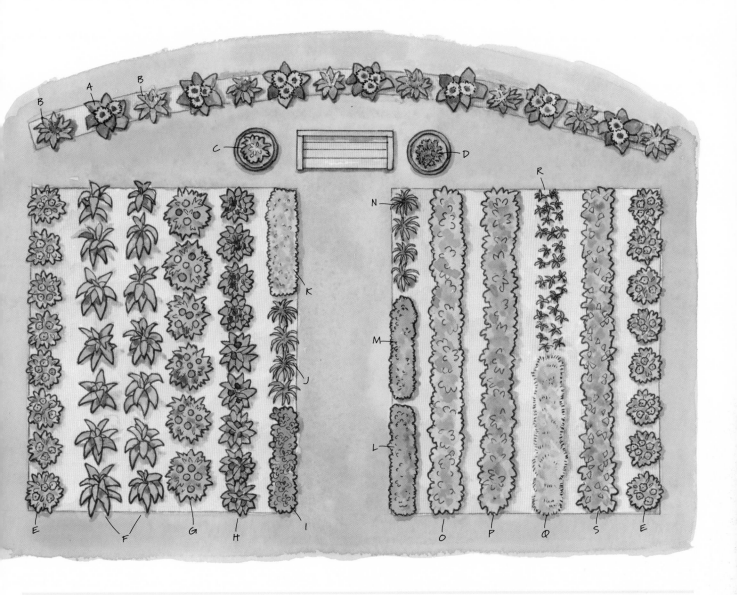

A COOK'S GARDEN

A: Sunflower

B: Amaranth

C: Sage

D: Rosemary

E: Calendulas

F: Sweet corn

G: Tomatoes

H: Peppers

I: Basil

J: Chives

K: Oregano

L: Parsley

M: Marjoram

N: Garlic chives

O: Lettuce mix

P: Spinach

Q: Carrots

R: Green onions

S: Beans

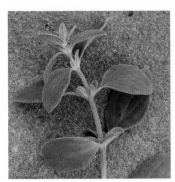

Marjoram, see page 206

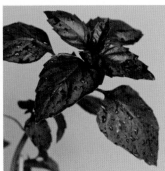

Purple basil, see page 176

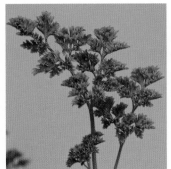

Parsley, see page 214

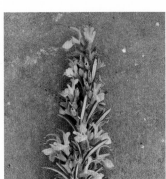

Rosemary, see page 219

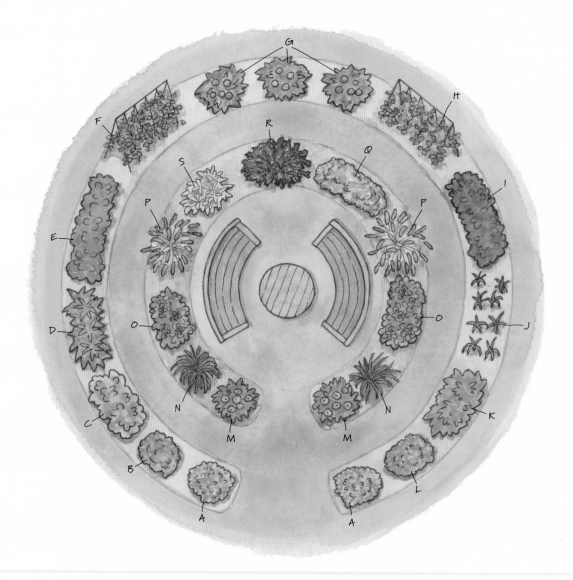

A CHEF'S RETREAT GARDEN

A: Cilantro

B: Greek oregano

C: Lettuce mix

D: Cayenne

E: Turnips

F: Beans

G: Tomatoes

H: Peas

I: Beets

J: Onions

K: Spinach

L: Italian oregano

M: Calendulas

N: Garlic chives

O: Basil

P: Lavender

Q: Parsley

R: Rosemary

S: Sage

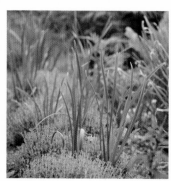

Garlic chives, see page 194

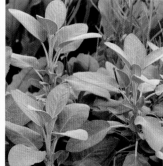

Sage, see page 221

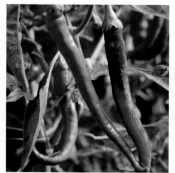

Cayenne, see page 182

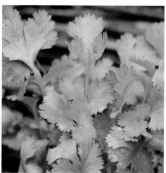

Cilantro, see page 185

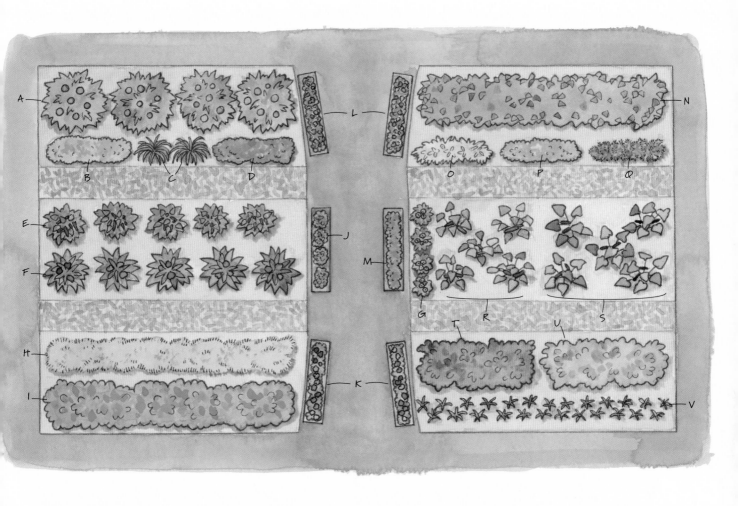

MR. MacGREGOR'S
VEGETABLE & HERB PATCH

A: Tomatoes
B: Oregano
C: Chives
D: Parsley
E: Hot chilies

F: Sweet peppers
G: Calendulas
H: Carrots
I: Lettuce mix
J: Basil

K: Violets
L: Nasturtiums
M: Cilantro
N: Beans
O: Sage

P: Thyme
Q: Rosemary
R: Summer squash
S: Cucumbers
T: Beets

U: Turnips
V: Green onions

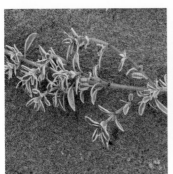

Silver thyme, see page 232

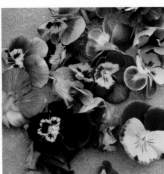

Violets, see page 236

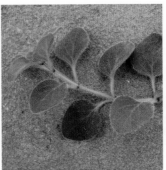

Oregano, see page 214

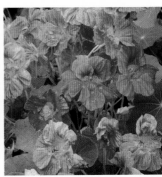

Nasturtiums, see page 212

Theme Gardens

Planting a theme garden is great fun. The motifs that you might consider are quite varied, and the design possibilities are nearly endless.

You could design an apothecary garden with beds devoted to herbs used to treat particular body systems. For example, you would plant herbs used for the respiratory system in one area, and herbs for the skin would be planted in another area.

The theme might also be gender- or age-specific, focusing on the plants for men's or women's health. These types of gardens would include herbs like lady's mantle and clary sage for women and turmeric and oats for men. The garden might be planted with herbs that delight children and would have plenty of lemon balm and chamomile. Another theme centers on culinary herbs, with all the cook's favorites, such as garlic chives, oregano, rosemary, and different kinds of basils. A scented garden would contain fragrant herbs: lavender, roses, mint, and of course lemon verbena — all are great for making into soothing hand creams or using in the bath.

Wildlife herb gardens are not only for human use, but also attract specific types of wildlife. A hummingbird garden contains a lot of bright orange, red, and pink flowers, such as you might get with agastache, monarda, and coyote mint. Other birds are drawn into gardens that have plants with abundant seeds for food, such as echinacea and lavender. The antics of birds are entertaining to watch, and insects are kept under control because they're part of the birds' diet. Butterflies are magical in the garden. Herbs in the carrot family (Umbelliferae) — dill, fennel, and parsley, for example — attract butterflies. Bees of all types should be welcomed in the garden; these creatures are fantastic pollinators. Bee-attracting herbs like catmint and motherwort are helpful additions in a wildlife garden. Bats and moths are also good pollinators and often will pollinate flowers that butterflies and bees do not. Bats, flying during their nightly forays, are especially fond of the passionflower vine. Don't forget to make a welcome spot for toads and salamanders, both of which eat a lot of pests, especially slugs.

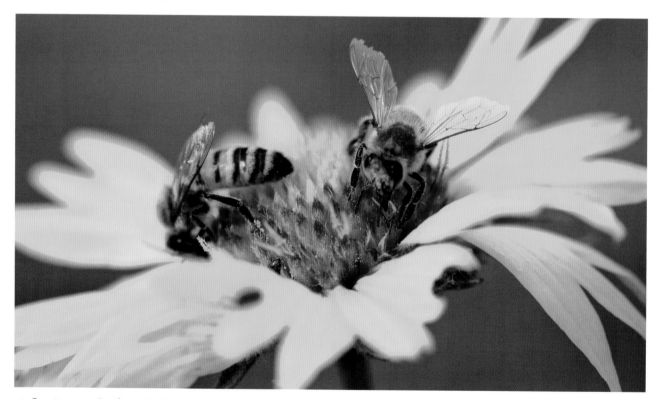

Create a garden for wildlife! Honeybees are welcome in the herb garden, as they pollinate flowers, helping to create good harvests of fruits and seeds. Welcoming the bees into the garden also means the beekeeper will be rewarded with a wonderful honey harvest.

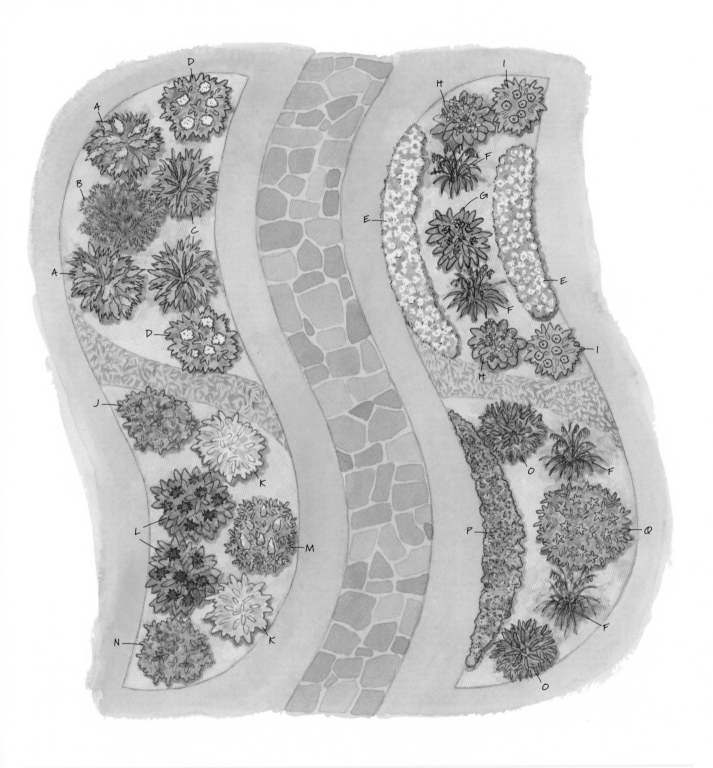

APOTHECARY HERB GARDEN

A: Goldenrod

B: Rosemary

C: Blue vervain

D: Lovage

E: Chamomile

F: Oats

G: Self-heal

H: Borage

I: Calendula

J: Spearmint

K: Sage

L: Monarda

M: Licorice

N: Peppermint

O: Skullcap

P: Thyme

Q: St.-John's-wort

PLANNING A THEME GARDEN

THEME GARDENS ARE A GREAT WAY TO ORGANIZE PLANTING. Medicinal theme gardens focus on the therapeutic effect of a group of herbs in order to treat or prevent a particular condition. For instance, marsh mallow and parsley might be planted in a urinary-care garden, as these plants are used to address conditions of the kidney and bladder. Herbs for the making of soaps, candles, cloth, and dye can be used to create a textile theme garden.

Herbs will settle nicely into a garden designed by theme. This chart gives ideas about what type of theme garden suits a specific herb.

COMMON NAME	LATIN NAME	GENDER-SPECIFIC	CHILDREN	CULINARY	SCENTED	TEA	MEDICINAL	WILDLIFE
Agastache	*Agastache rupestris, A. cana*			x	x	x	x	x
Angelica	*Angelica archangelica*	x women		x			x	x
Anise hyssop	*Agastache foeniculum*		x	x	x	x	x	x
Astragalus, Chinese	*Astragalus membranaceus*			x			x	
Basil	*Ocimum* species			x	x		x	
Borage	*Borago officinalis*	x women	x	x			x	x
Breadseed poppy	*Papaver somniferum*			x				
Calendula	*Calendula officinalis*		x	x			x	x
California poppy	*Eschscholzia californica*						x	
Catmint	*Nepeta × faassenii*				x			x
Catnip	*Nepeta cataria*		x	x		x	x	
Cayenne	*Capsicum* species			x			x	
Chamomile	*Matricaria recutita, Chamaemelum nobile*	x women	x	x	x	x	x	
Chasteberry	*Vitex agnus-castus*	x men, women					x	
Chives	*Allium schoenoprasum*		x	x				
Cilantro, Coriander	*Coriandrum sativum*			x			x	
Clary sage	*Salvia sclarea*	x women			x		x	
Comfrey	*Symphytum × uplandicum*						x	

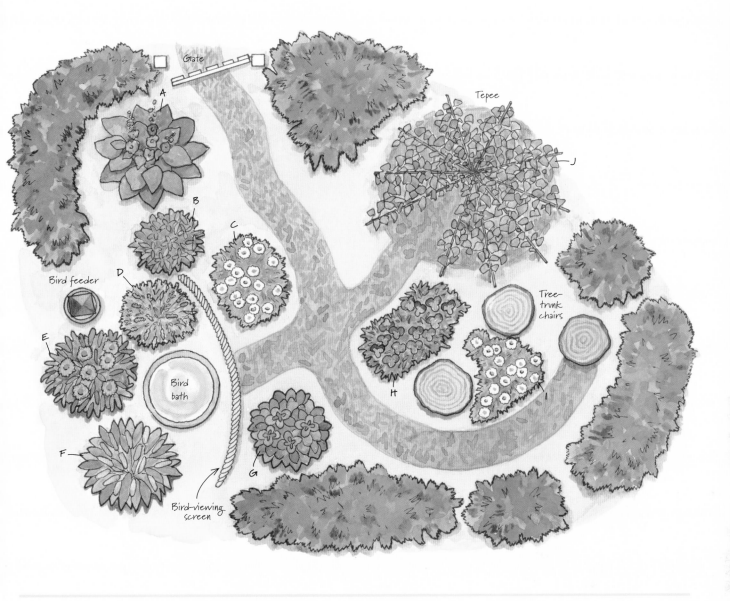

A CHILDREN'S HERB GARDEN

A: Hollyhock

B: Lemon balm

C: Chamomile

D: Lavender

E: Calendula

F: Anise hyssop

G: Basil

H: Violet

I: Roman chamomile

J: Pole beans

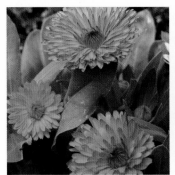

Calendula, see page 179

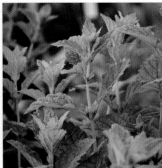

Lemon balm, see page 203

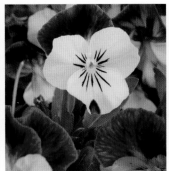

Violet, see page 236

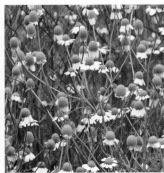

Chamomile, see page 183

Container Gardens

Many times a situation calls for planting herbs in containers or pots, or this may be the type of garden you prefer. There are many fabulous pots, in every size, shape, material, and color imaginable. Planting a container herb garden can be pure joy. For some people, such as apartment-dwellers, townhouse residents, and college students, this may be the only gardening option, aside from a community garden plot — but this doesn't mean their gardens won't be interesting and productive.

For others, like me, this method provides a mobile garden that can be rearranged at will. I *love* to incorporate planted containers into my other gardens, because I can give a garden another look or feel just by moving the pots to different locations. It also enables me to provide a much-needed splash of color to any area that is in a blooming lull at a particular time of the season.

> Most herbs grow very well when planted in containers.

I've found that most herbs grow very well when planted in containers. Clay, pottery, and ceramic pots are easy to care for and the plants seem to thrive in them more than they do in plastic pots (especially for longer-term growing). There are also many environmentally friendly types of containers nowadays, such as rice hull, wheat, corn, and paper fiber pots. These are great because you can compost the pots when they're no longer needed for growing.

Have fun with containers and don't limit yourself in what you try with them. My grandma once planted in an old pair of boots, partly because she needed a container and only had a limited budget, and partly because she thought it was amusing! One of my students used plastic wading pools that she drilled drainage holes into. She chose this approach because it was inexpensive and provided a large amount of growing space in a small area. She combined her veggies and herbs into these large, round swimming pool planters and all the plants grew vigorously.

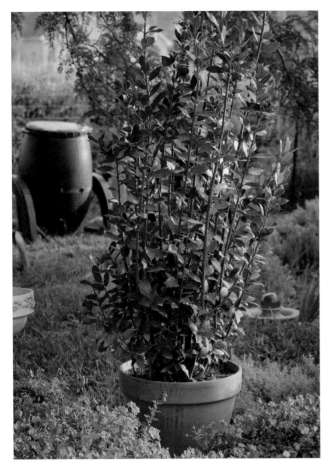

Herbs that won't survive a cold season, like this bay tree, can be kept in containers to facilitate taking the plant outdoors in summer and bringing it indoors for winter.

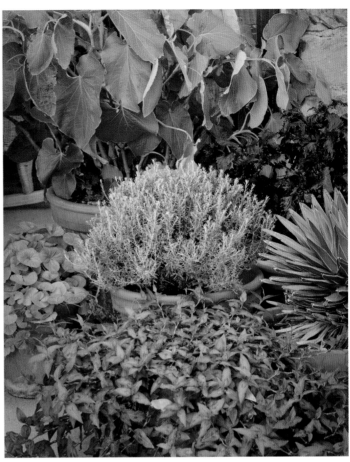

Growing herbs in containers allows you to create a green garden space on patios or decks, making these living areas comfortable and welcoming to everyone who gathers there.

I've also noticed that built-in planters have become very popular on decks, patios, even rooftops. These types of containers cannot be moved around easily, if at all, but they can be made quite large and give an appearance of a continuous green space when they're built into the perimeter of a patio or deck space. They sometimes act as living walls, with trellises to encourage plants to grow up rather than trailing down, thus providing screening and greater privacy from close neighbors where outside space is shared.

Rooftop gardens are a great way to create green spaces for city dwellers. And a business that has access to a rooftop or a courtyard garden can use it either as a gathering space for customers or as a small production space to grow fresh herbs and food plants for, say, a restaurant or small greengrocer. Really, the possibilities are only limited by one's imagination and willingness to put some energy into the project.

Windowsill and tabletop container gardens are a very enjoyable and viable choice for gardeners with no outside space whatsoever. Loft dwellers, college students, and seniors in assisted-living facilities can all take advantage of a windowsill or tabletop herb garden. Indoor herb growing is a great option, too, in climates that have a cold season, where gardening would otherwise be limited only to the warmest months. A great many herbs thrive indoors in bright indirect light, giving the gardener regular opportunities to harvest fresh herbs to use in cooking, as personal care items like bath herbs, and even for medicinal purposes. Certainly the green beauty of these living herbs in your home will make the heart and spirit feel enriched, and create a very welcoming space to gather, relax, rest, or enjoy the company of friends and family.

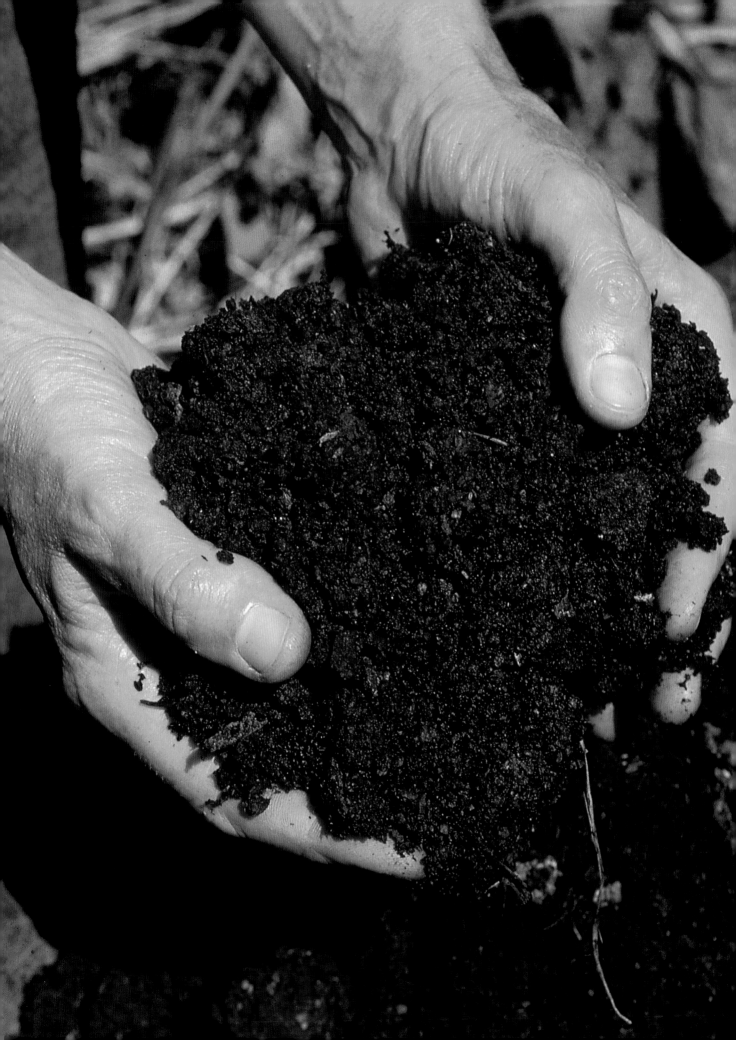

CHAPTER THREE

Secrets to Great Soil

The health of any plant begins with the soil. Most new gardeners think taking care of plants is all that's involved in growing herbs, but as an organic gardener, you'll need to cultivate healthy soil, just as you cultivate healthy plants. Evaluate the nature of your soil to determine how you can best improve and maintain it. Foster beneficial organisms that support the health of your soil, and use organic material, such as compost, to help maintain soil vitality. Nourishing the soil on a continual basis, using earth-friendly materials, is critical to growing the best-quality herbs. Plants utilize nutrients in the soil to become vibrant and healthy, and producing vital soil is the first important step toward a gorgeous and useful herb garden.

How Will Your Garden Grow?

Once the location has been determined and you know the size of your garden space, think about whether you will be growing in beds, rows, containers, or raised beds. This will help you decide how to treat the soil for maximum effect.

Bed or Row Planting

I prefer to grow in garden beds. This method enables me to maximize the space by using less of the area to accommodate pathways. It also means the growing areas won't be walked in, thus preventing the soil from becoming compacted. Less soil will be exposed to the elements, reducing its loss from wind and erosion.

I live in the high mountain desert of southern Colorado, where water conservation is critical. Bed cropping allows for drip-style or careful sprinkler irrigation, which uses less precious water while still meeting the growing needs of the plants. Even if you live where water is more abundant, you should be acting with a global consciousness so as to use as little of our water resources as possible.

Prepare the soil by digging up the beds and mixing in organic matter (see page 60 for more information on organic matter). Ideally, do this in the fall or early spring. Just before planting, till the soil again and then rake it smooth. Incorporate walking space into the area to allow for easy access to the beds. Proceed with planting in mid- to late spring.

If you must rely on flood-irrigating your garden, planting in rows may be your best choice. Some

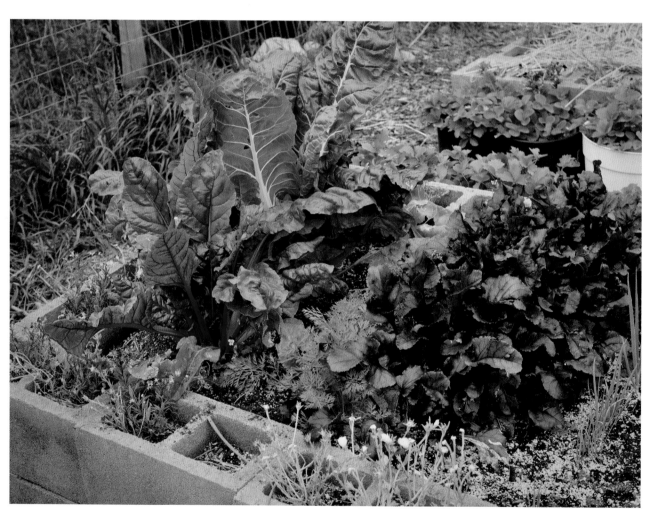

Create a raised bed for herbs and salad greens, using cinder blocks to form the planting box and compost-rich garden soil for the medium. This style of raised bed also provides easy access to maintain and harvest herbs at a comfortable height.

gardeners like row planting simply because it allows them to utilize a garden tractor, but I prefer to use a tiller or hand tools whenever possible. Using a tractor on more than a very occasional basis will compact the soil and make it more difficult for plants to develop an extensive root structure. That results in a lot more work for you when root harvest time comes and you're trying to dig them out of rock-hard soil. If you have decided to row-plant in your garden, incorporate mulching practices to help nourish the soil and hold in moisture. Mulching also helps prevent soil erosion and cuts down on the amount of weeds.

Container and Raised-Bed Gardening

Preparing planter boxes in the form of raised beds or growing in containers is also an excellent way to garden with herbs. If you have very limited space — a patio or balcony, for example — this may be your best or only option. In addition, containers allow for a better growing medium if the soil where you live is exceptionally poor or polluted and would thus make for poor-quality herbs.

For people who are physically challenged, containers or planter boxes make garden work a simpler task. They provide easier, safer access for those who use a wheelchair, a cane, or other aid. This type of garden may increase the comfort level of gardeners who aren't able to bend and stoop as much as a traditional garden requires. For this reason, those of us who are getting a bit older will find planter boxes and containers an ideal choice.

Fill containers and planter boxes with a good-quality soil. The soil should be light enough that it doesn't compact over time, heavy enough to hold moisture. Good container and planter box soil mixes are available at garden centers and nurseries as "planter's mix" and "perennial soil mix." Purchase these mixes by the bag or in bulk (cubic yard); the garden center or nursery staff will help you calculate how much you need.

SHARP SAND FOR WET CLIMATES

In climates that are very wet, humid, or extra cold, some gardeners incorporate sharp sand or gravel into the soil before they plant their herbs. These help the soil to warm a bit more than usual and improve drainage considerably. This simple step, although a lot of work initially to implement, may mean the difference between success in growing herbs like lavender and thyme — plants that would otherwise struggle in a wet or cold region — and a disappointing failure to make them happy.

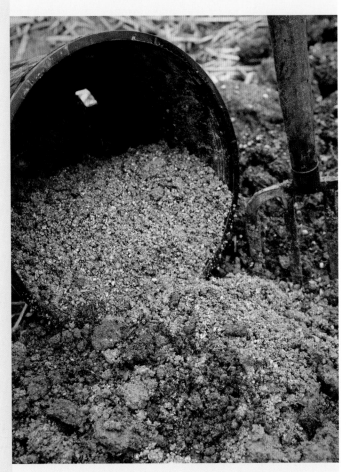

Adding sharp sand or gravel is an excellent way to improve drainage and raise soil temperatures in regions where the soil is heavy or winters are wet and cold.

Preparing the Soil

Now that the format of the garden has been determined, it's time to nourish the soil. If the soil is very rich and good, you certainly are a lucky gardener! Most of us will discover that our soil needs some type of nourishment. All garden soil must have caretaking to maintain its ability to grow healthy plants.

Adding Organic Matter

By far the most critical component of soil is organic matter. Organic matter consists of materials like leaves, manure, and cover crops that decompose in the soil and provide it with the nutrients necessary to grow healthy plants. Organic matter also offers soil "roughage," which helps maintain good soil consistency, making it possible for plants to develop a healthy root structure. Adding organic matter

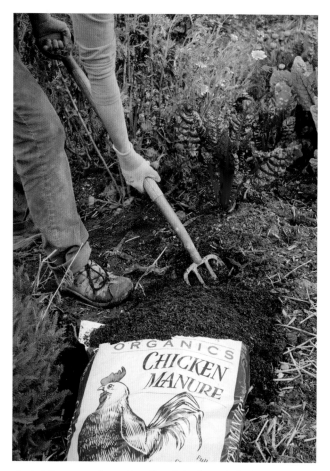

Adding organic matter, like dehydrated chicken manure, is a good way to increase the biological activity in the soil and the amount of nutrients available to plants.

improves soil health. As an ongoing process — one that must be repeated every year — it replenishes what plants deplete and will maintain healthy levels of nutrients.

To determine if your soil is of good quality, take a bit of the moist earth in your hand. Squeeze your hand into a fist. When you open the hand, the soil should crumble easily through your fingers when prodded, rather than forming a tight ball. If you have sandy soil, you'll need to examine it to see if there are bits of soil and composted organic matter mixed in with the sand. This sample, too, should crumble even after being squeezed.

For most plants, the ideal level of organic matter is between 4 and 5 percent. Send off a soil sample to your local Cooperative Extension Service to be tested so that you know if you need to add organic matter before planting your garden. Pick up a kit from the Extension Service — it will tell you how to prepare a soil sample for testing. Be sure to state what type of testing you would like to have done. In most cases, the soil will be tested for organic matter levels, nutrient levels, salt levels, and soil pH. The Extension Service will then send you an analysis of your soil, and recommendations for improving it.

Start with the Basics

Each year you will want to incorporate amendments into your garden soil. Organic matter (leaves, compost, manure) is best added to the soil in the late fall. If you can't add any in late fall, make it a point to add the organic matter in early spring. Use a wheelbarrow to transport the organic matter to the garden, and spread the material evenly on top of the soil. You can also use a manure spreader if you're tending a larger area.

The next step is tilling or digging in: Till as soon as possible once the organic matter has been spread over the soil. Delaying this step will result in nitrogen loss through its breakdown from exposure to the air.

Use Cover Crops

Cover crops, like organic matter, also help build good-quality soil. These are living "manures" that add vital nutrients to the earth. As cover crops grow and thrive, they protect the soil from wind and water erosion, at the same time providing much-needed food for wildlife.

The seeds of the cover crop are planted in the fall (or at the end of the normal growing season). For us in Colorado, that means late September to mid-October. In very early spring, or at least four weeks before the planting season begins, till the cover crop into the soil and let it sit for a week or two. After that time, till the soil again to prepare it for the actual spring planting of your herbs.

Common cover crops are grasses and legumes. Winter rye, oats, buckwheat, clovers, and alfalfa are all good choices. Short-term cover crops — such as buckwheat, winter rye, and oats — stay in place for only a season or two. If the garden is being left fallow for several seasons or even a few years, legumes, red clover, and alfalfa are good choices for the long term. All of these plants are deep-rooted and nitrogen-rich, excellent for replenishing the nutrients in tired soil.

Evaluating pH

A soil's pH level will indicate its degree of acidity or alkalinity. Plants are directly affected by pH, as this influences what nutrients are available to their roots. It also determines how deep a plant can root, as subsoils may have different pH levels. For these reasons, it's useful to know the pH of your soils.

Most plants grow best in a pH level between 6.0 and 6.5, providing there are adequate organic matter and nutrients available in the soil. Different soil components like sulfur and lime will raise or lower the pH level by increasing or decreasing acidity. As the soil pH changes, you will be able to detect changes in a plant's growth habits and health. Changing pH levels may also affect an herb's medicinal and nutritional potency.

We humans are not known to be very good soil caretakers when it comes to pH. By this I mean that when we try to adjust the pH to a level *we* feel is ideal, we often lose sight of what the plants need for the region they are growing in. Everything in a growing environment is interwoven: soil, available water, temperature, insect populations, and pollinators. The type of trees that are growing in your garden space will also influence the soil's pH.

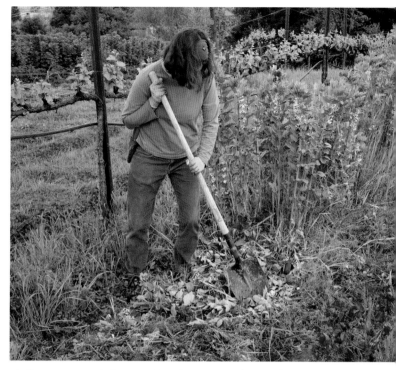

Cover crops of clover, oats, winter rye and many legumes can be dug or tilled into the soil, adding much-needed organic matter and helping to fix nitrogen in the soil.

In short, you will have better success growing herbs if you ensure that you have sufficient organic matter in your garden and then work *with* the existing pH level of the soil. The soil is integrated with all the other growing factors available to you; if you choose plants that can grow at the existing pH level, they will do well. If you manipulate the pH of the soil, you'll have to be really careful to get it right. Otherwise you risk creating an even more undesirable soil situation. Remember that there are a lot of environmental factors involved in addition to the soil's pH, and once you start the process of manipulating pH levels, you have to constantly maintain those new levels. This can be challenging, given that other factors are involved — like water quality, climatic conditions, and soil nutrition. Often we throw things *out of balance* more often than we keep things *in balance*. Learn what your soil pH is through a soil test (see page 60) and then work with what you've got, rather than trying to change it. If you would really like to grow an herb that needs a radically different soil than what you've got, consider growing it in a container.

Composting

One of the most important principles of organic growing is the use of compost. Compost begins as individual organic ingredients like kitchen scraps and garden trimmings. Combine these together in the right proportions, adding the working benefits of worms and microorganisms that process those organic ingredients, along with moisture and heat, and you have a process called composting. The end result is the efficient breakdown of individual ingredients to the point where they transform into a nutrient-rich source of organic material that both nourishes the soil, fertilizes plants, and keeps soil from compacting around plant roots. This same compost continues to nourish organisms, like beneficial nematodes and earthworms, which live in healthy soil.

Ingredients

Finished compost can be purchased by the bag or in bulk from your local garden center or nursery, making it immediately available and ready to mix into your garden soil. However, you may choose to start your own composting regime. You will want to incorporate into your compost a variety of ingredients. Soil, manure, small twigs and leaves, trimmings from garden maintenance, and vegetable or fruit scraps from the kitchen are all good additions to compost. After these items have decomposed, they will be added back into the soil of the garden or field as a nutrient-rich organic soil builder.

Compost Bins and Structures

To begin your compost, build a surrounding structure to contain the pile. You can create a compost pile without one, but I find that a structure helps to keep the compost ingredients together, so the decomposition process is more efficient. It also gives a tidier appearance.

There are several ways to build a structure. It can be made from wire, wooden pallets, cinder blocks, or a 55-gallon metal drum. Some people dig a pit in the ground and put their compost ingredients in the pit. You could forgo building a structure and instead purchase a ready-made compost bin or barrel from a garden supply shop.

Use wire, wood, or cinder blocks to form a cube or cylinder. Pasture wire and chicken wire work well, and can be formed into a tube and tied closed with baling wire or twine, Or, place four wooden pallets to form a cube and fasten the corners with wire. When the time comes to turn the compost pile, simply untie the wire and reverse the structure, sort of like turning a shirt wrong side out. Then retie the wire at the corners to secure the pallets into place, forming a new cube.

Cinder blocks will make the most permanent type of structure, when placed in a horseshoe shape of three sides and open in front for easy access. Turn the compost ingredients with a garden fork to facilitate the decomposition process.

Pit or Pile Composting

For pit composting, dig a hole in the ground. The hole should be 2 to 3 feet (0.6–0.9 m) deep and unlined. Add compost ingredients until the pit is filled sufficiently. Then cover compost with soil and allow the material to decompose. When the process is completed, use the compost as needed in the garden.

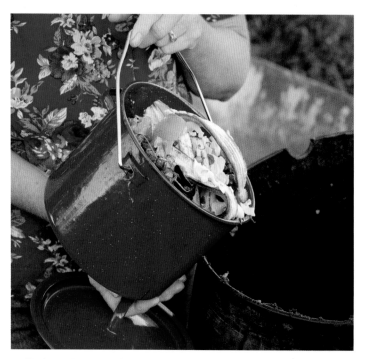

Fruit and vegetable scraps, along with yard waste, are excellent additions to the compost pile.

WHAT NOT TO USE IN COMPOST

In general, it's best to avoid adding meat and dairy products to the compost pile. A constant high temperature is required to break down meat and dairy products so that they can be used safely in a garden. It is extremely difficult to keep the compost temperature consistently hot enough, and if that high temperature is not maintained, those foods can become a health hazard. They also attract undesirable animal and insect visitors to the compost.

Along with dairy products and meats, there are a few types of plant materials that should not go into compost. Do not use succulent plants, like houseleek (also known as hen-and-chickens), because they don't decompose very easily. Annual and perennial weeds that have gone to seed are also best avoided. Never use plants that are infected with a virus or bacteria (see chapter 6 for more information on plant diseases). Do not add large branches to the compost unless they have been put through a chipper or shredder first. Lastly, human waste and pet waste are not appropriate ingredients for compost because of the health hazards they could introduce.

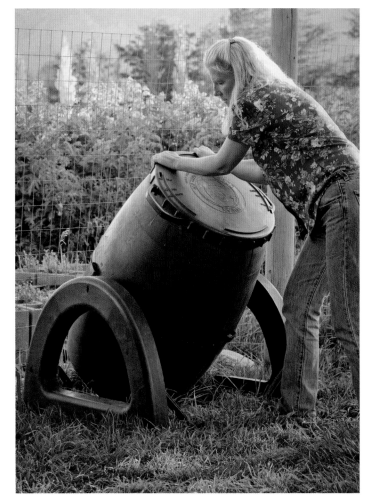

A rotating compost barrel makes composting easy for urban gardeners. Regularly add kitchen scraps and garden trimmings to the barrel, and rotate it often to stir the mix.

The simplest compost is a pile in a corner of the garden or field. This works fine if you are diligent about turning the pile and keeping it moist. It's not the most attractive type of compost, but it's certainly functional, and costs nothing to create.

Drum Composters

When choosing a drum for your composter, *never* select one that has been used to store toxic or petroleum-based substances. Whatever other drum you decide on, clean it with a hose that's been outfitted with a pressure nozzle. After rinsing well, fill it with water and an environmentally friendly cleaner such as a citrus-based detergent. Scrub the drum's interior with an old broom, then rinse thoroughly.

If you are making a compost bin from a 55-gallon metal drum, you will need to hire a welder to create a door of sorts in the side of the barrel. The door will provide access for adding ingredients and removing finished compost to be used in the garden. You will also need to create some holes in the ends of the barrel for air circulation. This type of bin works best if it can be put onto a horseshoe-shaped metal frame. The frame acts as a cradle, enabling you to roll the barrel to mix the compost. If you are using a plastic drum, be sure it is food-safe — that is, it does not contain chemicals that will leach into the compost.

Creating the Compost Pile

Once you have made a structure to hold the compost ingredients, you will begin adding the vital components to create compost. This is the best way I have found to layer the ingredients.

1. Place several small twigs in the bottom of the bin. These twigs will take some time to decompose; in the initial stages of your compost's life, they will form air pockets at the bottom of the pile, providing ventilation for the other ingredients.

2. Add a layer of soil, about 8 to 10 inches (20–25 cm) deep.

3. Cover the soil with a 4- to 6-inch (10–15 cm) layer of manure (for more information, see below).

4. Steps 1 through 3 comprise the early building blocks of your compost pile. Now you can begin layering additional ingredients. There are many choices for appropriate compost ingredients (see below). Utilizing a variety of components facilitates faster decomposition of the compost.

5. As you layer ingredients into the compost, add a 6-inch (10 cm) layer of soil and a 2- to 4-inch (5–10 cm) layer of manure about every 24 inches (60 cm) to ensure that you have incorporated all of the healthy elements of compost into the pile.

Manure

Use whatever type of livestock manure is available to you, as long as it is from a good organic source. (Feedlot livestock and poultry farm animals are often fed growth hormones and antibiotics, making their manure unsafe for your garden use.) Do *not* use dog or cat manure at all.

The more aged the manure is, the faster it will compost; fresh manure takes a bit longer to break down. Never put fresh manure directly on a garden; it will burn the plants and increase the amount of *E. coli* bacteria in harvested herbs.

Additional Ingredients

KITCHEN SCRAPS like vegetable and fruit trimmings, grains, eggshells, tea, and tea leaves are all good to use in compost. Again, avoid adding meat or dairy products to your compost pile (see What Not to Use in Compost, page 63).

LEAVES, GARDEN AND LAWN CLIPPINGS are very good ingredients for your compost. Whenever you weed, deadhead flowers, prune, or do other garden housekeeping tasks, add those trimmings to the compost. Be sure to mix grass clippings with other ingredients when adding them to the compost; large layers of grass clippings alone will mat, dry out, get very hot, and prevent water from moving through the compost efficiently.

Activating Compost

If you're anxious to have your compost ready to use as soon as possible, you can give the composting process a jump start by adding certain nitrogen- and mineral-rich organic ingredients at the start of the process that will be really good at breaking down and feeding the microorganisms. We call these ingredients compost activators. Garden shops offer compost activator products, which can be convenient, but it isn't necessary to purchase one: Consider making your own.

Nettle leaves, comfrey leaves, and seaweed are all excellent compost activators. Make a compost tea of any or all of these ingredients (see recipe on page 65) and add it to the compost once every three months. The tea supplies extra minerals and a rich source of nitrogen your compost will utilize to begin breaking down the other ingredients and making a supremely nutritious compost.

It is not absolutely necessary to use compost activators to create healthy compost, and you can easily proceed without them, but I find that using my surplus nettles and comfrey leaves as compost activators does get my compost really happening. Equally true is that it is not necessary to buy worms to add to your compost, although they are available for purchase from many garden shops. You can buy them if you want to, but if you are working your compost on a regular basis and are adding healthy ingredients to it, the worms will find their way into the bin on their own.

Working the Compost

It is important to turn compost once a month in warm and hot weather. During the cold winter months, the compost pile is not hot enough to decompose much, so turning is less important.

TURNING THE COMPOST can be done using a shovel or garden fork. I find it easier to work with a garden fork, but give both a try and see what you prefer. The goal is to flip the pile. Ideally you want all of the material on the top of the pile to become the bottom of the new pile and the material that is nearer the bottom to become the top. Everything in the middle usually stays in the middle, but it gets all mixed up in the process, which is perfect.

As you turn the pile, you may find that at the very bottom is a small amount of composted material: it will look like a rich, dark brown soil. That's the compost that is ready to use. Use it immediately or mix it back into the pile for later use. If you have a very large compost pile, such as might be the case on a small farm, you will need to use a tractor to turn it.

WATERING THE COMPOST is a key step, especially in arid climates, to maintain a hospitable environment for the microbes that do the decomposing. Compost should stay evenly moist; it should not be soaking wet, nor should it be dried out. I live in a very dry, hot, and sometimes windy region, and I need to water my compost about once a month during hot weather. In climates where there is more precipitation, you can water the compost less often. Simply water it with a hose, making sure that every part of the pile has been watered evenly.

Incorporating Compost into the Garden

Once the composted material is ready for use, it can be worked into the garden soil. If the garden will be freshly tilled, apply a 1- to 3-inch (2.5–7.5 cm) layer of compost to the top of the soil. Till or work the compost into the soil until it is well mixed. If you are adding compost to an existing perennial garden, apply a topdressing of compost ½ to 1 inch (1.25–2.5 cm) thick. Rake the compost into the soil all around the plants.

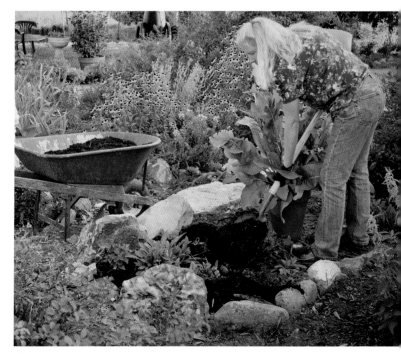

Topdressing with finished compost is an excellent way to add nutrients and organic matter to your soil. Simply spread the compost in a thin layer on top of the soil, working around the plants.

COMPOST ACTIVATOR TEA

To avoid skin irritation, be sure to wear gloves whenever working with fresh nettles. Don't let this mixture sit in the house while it's steeping — it doesn't smell very good! This makes enough activator for up to a 64-cubic-foot (1.8 m³) compost pile.

- 6 cups dried or 12 cups fresh nettles
- 6 cups dried or 12 cups fresh comfrey leaves
- 2 cups flaked or powdered kelp

Put all ingredients into a 5-gallon bucket and fill the bucket with water. Let the mixture sit in a warm place for 4 to 8 hours, then pour the contents of the bucket into the compost pile.

The ideal time to add compost is spring, but you can really incorporate it at any time of the year. Once you've added the compost, water the garden thoroughly. This will encourage the plants' roots to begin drawing up the nutrients the compost provides.

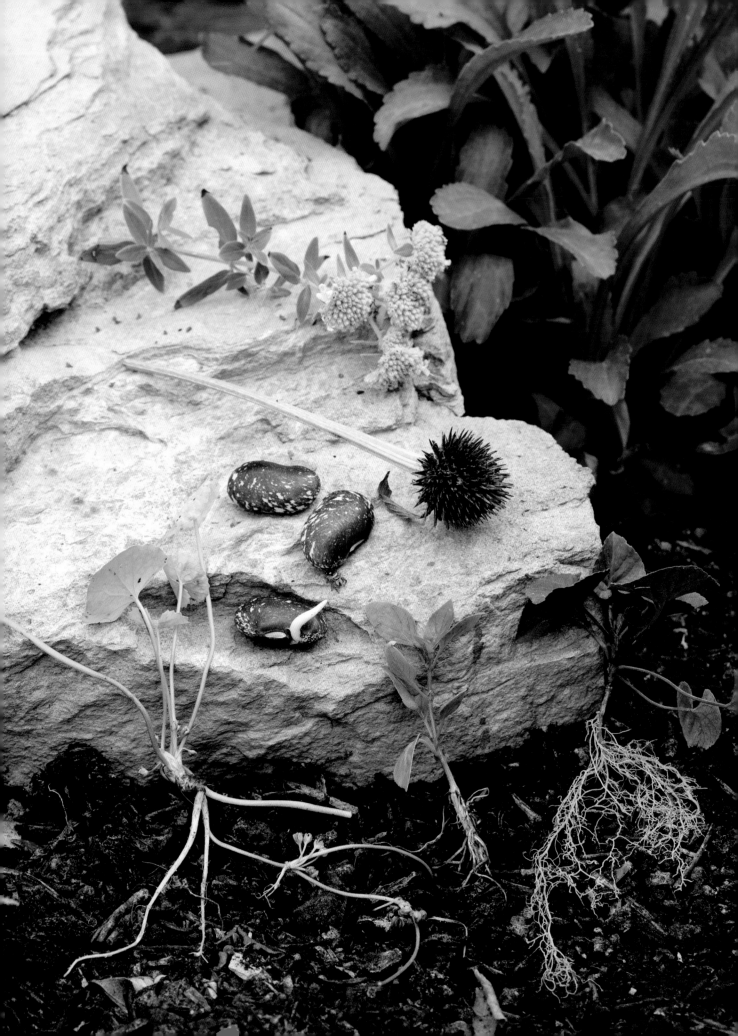

CHAPTER FOUR

Propagation Methods

When you're ready to start growing your plants, you'll first have to decide if you're going to grow them from seed or use some other propagation method, like cuttings or root divisions. Many of the herbs will be successful if you grow them in the same way that you handle vegetables or annual flowers, but far more of them will have at least one special requirement in order to sprout or root and begin a thriving life. Get acquainted with your chosen plants by browsing through chapter 10. You can also consult nurseries or other growers in your area for advice.

If you are new to growing herbs, remember that the *only* rule is that there are no rules. Open yourself to experimentation and flexibility. Many of the herbs — especially those closest to their wild roots — seem to hate rules, and they are ingenious at breaking them. Set aside technology for a moment and begin to think like the plant you want to grow.

Each Plant Is an Individual

The first step is to learn a bit about the individual plant. Learn as much as you can about where the plant might grow naturally — chapter 10 will provide more insight into each herb's personality traits. Also check wild-plant identification books; they are a good source of information about plants' natural habitats. In addition, I utilize geography books and naturalist guidebooks, and the Internet can also be a valuable resource. Knowing about each herb's natural preferences is the key to success in growing your favorite plants.

Ask yourself:

- What part of the world is it native to?

- Where would this plant grow if it could choose its ideal place?

- What type of climate exists where the plant comes from?

- What other plants grow in community with this plant?

- What types of animals and insects have a relationship with this plant?

Once you have an idea about a plant's natural growing environment, try to replicate that environment as closely as possible. As much as possible, provide the herb's desired temperature range. Offer some shade, if needed, and keep the plants evenly moist, but not soggy. (See chapter 3 for tips on getting your soil into the best possible shape.) Careful monitoring of changes in a plant's environment will yield consistent, positive results.

Choosing a Propagation Method

There are a number of propagation methods; the one you choose will be determined by the needs of each specific plant (see chapter 10 for individual plant requirements).

Whenever possible, I prefer to start my plants from seed, as I feel this gives me the strongest plants and preserves the plant's genetic identity. Plants grown from seed generally have very strong survival instincts that help them adapt to tough climates, critter interaction, insect pests, and disease.

However, plants grown from seed occasionally do not develop certain desirable characteristics, such as strong flavor, aroma, and medicinal value, and even cosmetic traits like flower or foliage color.

Some plants cannot be grown from seed reliably or even at all. Occasionally, plants do not produce viable seed, or the seeds consistently germinate too poorly. This is often the case with rosemary and comfrey. For plants that do not develop the desired characteristics (many mints, for example) seed growing is not the best choice. These plants must be grown from a cutting, root division, runner, or crown division. When plants are grown in this

> Knowing about each herb's natural preferences is the key to success in growing them.

way, the offspring is an identical clone of its mother plant. For example, we are used to peppermint having a very strong taste and fragrance. This is due to the high levels of volatile oils it contains. But peppermint grown from seed does not carry the desired levels of volatile oils and has a very weak minty taste and aroma.

Gotu kola and yerba mansa both multiply from their runners — essentially, this is the layering propagation method. Similar to strawberries, these herbs have runners that trail off the mother plant, and wherever the runner comes in contact with the soil, it puts down roots. For plants of this nature, layering is easy and effective.

Root and crown divisions are another way to propagate. In this method, the mother plant is lifted out of the soil and the roots are carefully separated and replanted in soil to create baby plants. Horseradish and comfrey are two herbs that are best propagated by divisions.

Keep in mind that *every plant is an individual with its own specific requirements*. Don't fall into the trap of lumping all plants into the same growing categories. Chapter 10 and the Propagation at a Glance chart on page 78 will give you more information to help you start your garden off right.

Growing from Seed

I am often told that starting plants from seed is just too difficult and intimidating. That does not need to be the case. Before you begin seed sowing, first determine where to get the seeds. Will you buy seeds or harvest, clean, and store your own from your garden year to year? Then, when you have your seeds, determine whether they will require special treatment prior to being sown.

Selecting and Purchasing Seeds

If your choice is not to save your own seed, you will need to buy seed from a reputable seed house. Large companies are not automatically quality companies. Seed companies, large and small, should be able to answer your questions to your satisfaction. Is their seed labeled correctly with common and Latin names? Has the seed been treated chemically in any way (avoid any with fungicides or antisprouting agents)? How long do they store seed? Is the seed fresh? Ask your supplier these questions *before* you buy.

There are a number of excellent seed companies, and I have listed many of my favorites in the Resources section (page 245). Each year I come across a seed house I wasn't aware of, and I always give new companies a try to see if the seeds perform well. Of course, I always look for organic seed choices whenever possible. When I do find an excellent seed source, I become a loyal customer.

I boycott seed houses that handle genetically modified/engineered seeds. I feel that propagating these seeds is unethical and dangerous both to the environment and to our bodies. As a medical herbalist, I believe that it's impossible to know how plants grown from such seeds will behave physiologically when they are ingested as foods or medicines.

Applying Seed Treatments

Some seeds will need extra treatment before you can sow them. This is where your previous research on the individual plant is most critical. What happens to that seed when it matures on a plant out in nature? Does it drop immediately to the ground or does the wind carry it off? Is it likely to be eaten by an animal or a bird? Will it spend several months exposed to the winter snow or a rainy season? Factors such as these will affect the germination of the seed. Put your mind in the place of the plant, and when you have thought about what the seed would experience in nature, ponder how you can duplicate those factors in your growing situation.

STRATIFICATION. If the seed would normally experience a period of winter with cold temperatures, ice, and freezing and thawing conditions, that seed will most likely benefit — indeed require — *stratification*. Stratification is the process of chilling or freezing moistened seeds to simulate winter. If the plant in its natural habitat would have to survive an icy winter, the seeds should be stratified in the freezer. Place seeds in a ziplock freezer bag with a few drops of water. Shake the bag to coat the seeds with moisture, then put the bag into the freezer for two to three months. Remove the bag from the

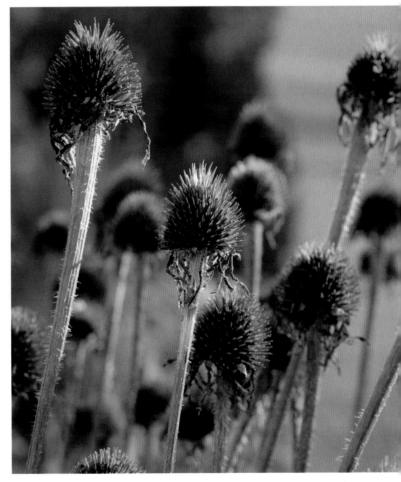

Many herb seeds will germinate more readily if they're treated before being sown. These echinacea seeds will respond well to stratification (cold treatment) before planting.

freezer once a month and allow the seeds to thaw for a few hours. Then return them to the freezer. This method, which is also called *wet stratification,* creates the freezing/thawing effects of cold climates.

If the seeds would normally experience a cold winter but not necessarily a frozen one, carry out the stratification in the refrigerator. In this case, put the seeds into moistened peat moss or sand in a ziplock plastic bag, place the bag in the fridge, and check it every couple of days. When the seeds start to sprout, plant them as usual. This technique is often referred to as *cold stratification.*

SCARIFICATION. Perhaps the seeds you want to germinate would experience some type of situation in their native environment that would cause the seed coat to get slightly damaged. This process allows moisture to more easily penetrate the seed and initiate germination. Maybe the wind would carry that seed across a gravelly or sandy surface, for example. Artificially inducing this process is

called *scarification.* There are several ways to scarify a seed. I lay a piece of coarse sandpaper in the bottom of a shoe box. I then place the seeds on top of the sandpaper and gently rub the seeds back and forth a few times. This will abrade the seed coat. Another method is to place the seeds in a small coffee can with some coarse sand. Cover and gently shake the can a few times; the friction of the seeds against the sand will cause scarification. For very large seeds or those that have an especially hard coat, you may have to nick each one with a small sharp knife. Use extreme care in this process; you don't want to injure yourself or damage the fragile embryo of the seed just inside the coat. The goal is to nick the seed coat without going any deeper.

SOAKING. Some seeds need to experience extended periods of wetness. In nature, this could occur in snow cover or a native habitat along a stream bank. This soaking time enables the seed coat to soften so that the seed may sprout more easily. If I think seeds will germinate more easily if soaked, I place them in a small bowl, pour hot water over them, and let them soak. Hot water is used because it softens

> Soaking enables the seed coat to soften so that the seed may sprout more easily.

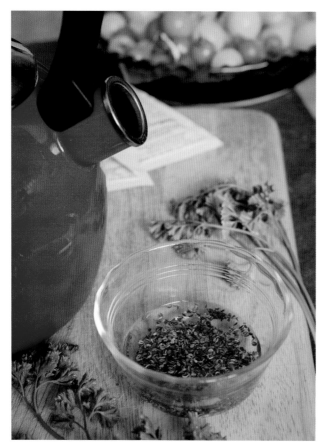

Parsley seeds typically take a long time to germinate, but soaking them in hot water prior to sowing will help them germinate more quickly.

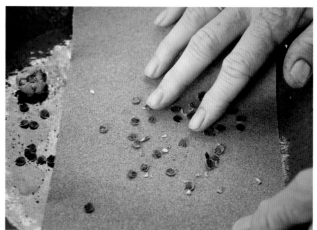

Hollyhock seeds can be rubbed lightly across sandpaper in a treatment called scarification. This scratches the seed coat, allowing the seeds to sprout more easily.

the seed coat more quickly; this is important, as simulated soaking will be for a shorter duration than the natural soaking process. The soaking time varies depending on the seed; refer to chapter 10 for more information. After the appropriate soaking time, sow the seeds immediately.

HYDROGEN PEROXIDE SOAKING. If you know that the plant you're propagating has seeds that usually get eaten and exposed to the digestive juices of an animal before germinating, consider a hydrogen peroxide soak. I use regular 3 percent hydrogen peroxide — the kind you might have in your bathroom cabinet for first-aid purposes. Many native dryland and desert plants seem to respond well to this type of treatment. The peroxide, like digestive juices, breaks down the seed coat a bit so that germination is easier. This type of soak should not be done for too long. Soak small or fragile seeds for only 15 to 20 minutes; larger or more durable seeds can soak for up to 45 minutes. Sow the seeds immediately after soaking.

Choosing a Soil Medium and Preparing the Seed Pots

Choose a soil medium that is not too heavy. You can purchase premade seed mixes or you can prepare your own using 4 parts soil, 8 parts peat moss, and 1 part perlite. Fill seed pots with your soil medium and water the pots well. I like to use a watering wand with a rosette sprinkler head for a soft, even water flow. (This waters thoroughly and evenly without washing the soil medium out of a pot.) Press the soil medium gently to eliminate any air pockets and to create an even sowing surface.

Step-by-Step Seed Sowing

As you are sowing the seeds, you should attempt to keep the spacing as even as possible. Seeds that fall in a clump will make transplanting more difficult, and these seedlings undergo more stress and shock when roots must be pulled apart during transplanting. Large seeds, like those of sage and hollyhock, are pretty easy to keep evenly spaced, whereas really tiny seeds like mullein and chamomile can be very difficult to space. If seeds are extremely tiny, mix 1 part seed with 2 parts cornmeal and then sow as usual, cornmeal and all. (The cornmeal acts as an

automatic spacing agent.) Now, gently tap the seeds onto the soil surface at the desired spacing.

One of the most important steps in sowing seed is to cover them to the proper depth. It is a common practice for people to plant their seeds too deep; these seeds will be unlikely to sprout. Most seeds should be planted to a depth that equals twice their diameter. Some seeds will require complete darkness, but most will need to be exposed to some light. I cover my seeds with vermiculite. Vermiculite allows light to penetrate, at the same time offering the seeds some protection and helping to maintain moisture in the flat.

Keep the Seeds Moist

Another critical step in germinating seeds is keeping them evenly moist (not soggy). They must never dry out! If they do, they won't sprout; if they have already sprouted and then dry out, the tiny seedlings will die. Take great care to keep your seed pots moist.

Since you soaked your seed pots thoroughly when you prepared them for sowing, it is usually only the surface soil that needs to have moisture renewed regularly. On a small scale, I find a spray bottle filled with water works great for this task; a gentle spray will give the seeds moisture without washing them out of the flat. In our greenhouses, I find a rosette watering wand held at shoulder height and moved evenly and slowly above the pots gently waters the seed surface.

Other Propagation Methods

Some plants can't be propagated from seed, either because they don't produce seed, the seed isn't viable, or the plants grown from seed will be missing a desirable trait, such as strong flavor. For example, comfrey doesn't produce seed; and rosemary produces seeds but usually the germination rate is extremely low. Other herbs have a unique characteristic like color variegation (such as lemon thyme) or extra-high amounts of volatile oil (such as peppermint and spearmint) that will not grow "true" when propagation is done by seed.

Tip cuttings, layering, root divisions, and crown propagation are other ways to start a new generation of plants.

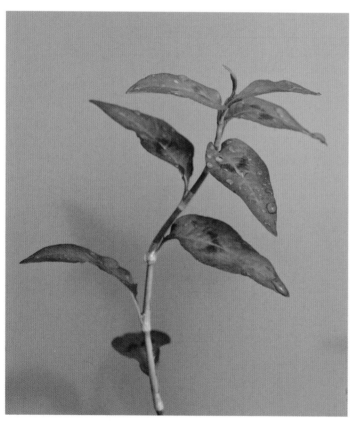

Vietnamese coriander is easily propagated from cuttings.

Cuttings

Cuttings are my second choice for propagating. Some herbs will be very difficult to root from cuttings but many will develop roots easily. Mints, Vietnamese coriander, and thyme are all easy to start from cuttings. For me, propagation by cuttings is usually easier than are other non-seed propagation methods.

PREPARATION. Fill small pots with the same soil medium you use for seeding. Water the pots.

After the pots are prepared, you will need a rooting hormone to get your cuttings off to a good start. Rooting hormone contains indole-3-butyric acid and 1-naphthaleneacetic acid, two naturally occurring plant growth hormones that stimulate sprouting along the stem nodes. There are three types of rooting hormone.

LIQUID CONCENTRATE ROOTING HORMONE is the one I prefer. Label directions give the appropriate dilution for the kind of plant you are trying to root. With this type of hormone, I can prepare the mixture as strong or as weak as necessary for the plant I am working with.

POWDERED ROOTING HORMONE is available at garden shops. Roll the cutting ends in the powder and then stick them into the soil. This type of rooting hormone, though convenient, is actually my least favorite because there is no way to adjust the level of hormone used. Some plants require little rooting hormone in order to produce good roots; other plants, especially those with woody stems, need a stronger rooting hormone solution. Vietnamese coriander roots easily with very little rooting hormone. However, rosemary and sage are woodier and benefit from a stronger solution.

HOMEMADE ROOTING HORMONE can be prepared from liquid kelp concentrate. Use 1 teaspoon of kelp concentrate per ounce of water. I find that kelp rooting hormone works pretty well for most cuttings, but some dryland native and desert plants don't seem to like this substitute. These arid-climate plants respond better to rooting hormone made from a very strong brew of willow bark tea. Use 1 teaspoon of bark per 1 cup of boiling water and infuse for at least 20 minutes before straining the bark out, allowing the tea to cool, and then proceeding as usual to dip your cuttings in the tea solution. If you make either of these homemade rooting hormone solutions, remember that they will keep for only two days, and be sure to refrigerate them when you are not using them. After two days you should prepare a fresh batch.

CUTTING TIPS. Take only one-third to one-half of the tender growth available. If you take more than that, you will increase the stress on the mother plant.

A quick rooting-hormone dip is fine for most plants. Use a small, thin stick to poke a hole into the soil, then stick the stem in the hole. Be sure that all peeled nodes are beneath the soil level. Remember to pinch the soil closed around the stem hole.

Put the pot of cuttings in a place out of direct sunlight. The area should be warm (68 to 70°F; 20–21°C), with good air circulation. Lightly cover the cuttings with a piece of shade cloth. Keep the soil evenly moist. Cuttings will root in 1 to 4 weeks, depending on the plant. You will know that the cutting has rooted in if it resists a *very* gentle tug.

Layering

If the plant you are working with has runners or offshoots, layering is the best method of propagation. These runners will root readily wherever a node has direct contact with the soil, resulting in plantlets all along the stems. Layering simply takes advantage of what nature already does.

PREPARATION. Fill a container with potting medium and water it in well. Unfold several paper clips and bend each into a simple horseshoe. Spacing them evenly, use the horseshoe clips to anchor the runners to the soil. Place the clips carefully so that every node or offshoot is firmly in contact with soil.

LAYERING TIPS. Set pots of layerings where they will be out of direct sunlight. The area should be warm (68 to 70°F; 20–21°C), with good air circulation. The layerings do not need to be covered. They will root in 1 to 2 weeks. Test for rooting by very gently tugging on a plantlet. If it has started to root,

it will not become dislodged by the gentle pressure. At this stage, clip the stem connection between the rooted plantlets with a pair of sharp scissors. When the herbs are ready to transplant, simply break apart the soil to create little plants with their own bit of soil around the roots.

Root Division

Whenever a plant has a branching root system, as with horseradish or comfrey, root divisions are a possible propagation method. Plants with a taproot — a single, long root rather than branching multiple roots — do not usually fare well by root division. This method will usually work for rhizomatous plants, such as ginger and turmeric, which have roots that grow laterally just under the soil surface, but again, research the individual plants before beginning to propagate in this way. It is always best to do root divisions in early spring or early fall, when the procedure is not quite so stressful for the mature plant.

Crown Propagation

Often a perennial plant, such as wood betony or self-heal, can be propagated by taking sections of the mother plant's root crown and planting those to create new plantlets. In this way the mother plant can remain in the garden happily growing but still yield a next generation of plantlets.

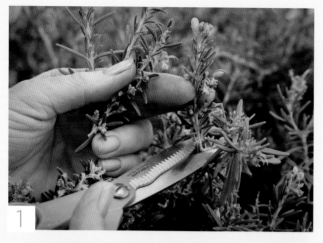

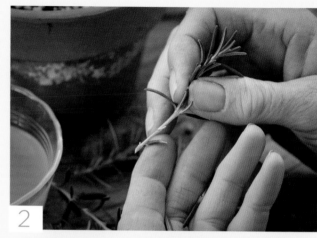

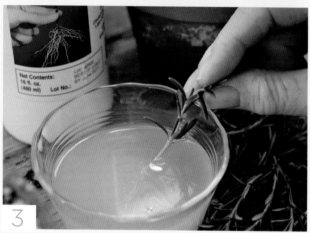

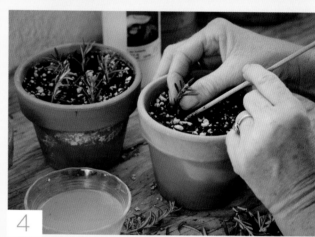

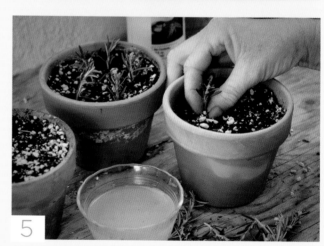

1) To take cuttings from the mother plant, snip off 1 to 3 inches (2.5–7.5 cm) of the tender tip growth.

2) Gently peel the leaves from the bottom two nodes, or joints, where they attach to the stem.

3) Dip the end of the stem into rooting hormone.

4) Stick the cutting deep enough into the soil medium so that all the stripped nodes will be under the soil surface.

5) With your thumb and first finger, gently pinch the soil up around the stem of the cutting.

LAYERING TO CREATE NEW PLANTS

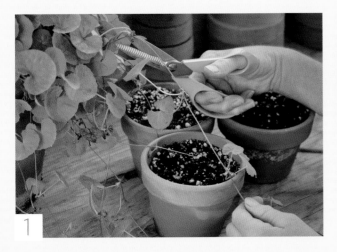

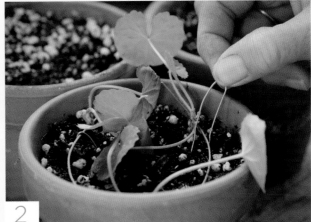

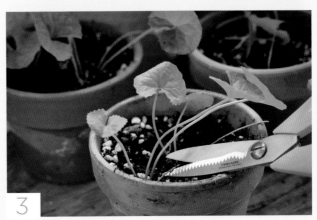

1) To layer in a pot, snip the runners near the point where they grow out of the mother plant. (To layer in the garden, lay a runner stem onto the garden soil where you would like the plant to root.)

2) Set the runner on top of the soil and secure with a bent, U-shaped paper clip.

3) Once the plantlets have begun to root well, snip the runner stem between the plantlets so each new plantlet can continue growing as an individual plant.

SOWING SEEDS

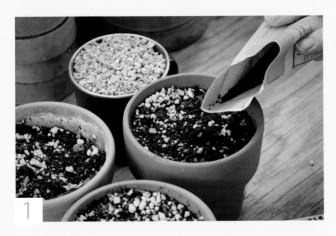

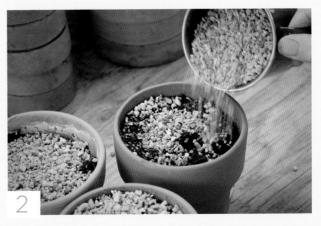

1) Once you have filled your pots by watering them in and gently pressing the soil to make a firm sowing surface, tap the seeds onto the soil at an even spacing.

2) Evenly cover the seeds at a depth that is approximately twice the seed's diameter. Keep seeds evenly moist until germination, or they won't be likely to sprout.

ROOT DIVISION

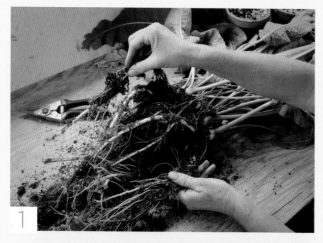

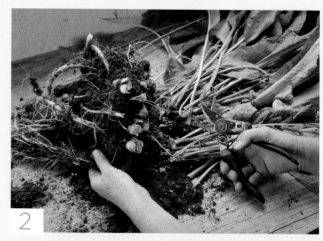

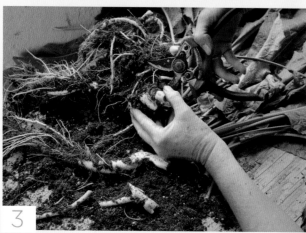

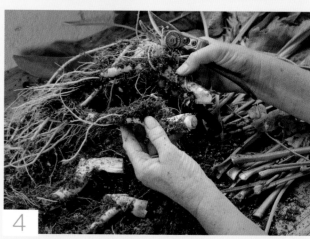

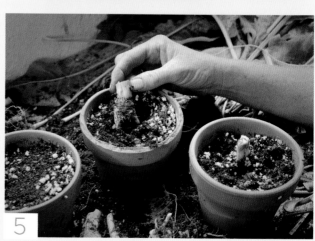

1) Carefully dig up the plant you want to divide and shake off excess soil from the roots.

2) Trim all the aerial tops from the root crown and discard them into the compost.

3) Turn the plant on its side, and using a sturdy pair of snips or a very sharp knife, slice through the root clump.

4) Make sure that each division has one or two roots attached to the crown.

5) Replant each division in the garden or in pots. Keep the soil evenly moist.

COMMON NAME (*LATIN NAME*)	PROPAGATION METHOD	WHERE TO START	SPECIAL TREATMENT
Sorrel, French, Red-veined (*Rumex acetosa, R. sanguineus*)	Seeds	Indoors, outdoors	Cold stratification
Southernwood (*Artemisia abrotanum*)	Cuttings, root divisions	Indoors, outdoors	Rooting hormone
Spearmint (*Mentha spicata*)	Root divisions, cuttings, layering	Indoors, outdoors	None
Spilanthes (*Spilanthes oleracea*)	Seeds	Indoors	None
St.-John's-wort (*Hypericum perforatum*)	Seeds	Indoors, outdoors	Cold stratification
Stevia (*Stevia rebaudiana*)	cuttings, seeds	Indoors	Rooting hormone; needs extra heat to germinate
Sunflower (*Helianthus annuus*)	Seeds	Indoors, outdoors	None
Sweetgrass (*Hierochloe odorata*)	Seed, root divisions	Indoors, outdoors	Wet stratification
Sweet woodruff (*Galium odoratum*)	Cuttings	Indoors	Rooting hormone
Thyme (*Thymus* species)	Root divisions, cuttings, seeds	Indoors, outdoors	Rooting hormone, cold stratification
Turmeric (*Curcuma longa*)	Root divisions	Indoors	Needs extra heat to root
Valerian (*Valeriana officinalis*)	Seeds	Indoors	None
Vervain, Blue vervain (*Verbena* species)	Seeds	Indoors	Cold stratification
Vietnamese coriander (*Polygonum odoratum*)	Root divisions, layering, cuttings	Indoors	None
Violet (*Viola* species)	Seeds	Indoors, outdoors	Wet stratification
Watercress (*Nasturtium officinale*)	Seeds	Indoors, outdoors	None
White sage (*Salvia apiana*)	Seeds	Indoors	Cold stratification; needs extra heat to germinate
Wood betony (*Stachys officinalis*)	Seeds	Indoors	Cold stratification
Yarrow (*Achillea* species)	Root divisions, seeds	Indoors, outdoors	Cold stratification
Yerba mansa (*Anemopsis californica*)	Seeds	Indoors	Needs extra heat to germinate
Yucca (*Yucca* species)	Seeds	Indoors, outdoors	Cold stratification, wet stratification

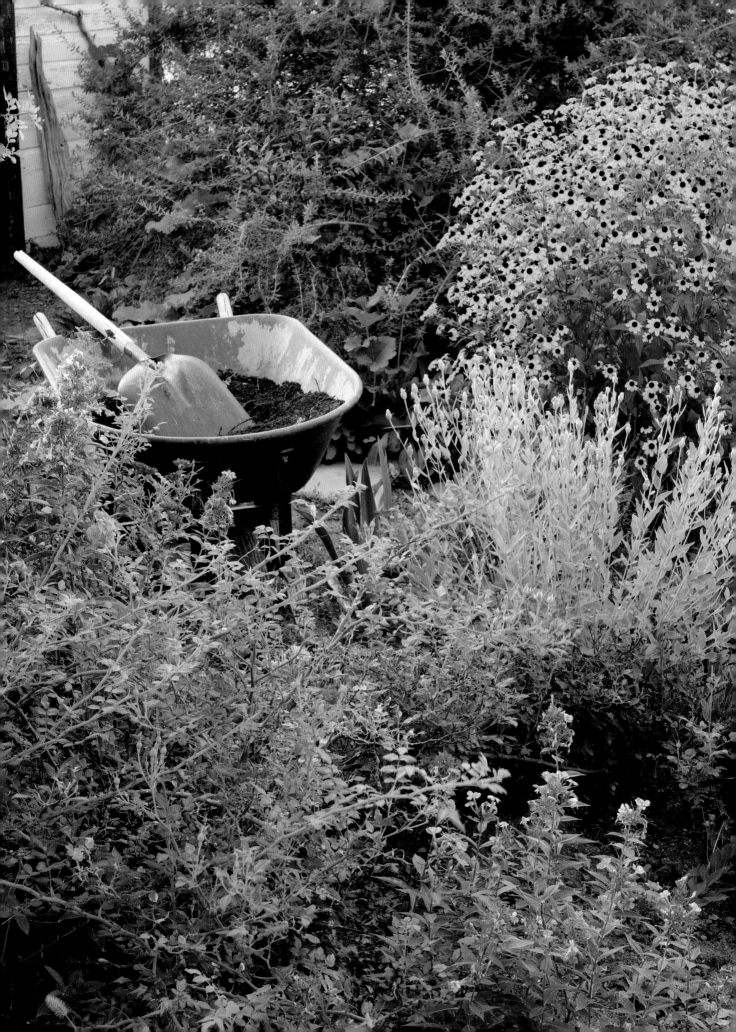

herbs but find them in your garden anyway, simply forage them out and put them to use in your cooking or medicine-making efforts.

Pulling Weeds

There are no two ways about it: Organic gardeners must pull weeds. The trick is to be efficient at the pulling so that you don't have to pull any more often than you want to.

Pull on a day when the ground is moist. Weeding is a much easier and faster task when the ground is damp. Grasp the weed as close to the ground as possible. Tug firmly on it to pull up as much of the root as possible. Some weeds have a complex root system and it is impossible to pull up 100 percent of their roots. Thistle and bindweed, for example, have root systems that are very difficult to pull up in one weeding. My husband, Chris, manages our farm, and it is his expert opinion that bindweed is really a great sleeping giant under the earth and pulling it amounts only to clipping the giant's fingernails, which will always grow again.

Do not get discouraged by persistent weeds; if you stay in charge of them, at some point they will begin to weaken and then eventually give you less of a problem. I find that if I spend 10 to 15 minutes a day, even with my extensive gardens, I can keep weeds under control and never have a weed disaster to deal with. Unfortunately, I *have* let my weeds get the upper hand on occasion. When this happens, I make a large pitcher of herbal iced tea for myself, and have a day of weeding frenzy to get things back on track.

Which Tools Should I Use?

There are several tools that I feel are invaluable in the task of weeding:

HORI HORI. Sometimes called a Japanese weeder, this is a 6- to 8-inch (15–20 cm), narrowly tapered hand spade with toothed edges. It easily digs, pries, and saws weeds out of existence. It is our primary tool of choice. It also doubles as a planting trowel and harvesting tool for roots and whole plants.

WINGED WEEDER. I have a hand-size winged weeder and one on a long handle to use as I would a hoe. This tool has a triangular blade that looks like a kite at the end of a curved neck. The long sides of the

SPECIAL WEEDING TIPS

It will make a big difference in your weed population if you can pull them out before they go to seed. Weeds have incredible survival instincts and they produce seed like crazy. Try to pull them out before the seed matures and you will be far ahead of the game.

Do not leave weeds that are in flower lying in the garden for later removal. Remember those survival instincts: Some weeds, like thistles, will still go to seed even after they have been pulled out! To prevent those unexpected weed seeds, remove the pulled weeds from the garden immediately.

Purslane is another great survivor, but in a different way. Also called portulaca, purslane is a succulent plant that will reroot where it is lying on the ground after being pulled out. Again, the key is to remove these weeds immediately from your garden area.

Once my weeds have been removed, including those like purslane, I put them into my compost barrel so that they can break down and become nutritious compost that goes back into the garden at a later time. If you have weeds with lots of seeds, you may wish to discard them in your trash. In our garden, any pulled weeds that we can't compost go into a big mucking bucket and are carried to our neighbor's chickens. The chickens forage through the weeds and eat up 99% of them, including the weed seeds. Problem solved. And instead of going to the landfill, the weeds are returned to the earth via chicken digestion.

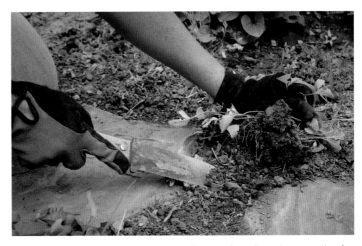

The hori hori, or Japanese weeding tool, makes short work of digging up weeds and getting the entire root system. It is an easy-to-use and very durable tool.

triangle are sharp. You work this tool just on the soil surface, going into the soil ½ to 1 inch (1.25–2.5 cm). The shape enables you to get very close to the base of garden plants, and the sharp edges cut off weeds as you go. This is a fast-weeding tool that also cultivates the soil a bit to keep it nice and loose.

TRADITIONAL HOES AND STIRRUP HOES are also useful for weeding. A traditional hoe has a long handle and a flat metal blade on a curved neck. As the tool is moved across the soil surface, the edge of the blade (which is usually sharpened) cuts off the weeds at the base of the stem. Stirrup hoes work in exactly the same way, but they are lighter because their metal blade isn't solid. This makes them a bit less tiring to use. All types of hoes do double duty as they also break up compacted soils.

HANDS. By far the best tools for weeding are your hands. Nothing is more efficient, because they can perform a great variety of functions.

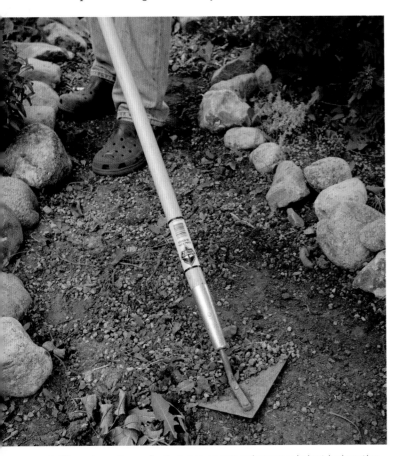

The winged weeder is great at removing weeds just below the surface of the soil. It is a lightweight tool that is faster and less tiring to use than a traditional hoe.

Protecting Plants with Mulch

Mulch serves many purposes in the garden. It can help keep weeds from becoming problematic. A good mulch retains moisture and warmth so that plants grow more vigorously and with greater water conservation. Mulch can also be used to create walking areas within a garden. The best part is that often mulch is either free or very inexpensive.

To apply a mulch, simply spread the material in a layer a few inches deep around the plants or in the walkways of your garden. Most mulching materials will last at least one growing season, and many of them will give you years of service.

Wood and Cloth Mulch

Many materials make great mulch. Recycled materials like cardboard and newspapers and even chipped branches can make great mulch. Wood-based mulch is readily available, slow to break down, and retains moisture quite well.

There are weed-barrier cloths that you can buy by the roll. These not only prevent weeds from growing through, but they also allow water to seep down to the plant roots. Because these barriers are made from black cloth, they absorb a lot of heat, helping to provide extra warmth for your plants. Although it is possible for the black cloth to absorb excess heat in summer, this problem is more common with black plastic.

If your weed-barrier cloth has been in place for many seasons, you may find that occasionally some weed seeds carried by the wind will land on top and try to grow. When this happens, it's best to pull those newly sprouted weeds before their roots get too established. By dealing with the situation at the start you'll avoid having it become a big problem.

Rock Mulch

In some areas, gravel and pebbles make good mulch. They also collect solar heat (especially dark-colored rock). A word of caution about black lava rock: It often collects *too* much heat and makes a space so hot that plants cannot survive, so use black lava rock with care.

CHAPTER SIX

Pest and Disease Control

Plant diseases and insect problems, fortunately, aren't usually as much of a concern for herb gardeners as they can be for vegetable and flower gardeners. My theory is that there is so much diversity among these plants that they become less attractive to pests. Diseases often focus on more homogeneous groups of plants; diversity would seem to be a great ally. Nonetheless, every gardener must deal with pests and diseases at one time or another.

Before you take matters into your own hands, though, remember that nature can play a huge role in keeping your garden healthy. Always try to enlist her help before you take other steps to control pest or disease challenges. I have learned that quite often nature already has a great solution if I can be present enough to enlist her as my ally in the garden.

Identifying Plant Diseases

Plant diseases can be very intimidating. It's frustrating to have to identify the problem and determine how to control it. There are many kinds of plant diseases; in this chapter I will be offering only a basic look at some disease categories. Use a good resource book or the local Cooperative Extension Service for additional information.

Disease prevention will always be your best tool. I encourage you to practice it seriously and become an expert at warding off the problems rather than fixing them. The following is a general overview of fungi, bacteria, and viruses, the three main disease categories.

Fungi

Fungal diseases are the most common plant diseases. There are many different fungal diseases, but they all fall into one of two groups: soilborne and airborne. Both types are reproduced by spores, which can be spread by air; water; contaminated soil, tools, and pots; even animals and humans.

Most fungi need warm temperatures to thrive, but a few actually favor cool temperatures. All are influenced by moisture. Keeping plants well drained and providing good air circulation by weeding, ensuring that the herbs are appropriately spaced, and practicing crop rotation are your best means of prevention.

SOILBORNE FUNGI, as their name implies, live in the soil and will often attack the roots and crowns of plants. To destroy this type of fungus, remove the affected plants and the surrounding soil, if possible. Plastic laid over the soil for several weeks during the hot part of the growing season will help "bake" the spores and kill a fungus remaining in the soil. Discard the plants into a *hot* compost pile, or dispose of them with your rubbish. You can also try sealing the diseased plants in a plastic bag and leaving it out in the sun, and even burning the plants — if your town permits.

COMMON FUNGAL DISEASES

> **Botrytis,** an airborne and waterborne disease, is a gray fuzzy mold on stems and leaves that causes the stems to cave in on themselves.

> **Damping-off** kills young seedlings by rotting them at the soil line. This fungus is transmitted through air and soil.

> **Downy mildew** is an airborne disease and shows up as white to purple fuzz, turning black, on the undersides of the leaves and on the stems. It usually kills a plant quickly.

> **Powdery mildew** is a white to grayish fuzz on the leaves, shoots, and other aerial parts of a plant. It is airborne and causes poor growth and lower yields, but does not kill the plant.

> **Rust** is both airborne and waterborne, and shows up as orange and white spots on leaves and stems. A plant becomes weak and yield is reduced, but it won't necessarily die.

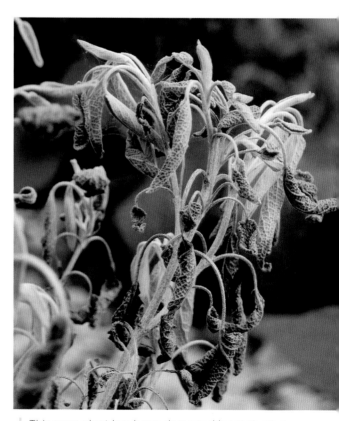

This sage plant has been damaged by root rot, a common soilborne fungus that is brought about by cultural conditions like overwatering and poor air circulation.

There is a type of beneficial soil fungus, mycorrhizal fungus. It affects plant roots, but in a helpful way: It helps to improve a plant's nutrient absorption and it assists the plant in coping with drought conditions.

AIRBORNE FUNGI attack the aboveground parts of a plant. To help control it, carefully prune away the affected plant parts and spray the plant with a fungicide treatment. If it is badly affected, you may need to sacrifice the entire plant to a hot compost pile or discard it with your rubbish.

Use superior oils — very light and purified horticultural oils that suffocate fungal spores and even soft-bodied insects without being absorbed by the plant — to help prevent spores of airborne fungi from reproducing and penetrating the plant parts. Baking soda sprays and garlic sprays are sometimes effective for airborne fungi if the problem has not become too widespread.

Bacteria

Fortunately, most bacteria found with plants are of a beneficial nature and actually help to increase soil fertility. Damaging bacteria that cause plant diseases occur in very warm and moist environments, which is why tropical and greenhouse gardeners have more difficulty with them than do gardeners in moderate climates.

The cells of bacteria are large enough to see under a basic light microscope and are mainly rod-shaped. In the right circumstances, these cells are capable of reproducing themselves every 30 minutes, so bacterial diseases can spread rapidly. This is facilitated by water, insects, contaminated tools, and animals, and by touching other infected plants. The bacteria infect the plant through wounds (such as pruning cuts) and natural openings.

Once again, prevention is your best defense. Keep tools clean and control insect-pest populations. Water can be a carrier of bacterial diseases, so make sure that water draining away from infected plants will not be wicked up by a healthy plant nearby. Just touching an infected plant and then handling a healthy one can spread the problem, so wash your hands and gloves after working with bacteria-infected plants.

NATURAL FUNGICIDES

Fungal infections in plants are the direct result of cultural conditions not being ideal. They can be stubborn to address, but if they aren't too advanced, and one is diligent, successful treatment with a natural fungicide like horsetail or baking soda can be very effective. In addition to using the natural fungicide, make sure that the plant has good air circulation, no dead or dying foliage lying on the soil at its base, and watering is done in the morning so that foliage has time to dry before cool night temps arrive.

Baking Soda Spray

This treatment can be helpful in controlling powdery mildew. Castile soap and Ivory are good choices for the dishwashing liquid, but almost any other kind will work, provided it's unscented and doesn't contain degreasing agents (these can be harsh solvents that dissolve the volatile oils plants contain in their foliage and flowers, and which are one of the plant's survival tools to protect itself from being eaten by insects or other critters, and from climatic extremes). You'll get two or three treatments from this recipe.

- 1 **teaspoon baking soda**
- 1 **quart warm water**
- 1 **teaspoon dishwashing liquid**

Dissolve the baking soda in warm water and add the dishwashing liquid. Mix well, then pour into a spray bottle. To use, spray plant thoroughly, especially the undersides of leaves. Space treatments three to five days apart.

Horsetail Spray

This is a natural fungicide that is effective on powdery mildew, botrytis, leaf spot, and other fungal diseases. Success with this spray varies, so you'll need to experiment a bit to see which plants and diseases it will be most effective in treating.

- ¼ **cup dried horsetail**
- 1 **gallon water**

Combine the horsetail and water in a large pot. Bring to a boil, reduce the heat, and simmer gently for 20–30 minutes. Remove from the heat; strain. To use, combine ¼ cup horsetail brew and 1½ cups water in a spray bottle or mister. Spray on affected plants. Repeat application every one or two weeks if symptoms persist.

Finally, practice crop rotation. This decreases the possibility that further plantings of the same crop will become infected.

Suspect bacterial infection if a plant wilts dramatically despite being in moist soil. Sometimes plant tissue will have mushy or slimy areas, especially within the stem wall. Some plants even develop cankers or galls (oozing growths on leaves, stems, or roots). Once plants have become infected with a bacterial disease, prune away the affected parts (remember to disinfect your snips or scissors between each cut). This may help, but if it does not solve the problem, your only alternative is to destroy the plants by discarding them with your rubbish or burning them.

A SIMPLE DISINFECTANT

To clean and disinfect tools and pots, wash them in a solution of 9 parts water to 1 part household hydrogen peroxide (3%). Rinse with a solution of 1 part vinegar and 9 parts water to remove any residues.

Viruses

Viral diseases are certainly the most difficult to identify, and there are no successful treatments once plants have become infected. Prevention is an absolute must, especially if you have an environment that is likely to foster viruses. Poor ventilation, standing water, extreme hot or cold temperatures, overabundance of pest populations, and contaminants such as chewing tobacco can all encourage the spread of viral infections.

Viral symptoms are tricky to discern because they can vary from plant to plant, depending on a plant's age and the growing conditions. It's even possible for plants to be carriers and show no symptoms. Occasionally, a plant is harboring a virus but the only signs of it are slow growth and eventual death — hardly the foolproof symptom picture I appreciate having.

Viruses can be spread in a number of ways, but water and wind are the primary culprits. It should be noted that viruses rarely live in weeds or plant pollens, so a virus won't be spread by bees, bats, or other pollinators. Leaf-chewing and sap-sucking insects, however, can spread viral diseases. As an insect bites an infected plant, it picks up the virus. When the insect bites into the next plant, it injects the virus (often in a concentrated form) into it. Among common virus-spreading creatures are aphids, leafhoppers, mites, nematodes, and whiteflies.

Propagating plants by cuttings or grafting with contaminated tools can cause an infection to spread, and tobacco users often carry the tobacco mosaic virus on their hands (from handling cigarettes, pipe tobacco, or chewing tobacco), unintentionally contaminating soil, seeds, and plants as they work.

I cannot stress enough how important the proverbial ounce of prevention is when dealing with plant diseases and insect problems. Keep those hands washed really well, and tools too. Ruthlessly eradicate all infected plants by pulling them out of the greenhouse, garden, or field. *Do not* compost them! Viruses can live for years in a dormant state in the soil or decaying plant material. Weeds are prime candidates for viruses, so keep up on your weeding tasks to decrease the possibility that they will become infected with a virus and spread it to your plants. Last, manage insect populations carefully to protect your herbs and other plants from contamination.

COMMON VIRUSES AND THEIR SYMPTOMS

> **Mosaic.** The leaves and fruits will show patches of mottling light green, yellow, and sometimes white. Flowers often become disfigured with unusual color variations.

> **Ring spot.** Leaves show rounded spots that are light yellow.

> **Leaf curl.** Leaves will begin to grow in a distorted fashion and curl for no apparent reason.

Let Mother Nature and Friends Help You

Before I discuss more aggressive ways to manage pest problems in the garden, I would like to remind you that there are lots of valuable allies nature provides to help you control pest problems. For example, cats help control rodents. Birds are great friends to have in the garden; they eat a variety of insects and are especially fond of caterpillars. Bats should be welcomed, too. They control evening-flying insects quite nicely. Salamanders have an appetite for insects, and nonpoisonous snakes and lizards are wonderful for eating both insects and rodents. As a bonus, nonpoisonous snakes often keep poisonous snakes away from your garden or field areas. And don't forget toads and frogs. These amphibians have a hearty appetite for insects and they provide an evening concert free of charge.

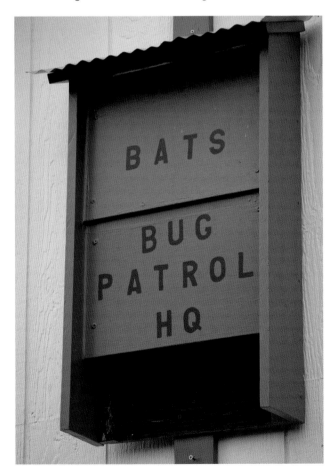

Welcome bats into your garden with a place for them to rest during daylight hours. Bats are extremely helpful in keeping insect-pest populations under control.

All of these creatures are assets I hope you will welcome into your garden space. They provide valuable services in your efforts to manage pests, and many of them, like salamanders, frogs, and bats, are experiencing habitat destruction and environmental hardships of their own. It's only right that we offer them our support in making a garden home available to them.

Chris and I are avid wildlife fans and we go to great lengths to welcome wild critters into our farm and garden spaces. After all, the wildlife were here before we were! Still, we do come across instances when we must take steps to prevent wildlife from eating our crops and garden produce, but this happens infrequently, as we learn how to work with the wild critters rather than automatically making every effort to keep them out of our garden space. Let me give you a few examples . . .

Rascally Rabbits

We have loads of cottontail rabbits here, and even a few jackrabbits. Many a visitor has expressed horror at the thought of wild rabbits pillaging the garden, feasting on my veggies, herbs, and flowers. No, I say. The solution to that problem is planting patches of parsley on the outer edges of my gardens. In that way I can please the rabbits and at the same time keep my garden safe and sound. The rabbits come to the parsley patches and nibble away at them. The parsley grows back quickly, leaving more than enough for my needs and plenty for hungry bunnies. The rabbits never bother to come farther into the gardens, so all is well. Cilantro also works to satisfy them, if you happen to have a somewhat shady garden instead of one in full sun.

Distracting Our Avian Friends

We have put up several feeding areas throughout our gardens for wild birds. We enjoy watching them and local Audubon Society members have said that our farm has an abundance and variety of bird species living in community here. That is affirmation to us of the benefits of working with wildlife rather than against it. Birds eat a tremendous number of insects and the result of encouraging them to be in my garden and yard space is that I have practically no pest insect problems worth addressing. There is one challenge for us specifically in having so many wild birds around: We grow perennial seed crops in our production field and the birds assume — and who could blame them — that the seed crops are planted to satisfy their taste buds. Of course, we cannot allow them to eat the seed crops, so we deal with that in two ways.

First, every year I plant a 100-foot-long wall of sunflowers specifically for the birds to eat. I always provide different sizes of sunflowers. The little birds, which cannot manage anything larger, have 'Autumn Beauty' and 'Velvet Queen' seeds, just the right size to eat. The larger birds enjoy the 'Fat Mama' and 'Tarahumara White' sunflowers, which produce huge heads filled with big seeds.

The second thing we do is put up bird flashing tape over the top of the scabiosa and gaillardia seed crops to discourage the birds from eating their seed heads. The result is that we enjoy having zillions of wild birds year-round, few pest insect problems, and fine yields from our seed crops for our seed customers. Everyone is happy!

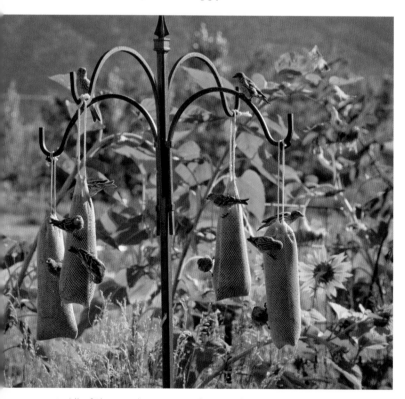

All of the gardens on our farm include bird-feeding stations. Birds are an important part of our insect pest control but we must also distract them from our fields of mature seed crops.

Dealing with Deer

Deer are another reality at our home place. There is a herd of 22 to 27 deer that pass through our production field and our gardens twice daily on their way to drink from our ponds. Neither Chris nor I really like fences, and the last thing we want to do is fence the wildlife out of our space. It's lovely to see the deer bedded down under our backyard honey

> I need to have a tall fence around my vegetable garden; the deer just cannot resist the lettuces.

locust tree, or to watch the fawns chasing each other around our farm stand building. In order to be able to enjoy the deer and still maintain our crops and my food gardens, we have compromised a little. In the production field, Chris uses a spray of rotten eggs and vegetable oil on three or four varieties the deer find tasty enough to persistently want to eat. Though we grow 52 varieties of seed crops, the deer seem pretty selective in what they have a taste for. Every week or two, Chris sprays those select varieties, and the rotten egg smell repels the deer from those plants.

I have come to the realization that if I want salad greens, I need to have a tall fence around my vegetable garden; the deer just cannot resist the lettuces. Aside from those two things, though, our gardens, including my herb garden, field crops, and our yard space, are freely open to deer. They hardly ever bother the herbs or other plantings. Perhaps the variety in tastes and smells is more confusing than appealing to them, but the deer pass through without nibbling too much. They do eat my tulip flowers, which I believe is the same as deer candy, so I have learned to plant daffodils and crocus instead. It is a small sacrifice in order to have the pleasure of the deer as part of our lives.

Don't Forget the Pollinators

While we're talking about wildlife and their role in the bigger picture, I want to mention the huge importance of pollinators. Without pollinators — wild varieties like hummingbirds and wasps, livestock varieties like honeybees — our world would be quite uninhabitable.

Pollinators are critical to the plants' production of fruits, nuts, and seeds. Without fruits, nuts, and seeds, no new generations of plants would grow in the wild or in our fields, gardens, and other green spaces. Without pollinators, we would have almost nothing to eat. The entire food chain depends on the successful work of pollinating creatures. I encourage you to go out of your way to make them feel welcome in your garden. Many of them, such as bats, do double duty because they not only pollinate night-blooming plants, but they also eat scads of insects. Bats pollinate passionflowers and are ravenous mosquito eaters, which helps to prevent the spread of illnesses like West Nile virus in humans and birds and sleeping sickness in horses.

If pollinators are not present, or if the right pollinator for a specific plant variety is not coexisting with the plant, there is nothing left but for humans to hand-pollinate the flowers. Chris has been granted the honorable title of Mr. Honeybee by the young schoolchildren who visit our farm, because he must hand-pollinate the hibiscus flowers every day during the blooming season in order for them to produce viable seed. Chris took on this job because we do not have a native pollinator that is interested in doing its bit with the hibiscus flowers, and honeybees won't pollinate the flowers either. So, in the morning, Chris takes his soft paintbrush and gently pollinates each new flower. This is crucial for a successful crop, but it is very time-consuming and labor-intensive. How we wish there was a pollinator creature that could do this work for us!

Beneficial Insects

Working with beneficial insects is another effective way to control pest insects if you educate yourself as to which beneficial insects stalk which pest insects. When you get a balance of beneficials in

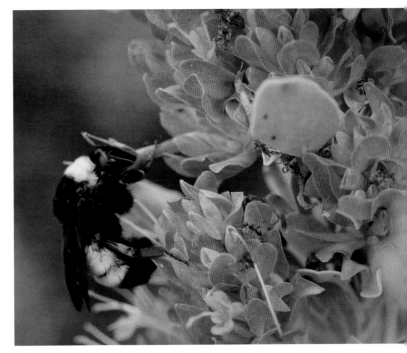

Pollinators like this Colorado native bumblebee are essential to the process of growing herbs and food plants.

your space, the pests nearly disappear. There are a number of excellent beneficial insectary houses that raise and sell these creatures (See Resources, page 245). They really know what they're doing with these bugs! Chris and I have found them wonderfully helpful in identifying what pest problems we have in the greenhouse, cold frames, and gardens and then determining which beneficial insects we should introduce.

I infinitely prefer to control insect problems this way rather than spraying with a pesticide — even approved certified organic pesticides. Spraying tampers with the ideal environmental balance, even when done properly, using safe preparations. I'll concede that it's more desirable to spray than to have an insect problem, but I feel it's always better to let nature handle her own difficulties, with my support, whenever possible. Besides, spraying takes a lot of time that I would rather spend doing something else in the garden. That being said, if you find the need to handle a pest problem by spraying, look for specifics in each entry in Insect Management (see page 103).

A GUIDE TO BENEFICIAL INSECTS

BENEFICIAL INSECT	PEST INSECT IT PREYS ON	OTHER BENEFICIAL EFFECTS
Aphid midge	Aphids	
Assassin bug	Flies, caterpillars	
Beneficial nematode	Root weevils, crown and stem borers, fungus gnats, shore flies	Excellent compost worker
Braconid wasp	Elm beetles, cabbageworms, hornworms, aphids, houseflies, horseflies	
Bumblebee, honeybee		Excellent pollinators
Centipede, millipede	Soil-dwelling mites, soil-dwelling larvae	Help decompose dead plant material into compost
Damselfly	Aphids, leafhoppers, thrips, small caterpillars	
Lacewing	Aphids, corn earworms, tomato fruitworms	Excellent general predator
Ladybug	Aphids, soft-bodied pests, spider mites, soft scale, mealybugs	
Parasitic wasp	Aphids, whiteflies	
Praying mantid	All the insects it can catch, both pests and beneficials	
Predatory mite	Spider mites, thrips	
Soldier beetle	Grasshopper eggs, caterpillars, beetle larvae	
Spider (all types)	Many kinds of insects	
Spined soldier bug	Caterpillars, grubs, Mexican bean beetle larvae	

Insect Management

The topic of insect management is very broad. The first step is proper identification of any insects you see on your plants. Some of them will likely be problematic and require a control of some sort, but you will also learn that many of the insects are beneficial and great helpers in caring for your garden. It's wise to learn the difference and then take advantage of those insect helpers.

As for plant diseases, invest in one or two good reference books (see Recommended Reading, page 246) to make the tasks of identification and treatment much simpler.

The list of pest insects seems very long, so for the sake of space and what is most relevant to herbs, I mention only the most common problem bugs. As I mentioned earlier, beneficial insects can often help you manage a pest situation, and I hope you will try that approach first. Natural preparations are a possibility as well. I make suggestions for both control methods under the listing for each pest. For more in-depth information about treating difficult pests, please refer to a good resource book. The art of plant pest control is indeed a topic for a whole book.

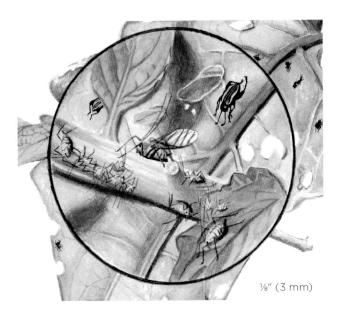

⅛" (3 mm)

wasps, damselflies, parasitic wasps, beneficial nematodes, ladybugs, and lacewings. Check with your local garden center for more information, or contact one of the companies listed in the Resources section (see page 245).

Soap sprays coat the aphids' bodies, effectively suffocating them. Neem tree extract is another effective control. We use a brand called NeemX, which qualifies for organic certification regulations (not every brand of natural insecticide meets organic standards, as they often contain inert ingredients that are not earth-friendly). Another recommendation for aphids is a garlic-oil spray. You can also plant garlic near the plants that seem especially susceptible to aphids. This preventive measure offers the plants additional protection.

Aphids

WHAT THEY LOOK LIKE: There are many types of aphids — black, red, white, green, even golden — and different ways to deal with them. This insect is oval or tear-shaped, with two "tubes" protruding from the back end (this is how it gives birth to live young). Aphids have six tiny legs and a pair of antennae. Some have wings.

WHAT THEY DO: Aphids suck the juice out of plant stems, leaves, and flowers. They excrete a sticky substance that may foster mold growth, and can even spread disease as they travel from plant to plant. Plants become deformed as aphids feed on them.

HOW TO TREAT THEM: I find it best to have a few different tricks in my bag when dealing with aphids, as they tend to develop resistance to control methods. Many beneficial insects help control aphids. Among these are aphid midges, braconid

Beetles

WHAT THEY LOOK LIKE: As with aphids, there are many types of pest beetles. These insects have hard-shelled, oval-shaped bodies between ¼ and 1 inch (6 mm–2.5 cm) long. Color also varies, but most beetles are some shade of black, blue, or brown. They have tiny heads in comparison to their bodies. Some beetles that tend to create problems with herbs are blister beetles, flea beetles, and Japanese beetles.

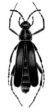

¼"–1"
(6 mm–2.5 cm)

WHAT THEY DO: Beetles are chewing insects that eat stems, leaves, and flowers. They prefer tender new growth, but will also consume older growth.

Beetles, continued

HOW TO TREAT THEM: Beneficial insects that offer some protection from various types of beetles are parasitic wasps and beneficial nematodes. Natural pesticide preparations for beetles are soap sprays, bug juice made with beetles (see recipe, page 109), and neem tree extract.

Cabbage Loopers

WHAT THEY LOOK LIKE: This pest is a green, 1-inch-long (2.5 cm) caterpillar. Cabbage loopers have white lines on their bodies and curl themselves into a distinctive loop shape as they move.

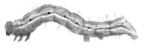

1" (2.5 cm)

WHAT THEY DO: Very destructive pests, cabbage loopers eat primarily leaves but will often attack the whole plant, chewing large holes as they go.

HOW TO TREAT THEM: If you are experiencing a large infestation of cabbage loopers, control them with beneficial parasitic wasps. Smaller populations can be nicely managed with a garlic-oil spray.

Corn Earworms, Tomato Fruitworms

WHAT THEY LOOK LIKE: This pest goes by a variety of names, but it is the same distressing creature. These 1- to 2-inch-long (2.5–5 cm), caterpillars are shades of green to brown with dark stripes and black legs.

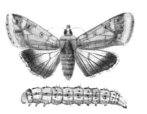

1"–2" (2.5–5 cm)

WHAT THEY DO: Corn earworms/tomato fruitworms create a lot of damage to fruiting plants like passionflower. The larvae burrow into fruits and flower buds, eating as they go. They also chew on leaves.

HOW TO TREAT THEM: Lacewings are helpful in controlling corn earworms and tomato fruitworms. Parasitic wasps are also quite good, and predatory insects such as assassin bugs and spined soldier bugs will all do their part to eradicate these pests.

Cutworms

WHAT THEY LOOK LIKE: These 1- to 2-inch (2.5–5 cm) caterpillars are gray or brown. They have many legs and often have a slimy appearance.

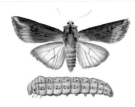

1"–" (2.5–5 cm)

WHAT THEY DO: A nocturnal insect, the cutworm does its damage at night. It will chew through an entire plant stem just above the soil surface and then eat off all of the tender new growth.

HOW TO TREAT THEM: Try beneficial nematodes for cutworms. Once nematodes have been introduced into the garden, you should see positive results throughout the growing season — without repeat applications.

Earwigs

WHAT THEY LOOK LIKE: Long, narrow, semihard-shelled bodies characterize the hungry earwig. This insect is brown and sports a set of pincers on its rear end.

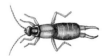

½" (1.25 cm)

WHAT THEY DO: Earwigs eat nearly everything in their path. All types of plants and plant parts satisfy their diet.

HOW TO TREAT THEM: I have just one method to control earwigs and it works incredibly well. Roll up sheets of damp newspaper into moderately tight logs and lay them around the base of the plants you are having trouble protecting. Do this in the early morning and then collect the logs in the early evening. Throw the paper logs into the trash, for they will be loaded with earwigs that have crawled into them throughout the hot part of the day. Repeat as necessary.

Fungus Gnats and Shore Flies

WHAT THEY LOOK LIKE: These tiny, flying, gnatlike creatures are often a problem for indoor gardeners. They are black, and some have dots on their wings. They actually resemble very small houseflies.

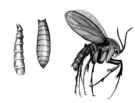

⅛" (3.2 mm)

WHAT THEY DO: Fungus gnats and shore flies signal that sanitation and/or watering practices need to be improved. They lay their eggs in the soil, and the larvae find a perfect home under fallen leaves and other decaying plant debris.

HOW TO TREAT THEM: Always remove all fallen or yellowing leaves. Next, make sure you are not overwatering or leaving water to stand in pot trays.

If you do have a problem, treat the plants with neem tree extract, garlic spray, or beneficial nematodes. Water the nematodes into the soil, where they will eat the larvae of many pest insects.

Grasshoppers and Crickets

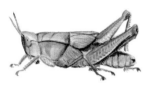 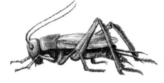

| length varies | length varies |

WHAT THEY LOOK LIKE: Grasshoppers can grow quite large — some are several inches long. They all have long back legs and big eyes. Colors range from greens and yellows to browns and blacks. Some have wings and can fly.

Crickets are black with long legs and antennae. These fast-moving insects make a distinctive hopping movement. They are generally 1 to 2 inches (2.5–5 cm) in length.

WHAT THEY DO: Grasshoppers and crickets eat a wide variety of plants and are especially fond of alfalfa, comfrey, and lemon balm. They are chewing insects that feed on leaves, buds, and flowers.

HOW TO TREAT THEM: I find grasshoppers and crickets difficult to control. They're ferocious eaters and aren't easily affected by natural control methods. Chris and I use beneficial nematodes initially to control the grasshopper population. Birds are also a fantastic ally because they adore a grasshopper meal and can eat a lot of those little critters. If you keep livestock, young turkeys will make a serious dent in your grasshopper and cricket populations.

Nolo Bait, an insect-specific bacterium injected into bran, is a long-term commitment to keeping the grasshoppers and crickets under control. It takes awhile to have an effect, but if you stick with it, you will not only help your current problem but you will also be making an impact on next year's "crop" by influencing the pests' reproductive cycle. Nolo Bait works by making grasshoppers and crickets

lethargic, thus leaving them prey to others of their kind. It also prevents them from reproducing.

Neem tree extract is very helpful against these pests in two ways. First, the pests don't like the taste of it, so they are deterred from eating your plants. Second, if they do indulge in a meal, the neem saps them of energy and they soon stop eating. As grasshoppers become sick, other grasshoppers will cannibalize them and in turn become infected with the oil. Neem tree extract has definitely saved some of our young, early-spring plants when the grasshoppers were feasting faster than the plants could get established. Without this control, we would have lost some important crops.

Leafhoppers

WHAT THEY LOOK LIKE: Another hopping and flying creature, a leafhopper has a soft body and wings. The insects are usually green, brown, or yellowish, and have very large eyes.

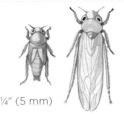

¼" (5 mm)

WHAT THEY DO: This insect sucks the juices from the stems and leaves of plants, spreading disease as it travels. Its saliva stunts and deforms plants.

HOW TO TREAT THEM: Predatory bugs and parasitic wasps may be introduced to control leafhoppers. Leafhoppers are carriers of plant diseases, so it's always best to check them before they become a large problem.

Soap sprays and neem tree extract sprays are both helpful in controlling leafhoppers before they get out of hand.

Leaf Miners

WHAT THEY LOOK LIKE: You would need a magnifying lens to see these tiny, black-and-yellow flying bugs, whose immature larvae actually cause the damage to plants.

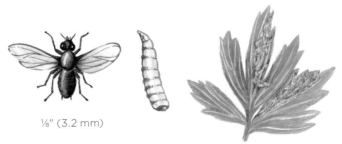

⅛" (3.2 mm)

WHAT THEY DO: Leaf miners cause a lot of harm to plant foliage as they tunnel through the leaves. The damage appears as white winding marks on the leaves that resemble a worm pattern.

HOW TO TREAT THEM: Control leaf miners with parasitic wasps. Once you have introduced parasitic wasps into your garden or greenhouse space, they should always be there, working hard to control pest insects.

Neem tree extract is also beneficial in managing leaf miners. We find that spraying the neem tree extract in the early evening gives the best results.

Scale

WHAT THEY LOOK LIKE: Scale are hard or soft round bumps that cluster on stems. They have no legs, wings, or other visible body parts. They may be white, yellow, red, brown, or black.

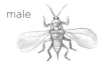

male   female

⅛" (3.2 mm)

WHAT THEY DO: These pests suck the juice from stems, fruits, and leaves. Scale may also inject toxins into a plant via their saliva. Rosemary is especially susceptible to scale.

HOW TO TREAT THEM: There are many different types of scale and some can be difficult to eradicate. Use parasitic wasps, soldier beetles, and ladybugs to help control this pest. Remember that scale spreads easily, so act quickly, at the first sign of a problem.

Dormant oil and superior oil sprays are also helpful in controlling scale. Use these solutions carefully and according to label directions. They are best applied when the sun is not at its most intense, to lessen the possibility of burning your plants.

Slugs and Snails

WHAT THEY LOOK LIKE: Soft-bodied and slimy, slugs have no shells, whereas snails are usually shades of gray, brown, or black and carry a shell on their back. Both have two antennae on their head.

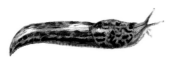
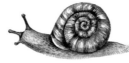

length varies   length varies

WHAT THEY DO: Slugs are very hungry creatures, and if left unchecked, they will quickly eat massive quantities of plants. Slugs and snails are especially fond of basil.

HOW TO TREAT THEM: You can control slugs and snails with a slug bait sold through organic growing supply sources (see Resources, page 245). It's toxic to them and a bit gory, but works really well.

You can also use a homemade remedy. Raw potato slices should work well; put them out in the evening and collect them very early the next day. Slugs will cluster on a potato for a feast and you will be able to eliminate a good number of them by discarding the slices. Or try lightly sprinkling wood ashes around the area where slugs are a problem. As slugs pass through the ashes, they become desiccated.

Spider Mites

WHAT THEY LOOK LIKE: Another very tiny insect that requires a magnifying glass to see, a spider mite looks like a miniature spider. These mites are red, green, or yellow.

less than ¹⁄₅₀" (0.5 mm)

WHAT THEY DO: Spider mites suck the juice from the undersides of leaves, thus weakening the plants. This pest causes yellow speckling of the leaves as it covers the plant with its tiny webs. The leaves will eventually turn yellow and fall off.

HOW TO TREAT THEM: I find spider mites one of the more difficult pests to deal with, partly because they are virtually invisible and also because they are persistent. A goldenseal grower once shared the following control method with me (goldenseal is especially susceptible to spider mite problems). When you see evidence of spider mites, sprinkle a light dusting of white sugar (yes, there's something good to do with white sugar after all!) on the soil and on the plants themselves. Ants will move in and eat the sugar and the spider mites. Once the sugar and mites are gone, the ants usually disappear again and all is well.

You can also use predatory mites to control spider mites. Unlike spider mites, predatory mites don't feed on plants.

Neem tree extract, soap sprays, and dormant oil sprays can all help you get rid of a spider mite problem. They aren't as effective as beneficial insects, however, because spider mites are tiny and they hide themselves in foliage. Give them a try, though: Thoroughly spray all the plant surfaces, and they'll do a good job.

Stinkbugs

WHAT THEY LOOK LIKE: This distinctive insect has a hard shell in the shape of a shield. It can be shades of green, brown, or black.

½" (1.25 cm)

WHAT THEY DO: Stinkbugs suck the sap from a plant, although they prefer the aerial parts of herbs. Their feeding leaves behind scarring. Too much stinkbug damage will weaken a plant and make it susceptible to other pests and diseases.

HOW TO TREAT THEM: One of the best ways to prevent stinkbugs from becoming a big problem is by cultivating around plants. Common weeds seem to attract these pests, so controlling weeds becomes your first line of defense. Parasitic wasps are also allies in managing stinkbug populations.

Thrips

WHAT THEY LOOK LIKE: Yellow, brown, or black, thrips are minute, bullet-shaped insects that are best seen with a magnifying lens.

less than ¹⁄₂₅" (1 mm)

WHAT THEY DO: Thrips suck juices from plant leaves and flowers. Their feeding leaves behind tiny white speckles that create an ugly, unhealthy appearance on a plant. Thrips can spread viruses as they travel from plant to plant.

HOW TO TREAT THEM: Controlling thrips is every gardener's and greenhouse grower's nightmare. They are really tiny, and they get down into the crevices of plants, making them almost impossible to control with natural pesticides. Beneficial insects are your best approach. Try pirate bugs, lacewings, ladybugs, and predatory mites against them. You can also make a dent in the thrips population by using sticky monitoring cards as insect traps. Thousands of thrips will be trapped on one sticky card alone.

If you do decide to work with natural pesticides, dormant oil sprays, neem tree extract, and soap sprays will make some inroads. Garlic-oil spray is also helpful.

Whiteflies

WHAT THEY LOOK LIKE: Whiteflies are very small, triangular insects with wings. As their name implies, they are totally white.

¹⁄₁₀" (2.5 mm)

WHAT THEY DO: Plants are weakened by whiteflies, which suck the juices out of the leaves and stems. In turn, a plant becomes more susceptible to other pests and diseases. After biting into an infected plant, a whitefly then spreads viruses to healthy plants.

HOW TO TREAT THEM: If you see whiteflies, address the situation immediately. Success in controlling them relies on doing something about the problem before it gets out of hand. Use either beneficial insects or a natural pesticide, but act immediately.

A small parasitic wasp, *Encarsia formosa*, is especially good at handling whiteflies. This wasp is so small you can barely see it without a magnifying glass, and it will not cause any harm to humans. Predatory beetles work well too. Sticky monitoring cards act as whitefly traps, catching thousands of them on a single card.

Soap or garlic sprays work fairly well against whiteflies. If the problem is still small enough, either should do the trick. Neem tree extract is also a possibility. If you have a severe whitefly infestation, however, the best thing to do is to get rid of the host plant, especially if the problem is indoors. Once these creatures get a foothold, they are extremely difficult to control with organic measures.

All-Natural Pest Treatments

There are numerous methods for controlling insect pests in the garden, field, or greenhouse. Prevention will always be your best approach, but if that fails, consider beneficial insects or nonchemical pest controls. Do your best to address problems when they begin; controlling pests at this point will be much easier and less expensive, and will require less time and energy.

Monitor your garden or greenhouse regularly to stay in touch with pest populations. If you're careful, you should be able to keep small problems from getting out of hand. It's a simple step toward keeping the garden healthy.

Monitoring Sticky Cards

You can purchase monitoring cards, sometimes called yellow sticky cards, to use as both a tracking tool and a trapping control method for insect pests. The cards are a bright, sunny yellow and are covered with a sticky substance that attracts and traps insects. Count the insects once a week and determine appropriate control methods based on which pests are causing problems. Because the cards actually trap insects, they are themselves a method of control.

> If prevention fails, consider nonchemical pest controls.

When you use sticky cards, there are a few things to keep in mind. First, always place the cards in the foliage area of the plants (don't place them high above plants; not all pests are flying insects). Second, put them in the same place in the garden from one week to the next. This will help you get an accurate picture of how well you are maintaining insect populations. Third, use a magnifying glass when looking at the cards, so that you can properly identify the insects. Keep a log of how many of each insect you see on each card from week to week: This gives you a tracking record and establishes whether any patterns exist.

Purchase sticky cards at a garden center or make your own. Here's how: Buy a package of bright yellow (insects are attracted to yellow) plastic picnic plates. Make a mixture of equal parts vegetable oil and honey. Smear a thin layer over the plates, front and back. Hang from a string, or clip with a clothespin to a wooden stake in the garden. Once a week, look at the plates and count the insects stuck to them. Then wash the plates, let them dry, and reapply the sticky goo, and you're set to begin a new week of bug catching.

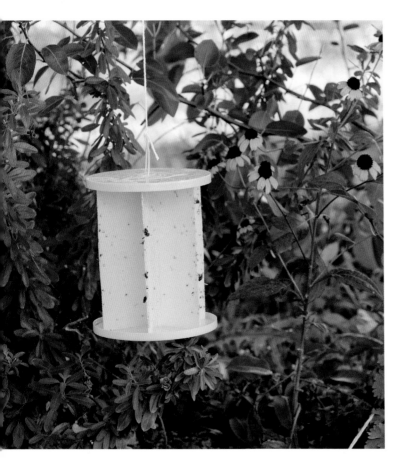

Sticky cards are good for monitoring pest insect populations and as a tool for trapping pest insects, many of which are attracted to the yellow color.

BUG JUICE

Many pests, especially beetles, will not feed on plants if they smell the dead of their own species. This preparation works especially well for Colorado potato beetles, Mexican bean beetles, and cabbage loopers. If there are virus-infected plants nearby, do not use this method; there is the potential of spreading viruses to healthy plants from the bodies of insects that fed on the affected plants.

1	cup pest bugs
3–4	cups water

1. Grind the pest bugs in an old blender. *Note:* Don't use the kitchen blender — go to a secondhand shop and purchase one to use just for preparing garden remedies.

2. Add enough water to get the ground insects to the consistency of milk. Strain the bug juice before putting it in the sprayer.

3. To use, spray the plants, covering all the surfaces. This should help repel similar pests from those plants for 3–4 weeks. Reapply in a month if necessary.

SOAP SPRAY

This broad-spectrum control method is used to treat spider mites, aphids, earwigs, whiteflies, mealybugs, thrips, and scale. It may also be helpful against ticks, beetles, and caterpillars. The spray works by both repelling insects and suffocating any that are already on the plants. It is just as effective as commercial insecticidal soap products that are available from your garden store. If you choose to purchase a soap spray, follow the label directions to prepare and apply.

1	quart water
1–2	teaspoons dishwashing liquid

1. Put the water in a large spray bottle and add the dishwashing liquid; shake to mix.

2. To use, spray over the entire plant, coating the surfaces well. Repeat every 5–7 days, as necessary, until pests are controlled.

GARLIC OIL

Most pests hate garlic, so this is an excellent control method. It's especially effective against aphids, whiteflies, spider mites, leafhoppers, squash bugs, and young grasshoppers. It's important to use mineral oil in this recipe, as it will not be absorbed by a plant.

Note: Some plants are sensitive to this spray, so do a test patch first. Spray one or two plants with the garlic oil. If the leaves turn yellow or brown within 24 hours, do not use the spray on that particular type of plant. If no burning occurs, go ahead and spray the remaining plants. This spray is best used around dusk; the oil content can provoke a "sunburn" reaction when the sun is hot.

6–8	cloves garlic, peeled and finely chopped
1	tablespoon mineral oil
1	pint water
1	teaspoon dishwashing liquid

1. Place the garlic in a clean glass jar and pour the mineral oil over it. Tightly cap the jar, then store at room temperature for 24 hours.

2. Line a strainer with a piece of cloth and then pour the oil mixture through it. Gather up the cloth and squeeze the remaining oil from the garlic. Discard the pieces of garlic and reserve the garlic-infused oil.

3. Combine the water and the dishwashing liquid.

4. To use, mix 1–2 tablespoons of the infused oil in a pint of the water-dishwashing liquid solution in a spray bottle or mister. Spray plant thoroughly.

ANT BAIT

This bait will attract ants of all kinds. Use it with caution around small children and animals, and do not inhale the dust when mixing. Mark the label with a skull and crossbones; it is poisonous. Be careful not to spill ant bait near the base of plants, as it will damage or kill the plants' roots.

3	cups water
1	cup sugar
3	teaspoons boric acid
	Cotton balls

1. Combine the water, sugar, and boric acid and blend well.

2. Fill each of three glass jars halfway with cotton balls. Pour 1 cup of the mixture into each jar and cover tightly. Punch small holes in the lids and label the jars clearly.

3. Lay the jars in the garden where ants are a problem. The ants will carry the mixture back to the anthill and it will destroy the colony. Replace the bait every 1–2 weeks, as needed, until ants are no longer a problem.

Natural and Homemade Organic Pest-Control Preparations

There are several all-natural pest-control preparations on the market, and you can certainly make some of your own. Remember that these are still pesticides, even though they aren't made from synthetic chemicals; they can be very toxic and should be used and stored appropriately.

Wear protective clothing (long sleeves and pants), waterproof boots and gloves, and serious eye protection when applying any type of pesticide. If you are using a sprayer, learn ahead of time how it works so you can apply any preparation safely and effectively. Do not apply anywhere close to children's or pets' play spaces, or water such as ponds and streams.

Remember that these are still pesticides, even though they aren't made from synthetic chemicals.

Read label instructions carefully before you begin to apply a substance, and never store it where children or pets can reach it, in open containers, or in containers that are not fully labeled. If you make the preparation yourself, you *must* label it completely with the preparation name and every single ingredient used. Also clearly mark containers with cautionary information if appropriate. Wait at least 24 hours before using a sprayed herb for any purpose.

Neem Tree Extract

Neem tree extract works in a number of ways: It kills some insects, acts as a growth regulator in others, and repels still others (they seem to dislike the taste). We use the brand NeemX, as it meets certified organic standards, and have found it to be very effective against beetles of many types, whiteflies, aphids, spider mites, thrips, leaf miners, mealybugs, and grasshoppers.

Use neem tree extract according to the manufacturer's directions. Generally, you spray it onto plants that are being eaten or otherwise damaged by certain pests. It acts in some capacity as a repellent, but when bugs ingest it, it will poison young, weak, or sick insects. If healthy insects ingest the extract, it disrupts their reproductive system and they are unable to reproduce.

Neem applied as a soil drench has a systemic effect on plants: Each plant draws up the neem into its leaves and stems, thus affecting the pest when it eats the plant. Neem may be toxic to some beneficial insects as well, but it does not seem to bother honeybees or spiders. Neem is not toxic to people or animals, and it is biodegradable.

Nolo Bait

This is a biological suppression bait for use on grasshoppers, locusts, and some species of crickets. Unlike chemical-based insecticides, Nolo Bait contains a naturally occurring spore, called *Nosema locustae,* that infects these insects. It is not toxic to humans, livestock, wild animals, birds, fish, or lifeforms other than grasshoppers and closely related insects.

The spore is injected into wheat bran, which grasshoppers like to eat. Most pest species of grasshoppers, particularly younger instars, will eat the bran; the resulting infection helps to control grasshopper populations without adverse effects on the environment. Depending on age and species, a grasshopper that eats even one flake of Nolo Bait can become infected. When sick, the insect eats less and less. Other grasshoppers often cannibalize the sick ones and thus become infected as well, spreading the disease among the population. In addition, infected females can pass the disease through their eggs, thus helping to control future generations.

Nolo Bait does not work rapidly, however. According to the Colorado State University Extension Service, the age and quantity of the insects influence how quickly you'll see results. Follow-up applications each year that grasshopper populations are on the rise will help manage the problem. Grasshoppers migrate over great distances; it is best to spread Nolo Bait where you need it frequently during the growing season. Ask the neighbors if they would like to participate; this will also improve your success rate.

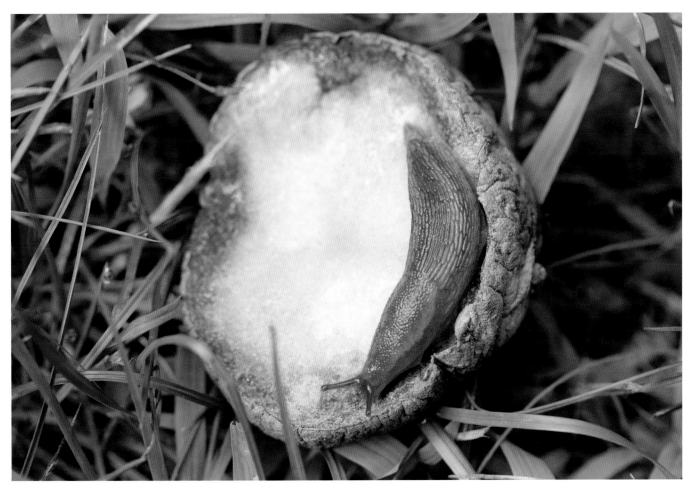

{ Slices of raw potato are an excellent way to collect and discard slugs in the garden.

Slug and Snail Bait

Although I know many methods to control slugs and snails, the one that works really well for us is potato. Just before dark, place large slices of raw potato on the ground where slugs are a problem. Slugs love these spud feasts and will munch happily all night long.

The downside of this method is that you must get up very early the next morning, just as traces of light appear. Gather up the potato slices into a box or can. They should be loaded with slugs (you may want to wear a pair of gloves if touching slimy slugs bothers you). Discard the "slug hotels" in the trash. Do this every day until you are no longer noticing slug-related damage. If you don't check the potatoes early enough in the morning, the slugs will have retreated back into the soil — and your plant roots — for the day. If you prefer not to kill the slugs, make

sure you transport them at least 200 feet (60 m) from the garden; slugs can travel quite a distance.

You can also purchase pelletized slug bait and sprinkle it on the greenhouse floor or on the soil in the garden wherever slugs and snails have become a problem (follow the directions on the package). The pellets work well, and are just the ticket for people who don't want to get up at the crack of dawn to deal with slug-coated potato slices.

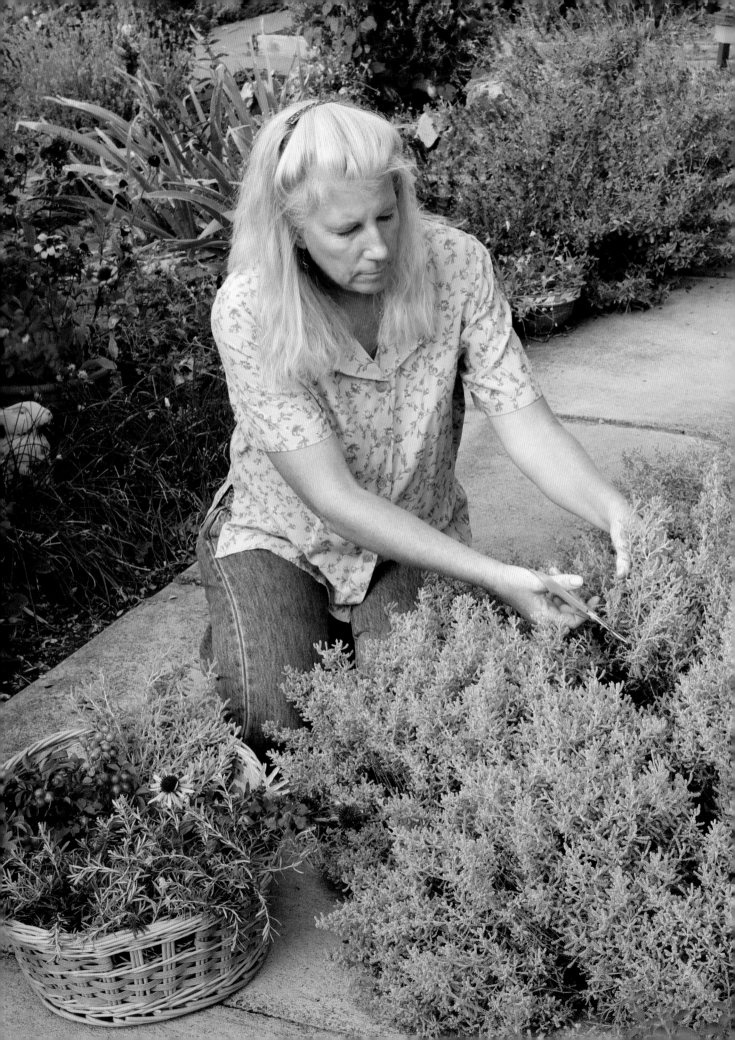

CHAPTER SEVEN

Harvesting from the Garden

Harvest is a time of abundance and prosperity, and there are many fantastic plants to utilize in the garden. Picking and preparing them as medicines and foods, personal-care preparations, even herbal bouquets will bring beauty, good health, and happiness into your home or workspace. Even many of the weeds I pull out of the garden may be used in a positive fashion as foods and preparations — even in compost. Enjoy your harvesting experiences. For me, this certainly is one of the most rewarding parts of growing plants and using them. As you harvest each plant, you will begin to think of all the different ways you will prepare it for use. There is no better definition of abundance and prosperity, in my opinion, than this time in the garden.

A Little Knowledge Goes a Long Way

It's important to learn as much as you can as you look forward to reaping what you have sown. If you know which types of tools work best for the plant part you are harvesting, your time will be spent very efficiently and enjoyably. Proper methods and good tools will cause the plants less stress as you are harvesting them.

Learn which time of the year is most appropriate to harvest certain parts of the plants. Harvesting at the wrong time can result in compromising the health of a plant. It's also true that harvesting in the wrong season may mean that the plant you picked is not as medicinally potent or nutritious as you would like it to be.

Once the plants have been picked, it is most helpful to know the best ways to process them. Have you ever thought about the difference between a fresh apple and a dehydrated one? Certainly both are good, nutritious foods, but the fresh apple has vitality, whereas some of the nutrients may have been compromised during the process of drying the fruit. This is a normal occurrence and shouldn't be viewed as a bad thing; after all, dried plants are perfect for use during the long winter. If you had a choice, however, wouldn't you opt to eat the fresh apple? Knowing which herbs are better used fresh and which are easier to use when dried is a great help during harvest time.

Good storage practices are important for maintaining a plant's potency as long as possible. Proper harvesting and storing of herbs is just as important to learn as proper growing techniques, especially when you plan to use these herbs for health and well-being.

Each part of a plant will have a harvesting method that works best for it. Roots should be dug up with a spade or garden fork. Flowers need to be picked gently to prevent bruising. Fruits and seeds must be picked when they are fully ripe, and some should even be gathered after a frost. Harvesting too early may influence the taste, fragrance, or medicinal potency of an herb. There are general guidelines that help the harvesting go more smoothly but, as is always the case with plants, remember that they are individuals, and each one may have its own specific requirements.

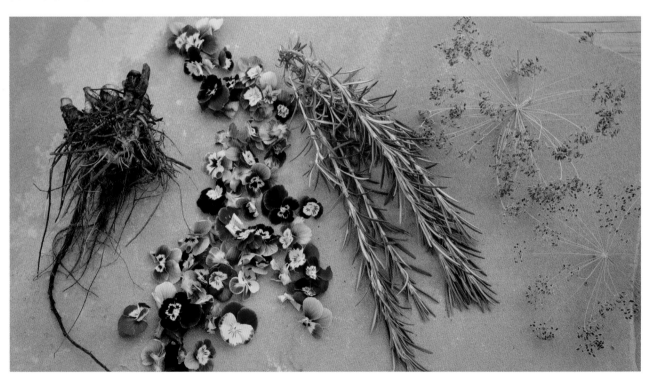

For each herb, you must consider which part of the plant should be harvested, at which point during the season, as well as which storage method is best. It's important to treat each herb as an individual in order to take full advantage of the uses it offers.

Knowing When to Harvest

As important as it is to know how to harvest each part of a plant, it will do you little good if you don't harvest it at the right time of the year. Annuals are not harvested at the same time as biennials or perennials. Roots are normally harvested at a different time from flowers, and so on.

Roots and Rhizomes

Roots, rhizomes, and bulbs are generally harvested during the spring or fall. Sometimes you will dig them in the winter months, if you live in an area where the ground does not freeze. Remember that whenever you harvest roots, you will be putting an end to a plant's life. Plant perennials and biennials accordingly, so you will have some roots to harvest and some to leave in the garden for next season.

ANNUAL ROOTS can be harvested at any point during their growing cycle, as long as this is done before the plant goes to seed. Once it has gone to seed, it will die and the root will be wasted.

BIENNIAL ROOTS should be harvested in the fall of the first year's growth or in the spring of the second year's growth. If you harvest in the spring of the first year, the roots will not be large enough to be valuable to you. If you wait until the fall of the second year, the plant will have seeded and then died, leaving you with pithy, woody roots that are not going to make a good food or medicine.

PERENNIAL ROOTS are best harvested in the spring, fall, or winter. If the plant is one that has flowers or seeds you would also like to use, harvest the roots when the other desirable parts are ready, for example while the plant is in flower or seed.

Whole Plants and Aerial Parts

Whole plants are harvested either when they are actively growing or when they are in flower or seed/fruit, depending on the requirements for the specific herb. The same is true for the aerial parts.

The flowers, buds, seeds, and fruits, of course, will be harvested when they are ready. As a general rule, berries and other fruits are picked in late summer or sometimes in fall, depending on when they ripen. Seeds are often harvested in early and late fall, but some seeds will ripen earlier; you must keep a close eye on them if you want to harvest the seeds before the plant disperses them into the air or onto the ground.

With a digging fork, you can usually harvest roots and rhizomes without damaging them and without leaving behind a huge hole in the garden.

AT-RISK AND ENDANGERED WILD ROOTS

One of the reasons many plants, such as echinacea, goldenseal, and yerba mansa, have become at-risk or endangered is improper and unethical wildcrafting (harvesting in the wild) that results in the roots and rhizomes being dug up during the wrong season. Some wildcrafters harvest perennial roots and rhizomes during the early spring to satisfy eager customers. Thus a plant is not allowed to flower and reproduce seed for that year, and this in turn jeopardizes self-propagation. When a plant becomes at-risk or endangered, it must be given every possible opportunity to survive; at-risk perennials especially should be allowed to produce seed. Gardeners can help by growing these plants in their own gardens, eliminating the need to harvest them from the wild. Making your own herb products, or buying those whose labels state the plants have been cultivated or ethically harvested, will also help protect endangered plants.

The Tools for the Job

Choose good-quality tools for harvesting; they greatly influence how pleasurable your harvest experience is! I consider my equipment an investment and I save money until I can afford a good-quality tool. I'm not suggesting that you need anything fancy, just that what you buy be well made.

What to Use and When to Use It

Although you should experiment to ascertain which tools work best for you and your plants, here are a few of my favorites:

NEEDLE-NOSE SPADE. I find this tool, which some garden stores call a nurseryman's spade, indispensable for harvesting whole plants and roots.

GARDEN DIGGING FORK. My absolute favorite root-digging tool is a garden digging fork. Buy one that has strong prongs that won't bend easily. I have an old one that belonged to my great-grandfather and the prongs on it are long with sharp points. It's fantastic for lifting out even some of the longest taproots. It's worth mentioning that a digging fork is different from a pitchfork, used for moving hay and straw. Pitchfork prongs are not strong enough to dig out roots without bending.

HAND SNIPS. A high-quality pair of harvesting or pruning hand snips is critical for every gardener. Choose a sturdy pair that will last a lifetime, replacing the springs and blades as needed. I have to replace blades annually and the springs every five years, but my snips get quite a workout. Buy a pair that is the right size for your hand and be sure to determine whether they are right- or left-handed snips. It is important to get a good pair with a proper fit so that you don't injure your hand while using them. Poor snips are easy to find; it's worth the trouble to seek out good ones.

SCISSORS. I always carry around a small pair of scissors. These easily fit in a harvesting basket or utility belt, making them readily available for all types of plant work throughout the day. I use them for everything, from pruning to harvesting.

FLOWER HARVESTING RAKE (sometimes called a chamomile rake). This helpful tool combs small, delicate flowers from plants without bruising them. My flower rake was originally a luxury tool for my garden shed, because I could do the same work by hand-picking and the rake was a bit out of my tool budget. However, I'm thrilled that I made the investment because it is used constantly, not only for harvesting flowers, but also for harvesting some types of seed, such as milky stage oatseed.

HANDS. Finally, I would like to put in a positive word for hand-picking. Sometimes there's no tool that works better than the human hand. Flowers, seeds, and fruits, for example, need the careful harvesting provided by hands.

Garden scissors are perfect for cutting tender stems from herbs like rosemary.

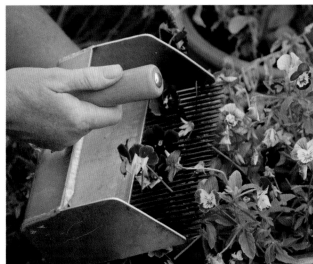

A flower rake (sometimes called a chamomile rake) gently frees flowers from the plant without damaging them.

Harvesting Roots, Rhizomes, and Bulbs

The underground parts of a plant often require the most energy to harvest, as they must be dug up. Use caution, though, or you may end up chopping off a valuable piece of root or piercing a fat juicy bulb. I loosen the soil around the root area and then gently lift the root out of the soil with a garden fork or needle-nose spade. A broad shovel won't work as well as a long spade will.

We grow in strong clay soil in southern Colorado, so I find it easier to harvest underground parts on a day when the soil is evenly moist rather than very dry or soaking wet. If the soil is too wet, it is nearly impossible to extract roots from that clay. If the soil is very dry, trying to get a spade or fork into it is like trying to penetrate concrete.

If you look closely at roots, you will notice a definite line where the plant begins to grow out of the soil. This is where the stems and leaves emerge from the roots, and it is called the root crown.

Drying Roots

You can dry roots in their whole form, chopped into small chunks (1 to 2 inches; 2.5–5 cm), or sliced. Whenever possible, I dry all of my plant parts whole. Whole dried plants will store better and maintain potency, flavor, and fragrance levels longer than will sliced or cut plants. Some roots, such as yucca and burdock, should be sliced before drying; once they have dried, they become extremely hard, and it will take a very strong piece of equipment (like a milling machine) to cut them up.

Lay out the whole, sliced, or chopped roots on a nonmetal or stainless steel screen (old nylon window

HARVESTING ROOTS

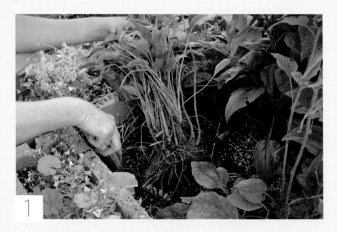

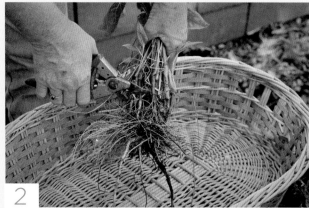

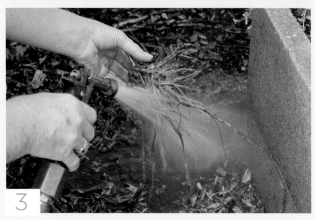

1) Carefully dig up the plant (in this case, echinacea), keeping as much of the root ball intact as possible.

2) Once the roots are out of the ground, trim off the tops or aerial parts of the plant to ¼ to 1 inch (6 mm–2.5 cm) above the root crown.

3) Separate the roots from the crown and gently rub the roots free of soil and stones. Wash well with a hose sprayer or faucet.

screens work nicely for drying plants) in an area that is out of direct sunlight and gets good warm-air circulation. Some roots and bulbs, like dandelion and garlic, can be tied with string and hung up in bunches to dry. Roots will take a week to several weeks to dry fully. They should feel brittle and snap easily in two. At that point, you can store them for later use. It is extremely important that the roots be completely dry before storage; even a small amount of moisture encourages the growth of mold. Garlic bulbs should have a couple of layers of papery outer skins when they are dry.

You can find more information on techniques for drying herbs under Drying for Optimal Quality on page 124.

FRESH-PROCESSING ROOTS

Wash the roots thoroughly. It is important that any manure or compost be cleaned off the roots to prevent contamination from *E. coli* or other bacteria. Process roots, rhizomes, or bulbs fresh as soon as possible. If it will be a few hours before you can begin processing, cool the plant part in a refrigerator or root cellar until you are ready to proceed, but for no longer than 48 hours.

Chop the roots into small chunks (1 to 2 inches; 2.5–5 cm) or grind them in a blender or food processor. Proceed as usual with your medicine making or whatever the intended use is going to be . . . maybe a component of a delicious meal.

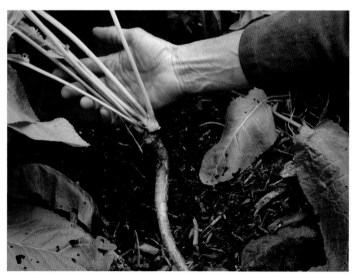

Horseradish root is harvested fresh and processed immediately to make horseradish sauce. It can also be made into an herbal vinegar that is quite helpful for clearing sinuses.

Harvesting Whole Plants

Harvesting whole plants is done in basically the same way as you do for roots, rhizomes, and bulbs. When harvesting a whole plant, first double-check whether the plant should be in flower or have formed seed at the time you harvest it (see chapter 10). To harvest a whole plant, use a spade or garden digging fork, penetrate the soil deep beneath the roots, and lift. Shake the plant to get rid of loose soil, then wash it clean of all soil and debris using a hose sprayer.

Whole plants may be dried using the screen method described under Drying for Optimal Quality on page 124, or by tying a rubber band or a slipknot around the roots of the plants and then hanging them upside down. It is important that hanging plants be spaced enough to allow for good warm-air circulation. Never hang them in direct sunlight, or the plant material will degrade quickly. Once dried, store the whole plants in a brown paper sack that has been taped closed at the top. You can also chop the plants into large pieces and store them in glass jars. The less the herb is chopped or ground, however, the more flavor, fragrance, and medicinal potency it will retain and the better it will store.

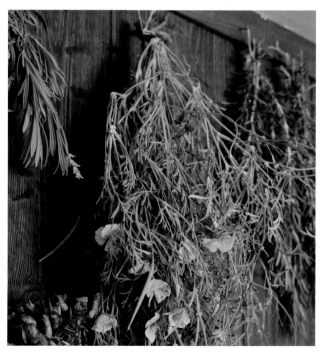

California poppy can be harvested as a whole plant while in flower and/or seed, and hung to dry for later use in tea and syrups,

Harvesting Aerial Parts

Often it is desirable to use all of the aerial parts of a plant. The aerial parts are the leaves, stems, flowers, and seeds or fruits. Harvesting can occur at any stage of the plant's growing season when any or all of these aerial parts are present. Check each individual plant's requirements to learn if it should be in flower or seed when it's harvested.

How to Harvest

To harvest aerial parts of an annual, I usually cut the plant just above the soil surface. When harvesting aerial parts of perennials, I cut the upper half to a third of the plant. This enables the plant to recover more easily and begin growing again sooner. I like to use a pair of sharp scissors, but good snips will work also. Use whichever tool you are more comfortable with.

Processing

After I have cut the aerial parts, I remove any dead or dying plant material and make sure the plant is free of dirt. If the plants have been grown properly and are healthy, I don't find it necessary to wash them, unless they've gotten muddy. But this is a judgment call for each of us. If you do wash your plants, be aware that you will be removing some of the water-soluble vitamins from the plant surfaces, as well as some of the volatile oils.

FRESH PROCESSING. I like to process many aerial plant parts for cooking or the making of fresh preparations. When cooking with fresh herbs, I pick them, then cook with them immediately. If you are making fresh preparations with any aboveground parts of the plant, try to process them no more than 24 hours after harvest time. It is best to get them put up within minutes of harvest. The sooner a plant is processed, the better and fresher it is. This makes a noticeable difference in your final product.

DRYING. Tie the plants into bundles and hang them upside down, or lay them on a nonmetal or stainless steel screen (never use aluminum screening to dry your herbs, as aluminum can alter the taste and medicinal qualities of the herb you are drying). If you dry aerial parts on a screen, be careful not to layer them too thick. A layer no more than

4 inches (10 cm) thick will let the plant material dry more evenly. It is critical to turn or toss the plants frequently to ensure even drying and prevent molding. Aerial parts, excluding the seeds (which will be firm and hard), will be brittle or crumbly when they are completely dry. Store dried plants for later use. Plants also dry easily when you put them loosely into shallow woven baskets. Toss the baskets gently every couple of days to facilitate air movement through the herbs. Basket drying is my favorite way to dry herbs.

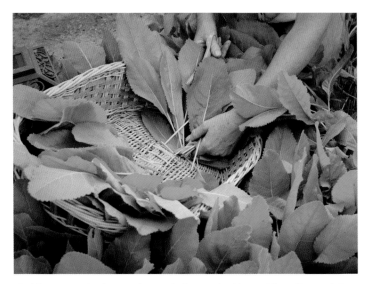

Like many herbs, costmary is harvested by cutting the aerial parts halfway down the stem and then bunching them together into small bundles that will be hung to dry.

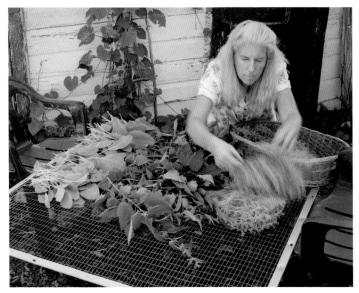

A good way to dry herbs is to set them out in a shallow layer on a screen, so that air can circulate through and around them. The aerial parts of costmary, nettle, and santolina all dry well this way.

Harvesting Flowers and Buds

I love to harvest herbal and edible flowers. Such a delicate but important part reminds me of all the vitality a plant a plant holds. Be gentle with flowers, as they bruise easily and will turn brown quickly if picked improperly.

How to Harvest

Normally I hand-pick flowers only. Sometimes, as is the case with chamomile, I harvest the flowering tops too, removing the flowers plus 2 to 4 inches (5–10 cm) of leafy stems. This type of harvesting is best accomplished with scissors. I use a basket to catch the flowers as I pick them, but my husband prefers a 5-gallon bucket, which he feels is sturdier and better protects the flowers. Using a flower rake to harvest them is another good way to help prevent bruising during the picking process.

Processing

Gently shake the flowers to remove any bugs or extra soil. Washing isn't necessary unless the flowers are muddy.

FRESH PROCESSING. If you plan to use the flowers fresh, immediately cool them in the refrigerator until you're ready to cook or process them.

Drying

To dry flowers, lay them out in a shallow layer on a nonmetal or stainless steel screen. Avoid direct sunlight and be sure that air circulation is good and temperatures are warm. I also like drying flowers in large, shallow baskets. Gently shake the baskets every day or so to redistribute the flowers, so that they all get exposed to the air and dry properly. I love the way baskets of drying flowers look and smell in my home. It's a beautiful and practical way to dry flowers and buds.

Once the flowers or buds are dried, put them into storage (see Proper Storage Methods, page 126, for information). I often dry extra baskets of flowers and buds, which I simply leave out in the house throughout the year to add color and fragrance. Because these flowers will gather dust and are exposed to the air constantly, I don't use them for cooking or making preparations. They are only to please the eye and nose.

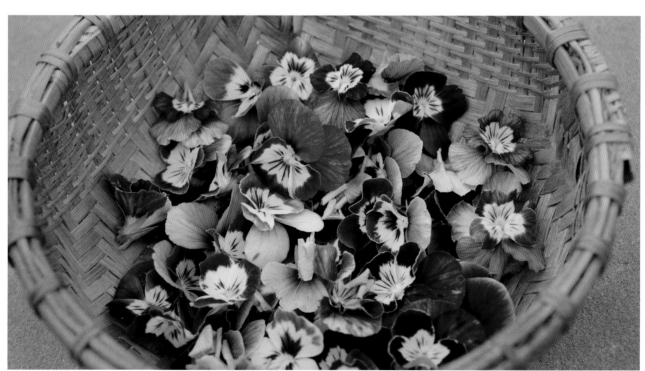

One of my favorite ways to dry herbs is in shallow baskets. It's an easy and attractive way to dry flowers like violas and chamomile, seeds like dill, and delicate tiny herbs like thymes.

Harvesting Seeds and Fruits

Most seeds and fruits should be picked when they are fully ripe. Occasionally a plant will be harvested when the seeds are still green. Check the individual plant's requirements in chapter 10 to know when to harvest its seeds.

How to Harvest

I usually hand-pick most seeds, but occasionally I use scissors or a flower rake to harvest entire seed heads. Pick fruits individually. It's best to place harvested seeds in a bucket, a close-woven basket, or a paper bag.

Processing

Organically grown seeds and fruits rarely require washing. Rinse any muddy fruits, but take care not to wash too much; excessive washing rinses away valuable water-soluble vitamins.

FRESH PROCESSING. Even though seeds and fruits may be fully ripe and appear dry when you harvest them, they are still considered fresh if they are processed immediately after harvest.

DRYING. I find it best to put seeds and fruits into a close-woven basket for a few days to a couple of weeks to let them finish drying. It's too disappointing to store fruits or seeds before they are fully dried and then see mold on them. Be patient; let them dry fully.

Once dried, seeds and fruits are best stored in paper bags or glass jars. The freezer presents optimum storage conditions for seeds. I often put seeds in a paper bag, place that bag into a freezer bag, and then put the whole package in the freezer. Fruits, on the other hand, may be stored at room temperature in a dry place, ideally in a glass jar.

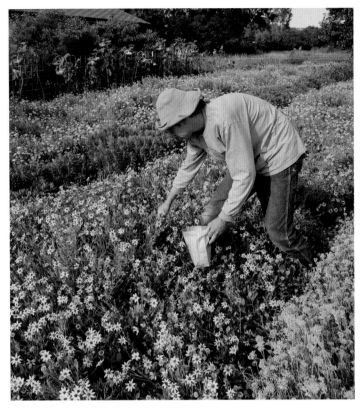

Every day Caleb picks chocolate flower seeds, as this plant produces new seed daily. The ripe seed heads are hand-picked and then allowed to dry in paper sacks.

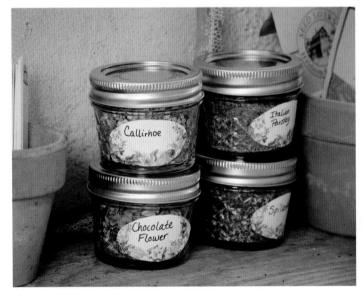

Once seeds are fully dried, they are cleaned and stored in tightly closed glass jars until they are ready to be used or planted. Stored seeds are best kept out of bright light and away from extreme heat.

Harvesting and Saving Seeds to Plant Later

When growing plants from seed, you'll have two choices for obtaining the seeds: buying seed from a seed house that provides good-quality stock or saving and cleaning your own seed. Both are good options, but in truth I think it is important to know how to save your own seed and do the cleaning process even if you opt never to attempt the task again.

Saving our own seed is a part of our ancestral traditions, just like growing our own food and preparing our own medicines. It is a skill that should be honored as a sacred part of our ability to care for ourselves. We should all endeavor to pass on this skill to our children, grandchildren, and future generations.

> Saving our own seed is a part of our ancestral traditions, just like growing our own food and preparing our own medicines.

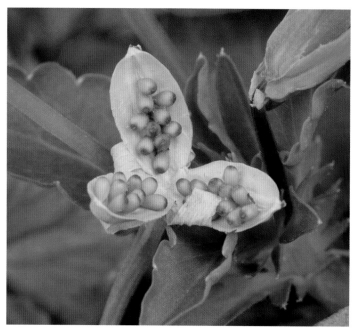

A viola seed pod opens to expose mature seeds. If allowed to stay on the plant, these seeds will scatter via wind and water. At this stage they are easy to harvest and save for later planting.

Another good reason to know how to save your own seed is the rising popularity of genetic engineering. Genetic engineering limits plant and animal diversity, gives inappropriate control or power to corporate entities and governmental agencies, and can have negative repercussions on health, nutrition, and healing. If you save your own seed from non–genetically engineered plants, you will be exercising your right to eat what you feel is best and make plant-based medicines, household items, and textiles from crops you feel are most appropriate for your needs.

The process of saving seed is not a difficult one, but in order to keep the seed viable, you must harvest, clean, and store it properly.

Harvesting

Harvest when the seed is ripe; look for seeds that are fully formed, showing evidence of a seed embryo inside (the seed should look plump). Ripe seeds usually have turned from green to another color — anything from brown, tan, black, and white to exotic colors like maroon and even speckled hues. The mature seeds may also have a somewhat dried appearance. If the seeds are fully ripe, pick them by hand or use a pair of snips or scissors. I like to gather my seeds in paper bags or tightly woven baskets. Do not use containers that are airtight, as these encourage the growth of mold if the seeds contain any moisture in or on them.

Cleaning

To begin the cleaning process, spread out newspaper on a table. A shallow cardboard box will also work nicely for this purpose. Seeds are normally contained within some type of shell, cone, or husk to protect them from wind and harsh weather or browsing animals or insects. You will have to dislodge the seed from that protective "house" and then attempt to remove as much of the chaff (the clinging bits of a seed's house) as possible. I use various-sized screens and baskets to accomplish this. As the seeds are sifted through a screen, they are separated from the chaff. It will be nearly impossible to remove 100 percent of the chaff, but don't worry; a bit of chaff doesn't hinder the sowing process much when you actually plant the seeds.

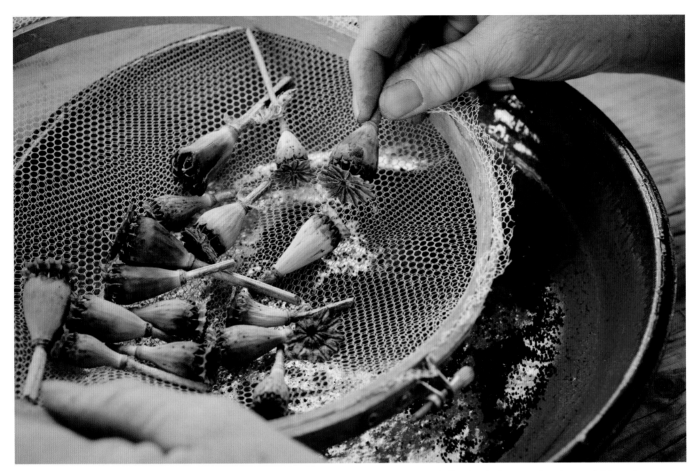

After seeds are fully dried, they can be cleaned. Place them over a newspaper or screen and sift the seeds out of the pods and husks. Discard any chaff, insects, or pieces of plant matter or dirt.

Storing

Once you have cleaned the seeds to your satisfaction, put them in a plain paper envelope. Label the envelope with the plant name, when and where the seed was harvested, and any other information you would like to remember. I sometimes note the elevation of the harvest location and weather conditions at the time of harvest.

If the seed is nontropical, it will stay viable longer if it is stored in the freezer. Put the envelopes in a plastic zipper-lock bag and put the whole package in the freezer. Stored in this fashion, seeds will often stay viable for several years. If the seeds are from a tropical plant, store them at room temperature in a dry place, protected from bright light. These seeds will also hold their viability for up to several years. For any type of seed, be sure to avoid excessive heat (over 100°F [38°C] for extended periods), bright light, and direct contact with moisture. Do whatever is possible to prevent pests like insects and mice from getting into the seed, too.

MAKE YOUR OWN SEED-CLEANING SCREEN

Be creative! Use sprouting screens, different-sized tea strainers and colanders, and old window screens for your seed cleaning. I create screens by using various sizes of fabric netting (available at fabric and craft stores) or different-sized nylon or noncorroding metal window screening (available at hardware stores). I stretch the netting or screening material between embroidery hoops (also available at fabric and craft stores) until they are taut. This gives me many different-sized, inexpensive cleaning screens to work with. If making screens does not appeal to you, you can easily purchase a set of seed-cleaning screens at an upscale garden center or from a mail-order gardening supply house.

Drying for Optimal Quality

There are a number of methods for drying plants, from hanging bundles to screen and basket drying to drying in paper sacks and cardboard boxes. Regardless of how you do it, be sure a plant is fully dry before storing or it will mold.

Attics usually work very well for drying plants; basements generally aren't good if they have poor air movement or are the least bit damp. I dry plants on our covered patio here in Colorado, but the climate is dry. People in areas with high humidity will have more difficulty. You may need to assist the process by setting up fans to improve air circulation and remove some of the moisture from the air. If plants are dried improperly, they may show signs of mold and mildew in the form of a white downy or black slimy coating. The plants will often smell musty or rotten; these plants must be discarded.

Please do not dry your plants in buildings where machine oils or other fumes will be present. Plants can absorb these substances, and that's the last thing you want if you plan to use them for health and well-being.

Hanging Bundles

If you decide to dry your herbs by hanging them upside down in bundles, it's important to pay attention to the size of the bundles. As you put together a bundle, look at the stems and be sure that the diameter of the bunch where the stems are tied together is no bigger than that of a pencil. This will allow for good airflow through the bundle, thus discouraging the growth of mold and mildew.

Tying herbs with a simple slipknot or a rubber band lets you keep the bundle together as it shrinks during the drying process. If you use string tied in a basic knot, stems will fall out as the plants shrink.

Harvesting herbs from your garden is a wonderful sensory experience. This rosemary is very fragrant and makes me feel hungry even as I harvest it.

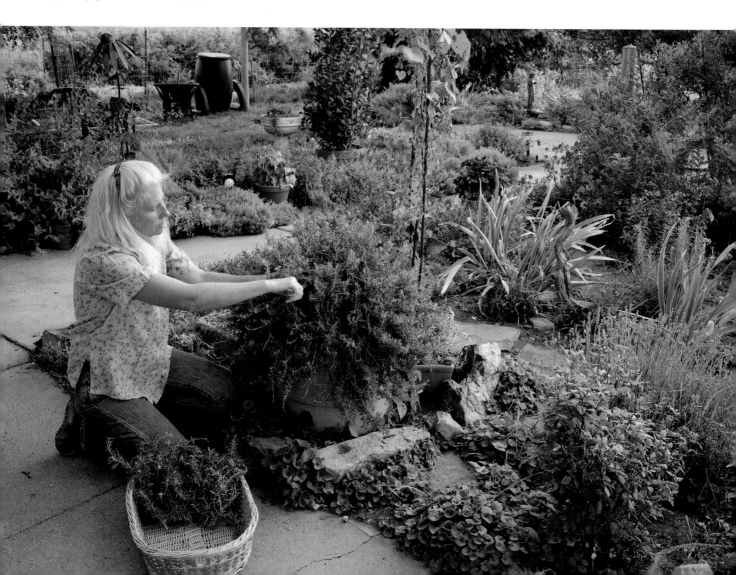

Don't hang bunches of herbs too close together; crowding produces poor air circulation. Bundles should be hung in an area that is protected from direct sunlight and moisture, where there is good warm-air circulation. Normally, bundles of herbs will dry in one to two weeks.

Screen and Basket Drying

When using screens to dry herbs, choose nonmetal (such as nylon) or stainless steel screening material. Aluminum screening can change the taste and fragrance of a plant as it dries, and there is also the potential that medicinal constituents will be altered. If you must use an aluminum screen, lay a barrier of cotton cloth or paper between the plant material and the screen. This will help protect the plants without preventing the movement of air.

Place the screen on blocks or hang it horizontally from the ceiling to allow air to move below, around, and above it. I simply prop my screen across two chairs. Place the screen out of direct sunlight and protect it from moisture. Plants will take from one to several weeks to dry on screens.

Basket drying is one of my favorite ways to dry small amounts of herbs. Select a basket that is shallow and has a weave big enough to let air flow through it but small enough that the plant material can't fall out. Gently toss baskets every day or so to redistribute the plants, allowing for even drying and air exposure.

Drying in Paper Sacks and Cardboard Boxes

If you're in a pinch and don't have any other way to dry your plants, or if you've gathered plants from a friend's garden and will be traveling for a few days before returning home, it's possible to dry plants in paper sacks or cardboard boxes.

The key to success with this method is to avoid putting too much plant material in each sack or box, and to leave the top open so that air can flow into the container. Check plants often to make sure they are not molding or mildewing. If you notice this happening, you probably have too much plant material in the container.

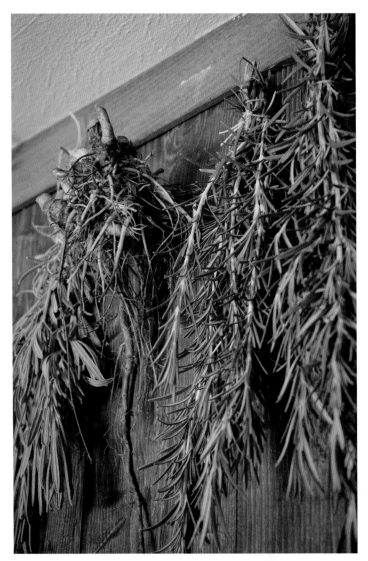

Hanging bundles of drying herbs add a beautiful touch to any space in your home that has good air movement, warm temperatures, and is not in direct sunlight.

WHAT ABOUT OVENS AND DEHYDRATORS?

I'm often asked if I dry my plants in a food dehydrator or in the oven. I don't want to expose my plants to any temperature that would be above that of normal warm air; heat can change or degrade a plant's constituents and nutrients. If you do choose a heat mechanism like a dehydrator, set it at the lowest temperature possible and check the plants often.

Gently shake the sack or box every day or two to redistribute the plant material and assist the drying process. Plants will usually dry in one to two weeks.

Testing for Dryness

Most plants, when fully dry, will be brittle and make a snapping or crackling sound when they are crushed. When this happens, your plants are ready to store; it's best to do so promptly to decrease their exposure to air and dust, which will degrade them more quickly.

Another way to test for dryness is to gently tear a piece of the plant material. If you notice any moisture beads forming along the tear, the plant needs to dry a bit longer. You can also place the edge of the tear against your upper lip, the most sensitive part of your body. If you feel any moisture there, let the plant dry a while longer before storing it.

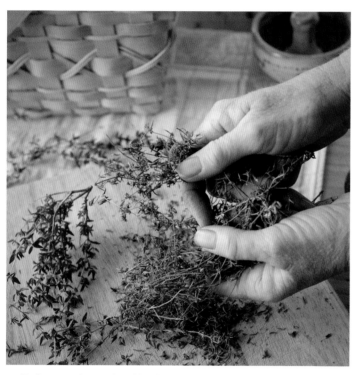
Before storing a dried herb, crumble a piece in your hand to make sure there is no moisture in it. This will ensure that it does not mold during storage.

Proper Storage Methods

Choosing the right container or location for storage can often affect how well your plants keep their potency, color, taste, and smell. Store dried plants in clean, airtight glass jars or paper containers that can be taped closed. Plastic and metal containers (except stainless steel) are unsuitable, although unchipped porcelain enamel (also called enameled metal) ones are okay. Most glass jars, such as canning jars, come with metal lids, but these are worry-free because the lids have a nonmetal coating. If you would like to store herbs in decorative tins, line them first with a paper bag or waxed paper to create a barrier between the plants and the metal.

Store dried plants in clean, airtight glass jars.

Where to Store

Keep storage containers out of direct light and away from extreme heat. Protect them, too, from moisture. Cabinets and pantries are good places to store herbs, but you can even set jars on open shelves, as long as they are not exposed to strong light or intense heat.

How Long Will They Last?

Properly dried and stored herbs will maintain their color; they should look vibrant and healthy. Their taste should be strong and their smell should resemble the scent when they were fresh. If your herbs do not meet these qualifications, discard them.

When properly stored, dried herbs will generally keep for a year. Ground and powdered herbs may have a shorter shelf life, four to six months, at which point just add them to the compost pile.

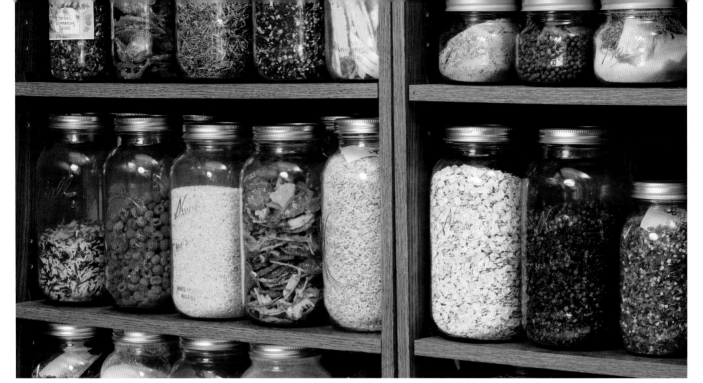

Dried herbs store beautifully in tightly closed glass jars, adding lovely colors and textures to the kitchen, while also being close at hand for cooking and making remedies.

Freezing Herbs

Another excellent way to store fresh-picked leaves of herbs is to freeze them. This is one of the easiest methods, and I find that herbs like basil, parsley, and chives, all freeze wonderfully. I generally do not bother to freeze roots, barks, and seeds or herbal edible flowers like calendula, heartsease, or nasturtiums, which don't hold their beautiful colors when frozen. I use these herbal parts either fresh or dried. Frozen herbs work best for later cooking or processing into some type of herbal preparation. The downside to freezing is that the herbs, once thawed, will be mushy and not very attractive to use as you would fresh in, say, a salad. Please refer to the harvesting guidelines chart on page 128 for information on which herbs are really good to freeze.

To freeze freshly picked herbs, simply shake them gently to remove any insects or bits of soil, put them into a freezer storage container, label, and freeze. If the herbs are muddy, rinse them gently first. Frozen herbs will keep about one year in the freezer if properly packaged.

You can also freeze herbs that have been puréed in a blender after they are picked. Pour the purée into ice-cube trays and put them in the freezer. Once the purée is frozen, pop the cubes out of the trays and transfer them into a freezer storage container. Label the container and return it to the freezer until you are ready to use the herbs. For example, when you want basil to make spaghetti sauce, just pull out as many frozen basil purée cubes you need and add them to the sauce while it's simmering. It is as easy as that.

Frozen herbs retain the flavor of fresh, along with the nutritional and medicinal value, and you have the convenience of having them when the garden is out of season. Anyone for pesto?

HERBS THAT STORE WELL FROZEN

The following are just a few of the ways that frozen herbs can be used.

> **Basil** — purée leaves and freeze for later use in pesto

> **Plantain** — freeze the whole plant to soothe insect stings and bites

> **Nettles** — freeze the aerial parts for use in soup broth

> **Echinacea** — steep the frozen root for an excellent winter tea to support the immune system

> **Mint** — freeze leafy stems, then add to chocolate chip cookie batter

HARVESTING GUIDELINES

COMMON NAME	LATIN BOTANICAL NAME	PARTS TO HARVEST	HARVEST TIME	BEST STORAGE METHODS	DRYING METHODS
Agastache	*Agastache rupestris, A. cana*	Flowering aerial parts	Summer to fall	Use fresh or dried	Hang in bunches, screen drying
Angelica	*Angelica archangelica*	Roots, stalks, flowers, seeds	Throughout growing season	Use fresh or dried	Roots and stalks on screens, flowers and seeds in basket
Anise hyssop	*Agastache foeniculum*	Flowering aerial parts	Summer to fall	Use fresh or dried	Hang in bunches, screen drying
Astragalus, Chinese	*Astragalus membranaceus*	Roots	Spring or fall	Dried	Screen drying
Basil	*Ocimum* species	Aerial parts	Throughout growing season	Use fresh, frozen, dried	Hang in bunches, screen drying, basket drying
Borage	*Borago officinalis*	Flowers, green or ripe seed	When flowers/ seeds are present	Use flowers fresh, seeds fresh or dried	Seeds in basket
Breadseed poppy	*Papaver somniferum*	Seeds	When seeds are ripe	Dried	Seeds in basket
Calendula	*Calendula officinalis*	Flowers	Summer to fall	Use fresh or dried	Basket drying, screen drying
California poppy	*Eschscholzia californica*	Whole plant	Summer to fall	Use fresh or dried	Hang in bunches, screen drying
Catmint	*Nepeta × faassenii*	Aerial parts with or without flowers	Spring through fall	Use flowers fresh, use aerial parts fresh or dried	Hang in bunches, screen drying
Catnip	*Nepeta cataria*	Aerial parts	Throughout the growing season	Use fresh, dried, or frozen	Hang in bundles, screen drying, basket drying
Cayenne	*Capsicum* species	Peppers only	When green or fully ripe	Use fresh, dried, or frozen	Screen drying, basket drying
Chamomile	*Matricaria recutita, Chamaemelum nobile*	Flowers, flowering tops	Summer into fall	Use fresh or dried	Screen drying, basket drying
Chasteberry	*Vitex agnus-castus*	Ripe berries	Late summer to fall	Dried	Basket drying
Chives	*Allium schoenoprasum*	Aerial parts with or without flowers	Throughout the growing season	Use fresh or frozen	Not applicable
Cilantro, Coriander	*Coriandrum sativum*	Aerial parts, flowers, ripe seeds	Throughout the growing season	Use aerial parts fresh, use flowers fresh, use seeds dry	Basket drying for seeds
Clary sage	*Salvia sclarea*	Aerial parts, flowers and flower husks	Throughout the growing season	Use fresh or dried	Hang in bundles, screen drying
Comfrey	*Symphytum × uplandicum*	Aerial parts with or without flowers	Throughout the growing season	Use fresh or dried	Hang in bundles, screen drying

COMMON NAME	LATIN BOTANICAL NAME	PARTS TO HARVEST	HARVEST TIME	BEST STORAGE METHODS	DRYING METHODS
Costmary	*Tanacetum balsamita*	Aerial parts	Throughout the growing season	Use fresh or dried	Screen drying
Coyote mint	*Monardella odoratissima*	Aerial parts with or without flowers	Throughout the growing season	Use fresh or dried	Hang in bundles, screen drying, basket drying
Cutting celery	*Apium graveolens*	Aerial parts	Throughout the growing season	Use fresh, dried, or frozen	Screen drying, basket drying
Dill	*Anethum graveolens*	Leaf, flowers, green and ripe seeds	Throughout the growing season	Use fresh, dried, or frozen	Hang in bunches, screen drying, basket drying
Echinacea	*Echinacea* species	Flowers, seeds, roots	Flowers in summer, seeds and roots in fall, roots also in spring	Use fresh or dried	Hang in bunches, screen drying
Epazote	*Chenopodium ambrosioides*	Aerial parts	Throughout the growing season	Use fresh or dried	Hang in bunches, screen drying, basket drying
Eucalyptus	*Eucalyptus* species	Leaves	Throughout the growing season	Use fresh or dried	Hang branches in bunches, screen drying — strip off leaves once dried
Fennel	*Foeniculum vulgare, F. vulgare* 'Rubrum'	Leaves, flowers, green and ripe seed, roots	Throughout the growing season	Use fresh or dried	Hang in bunches, screen drying, basket drying
Feverfew	*Tanacetum parthenium*	Leaves	Throughout the growing season	Use fresh or dried	Hang in bunches, screen drying — strip off leaves once dried
Garlic	*Allium sativum*	Bulbs	Late summer and fall	Use fresh-cured	Hang in bunches, screen drying — remove stems once dried
Garlic chives	*Allium tuberosum*	Aerial parts with or without flowers	Throughout the growing season	Use fresh or frozen	Not applicable
Ginger	*Zingiber officinale*	Roots/rhizomes	Winter in tropical climates or when container-grown	Use fresh or dried	Screen drying
Goldenrod	*Solidago* species	Flowering aerial parts	Late summer or fall	Use fresh or dried	Hang in bunches, screen drying
Goldenseal	*Hydrastis canadensis*	Roots	Spring or fall	Use fresh or dried	Screen drying
Gotu kola	*Centella asiatica*	Aerial parts	Throughout the growing season	Use fresh, dried, or frozen	Screen drying, basket drying
Heartsease	*Viola tricolor, V. cornuta*	Flowers and leaves	Throughout the growing season	Use fresh or frozen	Screen drying, basket drying
Hollyhock	*Alcea* species	Flowers, leaves and roots	Flowers and leaves throughout the growing season, roots in spring or fall	Use flowers fresh, use leaves or roots fresh or dried	Screen drying

COMMON NAME	LATIN BOTANICAL NAME	PARTS TO HARVEST	HARVEST TIME	BEST STORAGE METHODS	DRYING METHODS
Hops	*Humulus lupulus*	Strobiles (flowers), green or fully mature	Late summer or fall	Use fresh or dried	Screen drying, basket drying
Horehound	*Marrubium vulgare*	Aerial parts	Throughout the growing season	Use fresh or dried	Hang in bunches, screen drying
Horseradish	*Armoracia rusticana*	Roots	Spring or fall are best, summer is acceptable	Use fresh or dried	Screen drying
Hyssop	*Hyssopus officinalis*	Aerial parts with or without flowers	Throughout the growing season	Use fresh or dried	Hang in bunches, screen drying, basket drying
Lady's mantle	*Alchemilla vulgaris*	Leaves	Throughout the growing season	Use fresh or dried	Screen drying, basket drying
Lavender	*Lavandula* species	Aerial parts with or without flowers, flowers alone	Throughout the growing season	Use fresh, dried, or frozen	Hang in bunches, screen drying, basket drying
Lemon balm	*Melissa officinalis*	Aerial parts	Throughout the growing season	Use fresh, dried, or frozen	
Lemongrass, East Indian, West Indian	*Cymbopogon flexuosus, C. citratus*	Leaves	Throughout the growing season	Use fresh, dried, or frozen	Hang in bunches, screen drying
Lemon verbena	*Aloysia triphylla*	Leaves and flowers	Throughout the growing season	Use fresh, dried, or frozen	Hang in bunches, screen drying — strip leaves from stems once dried, basket drying for flowers
Licorice	*Glycyrrhiza glabra*	Roots/rhizomes	Spring or fall	Use fresh or dried	Screen drying
Lovage	*Levisticum officinale*	All parts	Roots in spring or fall, leaves, flowers, and seeds throughout the growing season	Use fresh or dried	Hang in bunches, screen drying, basket drying for flowers and seeds
Marjoram (sweet, za'atar, wild)	*Origanum majorana, O. syriaca, O. vulgare*	Aerial parts	Throughout the growing season	Use fresh, dried, or frozen	Screen drying, basket drying
Marsh mallow	*Althaea officinalis*	Flowers, leaves, roots	Roots in spring or fall, flowers and leaves throughout the growing season	Use flowers fresh, use leaves and roots fresh or dried	Hang in bunches, screen drying
Melaleuca, Tea tree	*Melaleuca alternifolia*	Leaves	Throughout the growing season	Use fresh or dried	Hang in bunches, screen drying — strip leaves from stems once dried
Mexican oregano	*Lippia graveolens*	Leaves while in flower or not	Throughout the growing season	Use fresh or dried	Hang in bunches, screen drying, basket drying — strip leaves and flowers from stems once dried

COMMON NAME	LATIN BOTANICAL NAME	PARTS TO HARVEST	HARVEST TIME	BEST STORAGE METHODS	DRYING METHODS
Monarda	*Monarda* species	Aerial parts with or without flowers	Throughout the growing season	Use fresh or dried	Hang in bunches, screen drying, basket drying — strip from stems once dried
Motherwort	*Leonurus cardiaca*	Aerial parts	Throughout the growing season	Use fresh or dried	Hang in bunches, screen drying
Mugwort	*Artemisia vulgaris*	Aerial parts	Throughout the growing season	Use fresh or dried	Hang in bunches, screen drying
Mullein	*Verbascum thapsus*	Roots, leaves, flowers	Roots in spring or fall, leaves and flowers throughout the growing season	Use fresh or dried	Screen drying
Nasturtium	*Tropaeolum majus*	Leaves and flowers	Throughout the growing season	Use fresh	Not applicable
Nettle	*Urtica dioica*	Aerial parts	Throughout the growing season	Use fresh, dried, or frozen	Hang in bunches, screen drying — strip from stems once dried
Oats	*Avena sativa*	Leaves (called the straw), milky stage seeds, ripe seeds	Throughout the growing season	Use fresh, dried, or frozen	Screen drying, basket drying
Oregano	*Origanum* species	Aerial parts with or without flowers	Throughout the growing season	Use fresh, dried, or frozen	Screen drying, basket drying
Parsley	*Petroselinum crispum, P. crispum* var. *neapolitanum*	Aerial parts, roots	Roots in spring or fall, aerial parts throughout the growing season	Use fresh, dried, or frozen	Hang in bunches, screen drying
Passionflower	*Passiflora incarnata, P. edulis*	Aerial parts with or without flowers and fruits	Throughout the growing season	Use fresh or dried	Screen drying
Pennyroyal	*Mentha pulegium*	Aerial parts	Throughout the growing season	Use fresh or dried	Screen drying, basket drying
Peppermint	*Mentha piperita*	Aerial parts with or without flowers	Throughout the growing season	Use fresh, dried, or frozen	Hang in bunches, screen drying, basket drying
Potentilla	*Potentilla* species	Aerial parts with or without flowers	Throughout the growing season	Use fresh or dried	Screen drying, basket drying
Prickly pear	*Opuntia* species	Pads, flowers, fruits	Throughout the growing sesason	Use fresh	Not applicable
Red clover	*Trifolium pratense*	Flowers	Throughout the growing season	Use fresh, dried, or frozen	Screen drying, basket drying
Rosemary	*Rosmarinus* species	Aerial parts with or without flowers	Throughout the growing season	Use fresh, dried, or frozen	Hang in bunches, screen drying, basket drying

COMMON NAME	LATIN BOTANICAL NAME	PARTS TO HARVEST	HARVEST TIME	BEST STORAGE METHODS	DRYING METHODS
Rue	*Ruta graveolens*	Aerial parts	Throughout the growing season	Use dried	Hang in bunches, screen drying, basket drying
Sage	*Salvia officinalis*	Aerial parts with or without flowers	Throughout the growing season	Use fresh, dried, or frozen	Hang in bunches, screen drying, basket drying
Salad burnet	*Sanguisorba minor*	Leaves and/or flowers	Throughout the growing season	Use fresh	Not applicable
Santolina	*Santolina* species	Aerial parts with or without flowers	Throughout the growing season	Use fresh or dried	Hang in bunches, screen drying
Savory, summer	*Satureja hortensis*	Aerial parts	Throughout the growing season	Use fresh or dried	Hang in bunches, screen drying, basket drying
Savory, winter	*Satureja montana*	Aerial parts	Throughout the growing season	Use fresh or dried	Hang in bunches, screen drying, basket drying
Self-heal	*Prunella grandiflora* subsp. *pyrenaica*, *P. vulgaris*	Aerial parts with or without flowers	Thoughout the growing season	Use fresh or dried	Screen drying, basket drying
Shiso	*Perilla frutescens*	Aerial parts with or without flowers	Throughout the growing season	Use fresh	Not applicable
Skullcap	*Scutellaria lateriflora*	Aerial parts in flower	During flowering only	Use fresh	Not applicable
Sorrel, French, Red-veined)	*Rumex acetosa*, *R. sanguineus*	Leaves	Throughout the growing season	Use fresh	Not applicable
Southernwood	*Artemisia abrotanum*	Aerial parts	Throughout the growing season	Use fresh or dried	Hang in bunches, screen drying
Spearmint	*Mentha spicata*	Aerial parts with or without flowers	Throughout the growing season	Use fresh, dried, or frozen	Hang in bunches, screen drying, basket drying
Spilanthes	*Spilanthes oleracea*	Aerial parts in flower	Throughout the growing season	Use fresh or dried	Hang in bunches, screen drying, basket drying
St.-John's-wort	*Hypericum perforatum*	Flowering tops (upper 3-4" of flowering stems)	During flowering only	Use fresh	Not applicable
Stevia	*Stevia rebaudiana*	Aerial parts with or without flowers	Throughout the growing season	Use fresh or dried	Hang in bunches, screen drying, basket drying
Sunflower	*Helianthus annuus*	Seeds	When fully ripe	Use dried	Basket drying
Sweetgrass	*Hierochloe odorata*	Leaves	Throughout the growing season	Use fresh or dried	Screen drying
Sweet woodruff	*Galium odoratum*	Aerial parts with or without flowers	Throughout the growing season	Use fresh or dried	Screen drying, basket drying

COMMON NAME	LATIN BOTANICAL NAME	PARTS TO HARVEST	HARVEST TIME	BEST STORAGE METHODS	DRYING METHODS
Thyme	*Thymus* species	Aerial parts with or without flowers	Throughout the growing season	Use fresh, dried,or frozen	Screen drying, basket drying
Turmeric	*Curcuma longa*	Roots/rhizomes	Winter in tropical climates or when container-grown	Use fresh or dried	Screen drying
Valerian	*Valeriana officinalis*	Roots	Spring or fall	Use fresh or dried	Screen drying
Vervain, Blue vervain	*Verbena* species	Aerial parts with or without flowers	Throughout the growing season	Use fresh or dried	Hang in bunches, screen drying — strip from stems when dried
Vietnamese coriander	*Polygonum odoratum*	Leaves	Throughout the growing season	Use fresh	Not applicable
Violet	*Viola* species	Leaves and flowers	Throughout the growing season	Use flowers fresh, use leaves fresh or dried	Screen drying, basket drying
Watercress	*Nasturtium officinale*	Aerial parts	Throughout the growing season	Use fresh	Not applicable
White sage	*Salvia apiana*	Aerial parts with or without flowers	Throughout the growing season	Use dried	Hang in bunches, screen drying
Wood betony	*Stachys officinalis*	Aerial parts with or without flowers	Throughout the growing season	Use fresh or dried	Screen drying, basket drying
Yarrow	*Achillea* species	Aerial parts with or without flowers	Throughout the growing sesason	Use fresh or dried	Hang in bunches, screen drying, basket drying
Yerba mansa	*Anemopsis californica*	Roots or whole plant	Spring or fall is best, late summer is acceptable	Use fresh or dried	Screen drying
Yucca	*Yucca* species	Roots, flowers	Spring or fall for roots, flowers when present	Use flowers fresh, use roots fresh or dried	Screen drying

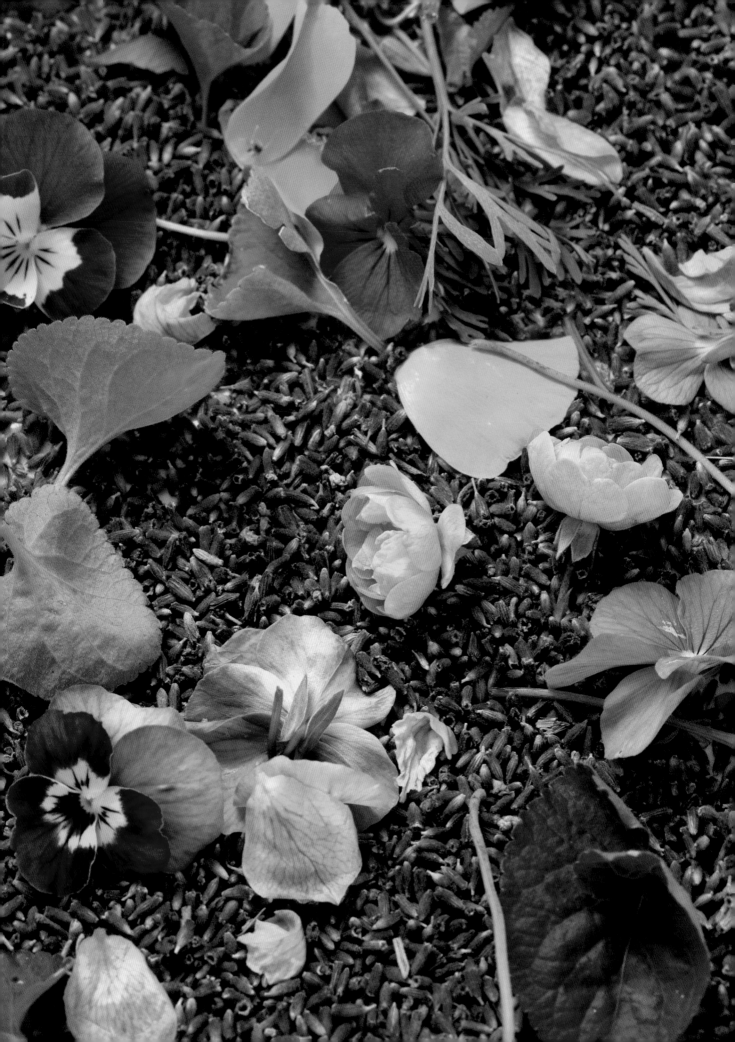

CHAPTER EIGHT

Making Herbal Preparations for Medicine and Personal Care

There are countless ways to utilize your garden herbs to make your own botanical medicines, hand creams, bath herbs, insect repellent, and other personal-care items. The recipes and directions in this chapter will act as general guidelines to enable you to make these items in your own kitchen. Remember that every plant used medicinally will have its own specific dosage recommendations and cautionary notes, so I recommend you invest in one or two reliable resource books for information on effective and safe usage (see Recommended Reading, page 246, as well as chapter 10). Whether you prepare these items for your own use or as gifts for friends and family, I'm sure you will enjoy the process and the feeling of empowerment you gain.

Choosing Utensils and Equipment

Preparing medicinal remedies and personal-care preparations in your kitchen requires that you give a few moments' thought to the utensils you will be using. It isn't necessary to buy fancy or extra equipment, but you will want to be sure that you have utensils that are made from appropriate materials.

Materials

Plastic should not be used at all when making or packaging herbal preparations. Only stainless steel or unchipped enamel is acceptable for metal containers. Avoid aluminum and copper pans at all costs; neither of those materials is conducive to good health. Glass and Pyrex containers and pans are the best. I like to use wooden spoons, but stainless steel spoons are also fine. Follow the same criteria for bowls and packaging containers.

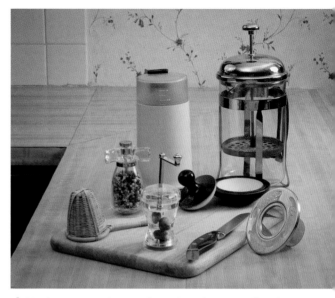

Having appropriate tools and equipment will make processing herbs much easier and more enjoyable. Choose high-quality tools that will last through many years of use.

Equipment and Utensils

You could stock your kitchen with a huge variety of pots, pans, spoons, and jars, but the truth is that you can make do with just a few items. Here are the equipment and utensils I keep on hand in my kitchen:

- Long-handled wooden spoons
- Several different-sized kitchen knives
- Different-sized strainers (at least three)
- One or two large kettles (I have one stainless steel and one Pyrex)
- A few saucepans, varying in size from 1 to 3 quarts (0.95 L to 2.84 L)
- A set of measuring cups and spoons
- Pint and quart canning jars
- Mortar and pestle
- Spice mill
- Blender (good quality is essential)
- Different-sized funnels
- Glass and glazed pottery bowls
- Wooden cutting board
- Cotton napkins (for use as straining cloths)

Homemade Remedies

The decision on which type of remedy you should prepare will ultimately be based on the plant, the person who will be taking the remedy, and the condition for which it is being used.

Infusions and decoctions are good for many types of herbs, but they require preparation time for each use. Vinegars, syrups, elixirs, and honeys are all pleasant and effective ways to use herbs, but they have a limited shelf life. Tinctures, on the other hand, have nearly unlimited shelf life and are convenient to use. Topical preparations like salves and ointments are neat, easy methods of applying herbs. Regardless of what type of remedy you prepare, each one can enhance your health and well-being.

Infusions and Decoctions

Infusions and decoctions are medicinal-strength teas, rather than beverage teas. Whether you infuse or decoct the plants is determined by the part of the plant you'll be using.

INFUSIONS are prepared from leaves, stems, and flowers. They are covered with boiling water and allowed to steep.

DECOCTIONS are prepared from roots, rhizomes, bark, and seeds, and are gently simmered in water.

As a general measurement, use 1 teaspoon of dried herb or 2 teaspoons of fresh per cup of water. Most herbal infusions and decoctions will keep for up to three days when stored in a tightly closed glass container in the refrigerator. Discard any tea left after that time and make a fresh batch.

Many teas may be drunk either hot or cold. Occasionally it is preferable to drink a particular tea at one temperature only, so see chapter 10 to learn more about the individual herb you plan to use. I feel strongly that you should not use a microwave oven to make or reheat a tea. Microwaves emit a small amount of radiation, and I don't think it's healthy to include that in your medicinal infusions or decoctions. It really takes only a short time to prepare these teas by a more traditional method (stove, electric coffeepot, or French press, for example).

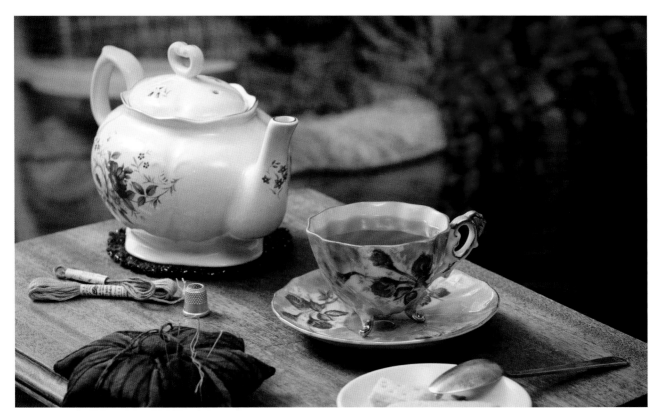

A cup of well-brewed herbal tea can be a potent medicinal preparation, as well as the perfect way to relax following a stressful day. In either case, it is a wonderful thing to make tea from herbs you harvested from your own garden.

TO PREPARE AN INFUSION: Measure the correct amount of herb into a heat-tolerant container. In a pan or teapot, bring the water to a boil, then pour the water over the herb. Cover with a lid and let the herb steep for 10 to 15 minutes. Strain out the herb, and you're ready to enjoy your infusion.

TO PREPARE A DECOCTION: In a pan or teapot, bring the water to a boil. Add the measured herb to the pan and reduce the temperature until the water is gently simmering. Let the herb simmer for 15 to 20 minutes, strain, and enjoy.

Preparing a Tincture

Traditionally, tinctures have been made by a process called maceration. This method can be used to prepare both alcohol and vinegar tinctures, as well as topical liniments.

You will need the following components to prepare the menstruum (the macerated plant and solvent):

- A clean 1-pint (473 ml) glass jar with a tight-fitting lid (canning jars work great)

- Approximately 1 cup of chopped fresh herbs or ¼ cup of coarsely ground dried herbs

- 1 pint of brandy or vodka (your choice; brandy is usually 75–80 proof, whereas vodka is generally 80–85 proof)

STORAGE. Tinctures with at least 25 percent alcohol content will keep indefinitely. They do not require an expiration date and can be used until they are gone. My friend Brigitte Mars is fond of saying a tincture is something you give to your grandchildren that they can pass on to their grandchildren, providing it has not been used up.

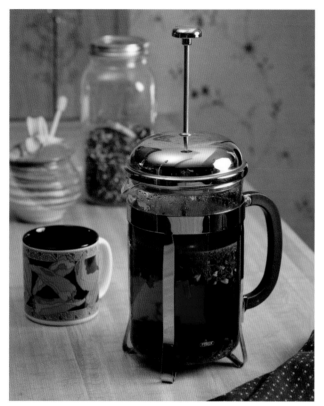

Nothing could be simpler than making an herbal infusion. All you need is a French press (or simply a bowl and fine-mesh sieve), the herbs, and boiling water.

GREAT HERBS FOR INFUSIONS AND DECOCTIONS

> **Peppermint–lemon balm** infusion will soothe an upset digestive tract.

> **Goldenseal root** decoction is a wonderful support for the liver.

> **Oat straw** infusion is beneficial to the nervous system.

> **Nettle** infusion can be used as a whole-body tonic.

> **Red clover blossom** infusion helps boost the immune system.

TERRIFIC TRADITIONAL TINCTURE HERBS

> **Chinese astragalus and spilanthes** make an excellent combination tincture for immune system support.

> **Skullcap and catnip** can be tinctured together for stress and anxiety.

> **Thyme, echinacea, and monarda** are a powerful trio for cold and flu symptoms.

> **Dill and peppermint** are a perfect tummy-soothing blend.

> **Echinacea and ginger** can be tinctured together to fight a virus.

> **Gotu kola, rosemary, and spearmint** are a great formula for clear thinking.

> **California poppy and passionflower** tincture will help relieve pain.

PREPARING A TINCTURE

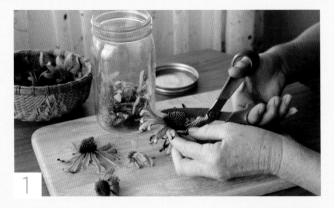

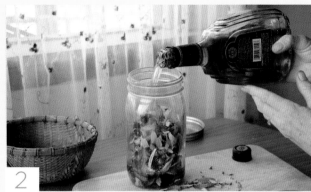

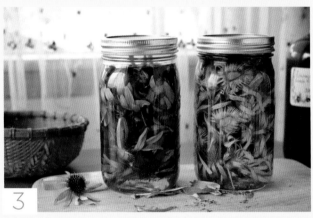

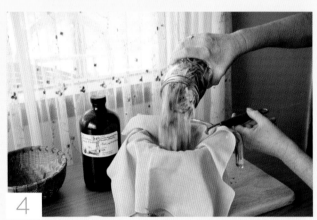

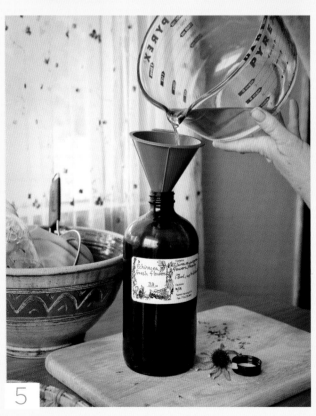

1) Cut up the herb material and place it in the jar.

2) Pour the alcohol over the top of the herbs until it reaches the shoulder of the jar. Put the lid on tight and label the container with all of the ingredients and the date. This is the menstruum.

3) Store the menstruum at room temperature for four to six weeks. Shake the jar vigorously every couple of days.

4) After four to six weeks, you can squeeze out the menstruum. Place a clean cotton cloth in the bottom of a colander or strainer. Put the colander in a pan or bowl. Slowly pour the liquid and herb material into the colander and let it drain for a minute or two, then pull up the corners of the cloth and squeeze the bundle until all the liquid has been removed. Add the plant material, called marc, to your compost pile.

5) Store your finished tincture in a clean glass bottle, tightly closed and fully labeled. For convenience, I keep 1- or 2-ounce (30–60 ml) labeled bottles of tinctures in the medicine cabinet, refilling them as needed from the larger bottles in my dispensary.

Vinegar Tinctures

To prepare a vinegar tincture, follow the same instructions for traditional tinctures (page 139), but use organic apple cider vinegar in place of the alcohol. Never use white distilled vinegar to prepare a vinegar tincture, unless it is certified organic. Other white vinegar can be processed using harsh, toxic chemicals that you will not want in your botanical medicines or in your body.

Vinegar menstruums should sit for two to six weeks, after which you can squeeze them out and begin using the tincture. Vinegar tinctures have a shelf life of one year from the date the plant was put into the menstruum. Make sure the expiration date is noted on the label.

NOURISHING VINEGAR TINCTURES

> **Oatseed** is fabulous for bone health.

> **Ginger and peppermint** reduce flatulence.

> **Chamomile and catnip** help to alleviate grumpiness in kids.

> **Thyme** tincture is a must for good intestinal function.

LINIMENTS TO LIVE BY

> **Yucca** will relieve joint pain.

> **Peppermint** is soothing to sore muscles.

> **Lemon balm** will help heal cold sores.

> **Lavender** is an excellent all-around soother.

> **Echinacea** makes a great antiseptic liniment.

> **Yarrow** liniment relieves itchy skin.

Topical Liniments

Although they are prepared in the same manner as traditional and vinegar tinctures, liniments are not taken internally but instead are applied to the skin.

Because they will be applied topically, I don't use brandy or vodka to prepare liniments; those alcohols feel a bit sticky on the skin. Instead, I use equal parts pure grain alcohol (the brand most readily available is Everclear) and spring water as the menstruum. If pure grain alcohol isn't available, you may substitute vodka; it will be a little tackier to the touch, but it will have the same medicinal value. I don't use rubbing alcohol in my liniments because it isn't a pure solvent, and I prefer not to have it absorbed into the skin.

Liniments are made exactly as you prepare tinctures; allow the menstruum to sit for four to six weeks. Liniments, too, have an indefinite shelf life.

SUNBURN RELIEF SPRAY

When spring and summer feel extra hot and the skin gets a little too pink for comfort, it's time to pull out the sunburn relief spray. This spray is soothing and cooling and it helps the skin to regenerate itself, so the burn doesn't linger and the skin doesn't suffer the consequences of too much exposure without a sun hat and protective clothing. This recipe makes 1 cup (237 ml) and will keep in the refrigerator for about two weeks if aloe juice is used, six months if you use witch hazel.

6 tablespoons (89 ml) either witch hazel extract or aloe vera juice
5 tablespoons (74 ml) lavender tincture
5 tablespoons (74 ml) calendula tincture
25 drops lavender pure essential oil (optional)

Mix all ingredients in a jar, close tight, and shake vigorously. Pour enough to fill a 2-ounce (59 ml) glass bottle fitted with a spray pump top (purchase from a mail-order supplier). Label, being sure to include an appropriate expiration date, along with directions to shake well before using and to avoid spraying in the eyes or mouth. This sunburn spray can be applied as often as desired for soothing relief. Store the 2-ounce bottle, and the larger jar for refilling, in the refrigerator.

I find that this spray remedy is also wonderful when used as a nourishing skin blend and feels great when applied to newly shaven skin.

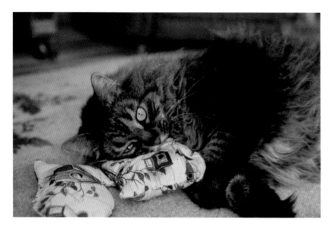

{ Treat your kitties to a catnip toy, harvested from your garden and handmade by you. They'll love you for it!

Catnip Toys

My cats, Pouncita, Professor Longhair, and Gwen-eviere have something to add to this chapter. They love herbs, and not just catnip (although that's by far their favorite treat). Their other favorites are oats in the grassy stage, valerian, and lemongrass. My parents' little dog also enjoys playing with a catnip pillow!

To be especially popular with your dog and cat friends, stitch up small catnip pillows as toys. You can also make little pillows filled with different herbs that are just like sleep pillows for humans; when these are tucked in the beds of cats and dogs, they repel fleas and ticks.

Cut one 6-by-8-inch (15-by-20 cm) piece of cloth. (Any natural-fiber cloth will do; to keep with the theme, perhaps choose fabric with an animal design.) Fold the cloth in half, with the wrong sides together, and stitch two edges (leave one end open). Turn the sewn cloth right side out. Put approximately ¼ cup of crushed dried catnip into the pillow and stitch the open end closed.

Insect-Repellent Bedding for Pets

Dried herbs and essential oils can help protect your pets from fleas and ticks. Add equal amounts of dried lavender flowers, cedarwood chips, and dried pennyroyal herb (*not* essential oil) to the stuffing of an herbal repellent pillow for a cat or dog. *Caution:* Never apply pennyroyal essential oil to a cat as a flea repellent. Cats clean themselves often and thus could ingest the oil, which can be fatal.

HERBAL HEATING PAD

We keep a huge basket of these heating pads at our house, and every bedroom has one. This is the best warmer my feet have ever known, and they're so popular, we've given them to many of our extended family. When it's especially chilly out, I've been known to "borrow" someone else's heating pad so I can have two body areas warm at the same time.

Cut a piece of cotton flannel into a 14-by-26-inch rectangle. Fold the flannel piece in half, wrong side out. Sew two and a half edges with very tight stitches. Now turn the "pillowed" cloth right side out and you'll have an empty, 12-inch-pillow-shaped cloth. Now comes the fun part!

Carefully pour 1 cup of dried lavender flowers and 2 to 4 cups of uncooked rice into the pillow. You want it full, but loosely so. Adjust the amount of rice and lavender to make the pad flexible and sort of floppy when you place it over a part of your body, such as your feet. It will more or less conform to your body's shape. Once it's just right, stitch the opening tightly closed.

You're done, and ready to use this great new heating pad. To warm the heating pad, place it in the microwave for 3 to 4 minutes on high. Adjust the heating time to how hot you like a pad. I usually heat mine for 3 minutes exactly. Put it over your sore muscles, stiff neck, or freezing feet; it will stay warm for hours of comfort.

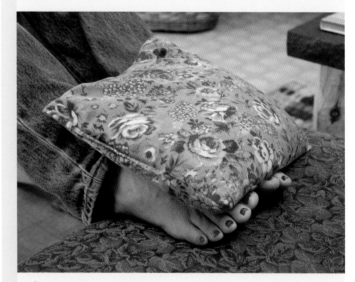

{ Herbal heating pads are considered mandatory herbal equipment at our house. On winter nights we heat them up and use them to warm cold feet or hands.

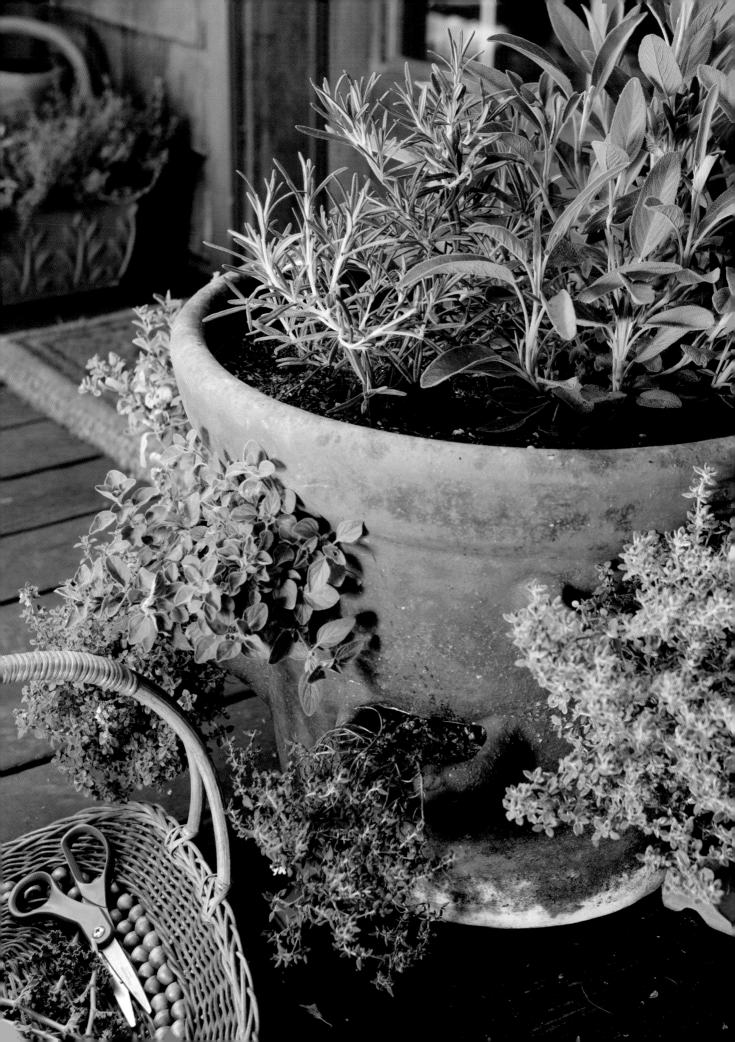

CHAPTER NINE

Cooking with Herbs

Cooking with herbs, especially fresh-picked from the garden, is definitely one of the great pleasures of life. Yes, you can purchase jars of herbal seasonings or small packets of fresh herb sprigs at nearly any grocery market. Indeed, in Denver, like most other cities, we have shops that specialize in herbs, spices, and uniquely blended teas. It is great fun, I must admit, to make a field trip of driving to the city to visit one of these little shops. What a pleasure to discover a new herb or spice that will not grow in my garden.

Still, shopping at the market for herbs is just not the same as being able to step out my back door and harvest them fresh from my garden, or cutting a few sprigs from herb pots growing on the kitchen countertop. It is so easy, and with a moment's notice I can add homegrown herbs to my cooking. Now that's definitely the magic of cooking with herbs.

Start in the Kitchen

Few things bring as much pleasure as delicious food prepared with simple ingredients. Herbs and spices play a significant role in my cooking. I use only the highest quality, freshest herbs and spices when I must purchase them; however, I much prefer to grow my own herbs. This enables me to harvest, dry, and store them myself. I keep a large stock on hand so that I can mix and blend them into delicious seasonings whenever I want. Living and working on our farm brews up a mighty appetite for well-seasoned food. The recipes that follow are enjoyed by my family, and I often package them in beautiful containers to give to friends on special occasions.

I encourage you to experiment with these recipes. Adjust them to your tastes as you cook delicious food in your own kitchen.

GARLIC AND HERB SEASONING BLEND

The perfect seasoning for breads, pasta, and vegetables like cauliflower or turnips. Absolutely delicious!

YIELD: approximately 1 cup

- 2 tablespoons dried basil (consider using Thai basil in place of sweet basil)
- 2 tablespoons dried marjoram
- 2 tablespoons dried oregano
- 2 tablespoons dried parsley
- 2 tablespoons dried rosemary
- 1 tablespoon dried onion flakes
- 1 tablespoon dried thyme
- 1 tablespoon sea salt
- 2 teaspoons garlic powder
- 1 teaspoon freshly ground black or white pepper

Combine all ingredients and store in an airtight glass container until ready to use. Remember to add a label that includes an expiration date of one year. Store away from excessive heat and out of direct sunlight.

BOUQUET GARNI

This little bag is one of the simplest ways to season soups, stews, and meat dishes. Just add one bag to the pot or baking dish while cooking, then remove it just before you serve.

YIELD: 8 seasoning bags

- ½ cup dried parsley
- 8 teaspoons dried basil
- 8 teaspoons dried oregano
- 8 teaspoons dried rosemary
- 16 dried bay leaves
- 48 dried black peppercorns
- 1 clove of garlic

Cut eight 3-inch squares of cotton or cheesecloth for the bags. (You can also use pre-sewn cotton tea bags, available from a natural foods store or mail-order supply source.) Lay each square on a flat surface. Into the center of each place 1 tablespoon parsley, 1 teaspoon each of basil, oregano, and rosemary, two bay leaves, and six peppercorns. Gather the corners and tie each with a piece of cotton string, but don't make the knot too tight.

Store bouquet garni bags, without the garlic, in an airtight glass container until ready to use. Label the jar with the ingredients and an expiration date of one year.

To use, take a bag from the glass container, untie the string, add one clove of garlic, and then tie it up again, this time tightly. Put the bag in the cooking pot as you're preparing your favorite soup recipe, or add it to the baking dish with chicken and vegetables.

Follow your recipe for cooking times, and just before serving remove the bouquet garni bag and serve your meal as usual. Discard the herbs from the bag into your kitchen compost tub and launder the cloth bag so that it is ready for use again another time.

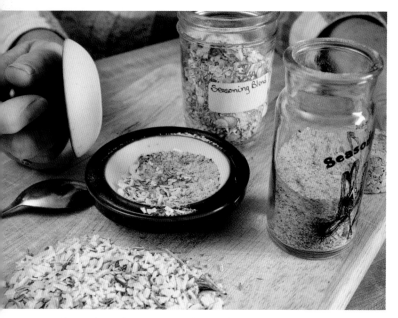

A pestle and mortar are the perfect tools for turning blends of coarsely cut dried herbs into a fine powder perfect for sprinkling into your cooking pot.

Not Your Ordinary Seasoning Blends

Consider creating a wide variety of seasoning blends to use in many different ways. They will be great substitutes for traditional salt and pepper in your diet. You can use them in predictable ways, such as Whole Grains Poultry Seasoning in your turkey dressing, and Italian Seasoning (goes without saying) on your home-baked pizza or calzone. The basic seasoning blend is tasty as a salt substitute and is delicious sprinkled over a leafy green salad.

Occasionally you may even want to be outrageous in your seasoning blends and try adding them to your garlic bread, even your popcorn! Next time you make a batch of popcorn, toss it lightly with melted butter or olive oil and then sprinkle it generously with one of these blends, adjusting to your personal taste. You may think about purchasing some inexpensive pepper mills and filling them with an assortment of homemade seasoning blends. Keep them on the counter or table for easy access. Following are three of my favorite seasoning blends.

BASIC SEASONING SALT

Serve this in place of regular table salt. It's a tasty way to decrease the amount of salt in your diet.

YIELD: approximately 1 cup

- ½ cup coarse sea salt
- ¼ cup dried granular kelp
- 1 tablespoon dried thyme
- 2 teaspoons dried garlic granules

In a blender or spice grinder, process all ingredients until the mixture reaches the desired consistency, a coarse grind or a finer powder. Store in an airtight glass container and label with an expiration date of one year. Fill a saltshaker and refill from the storage container as needed.

ITALIAN SEASONING

This is a great way to zip up any pasta dish or even popcorn! It's good on pizza too.

YIELD: approximately ¾ cup

- ½ cup dried parsley
- 4 tablespoons dried onion flakes
- 1 tablespoon dried oregano or marjoram
- 2 teaspoons dried minced garlic
- 1 teaspoon red pepper flakes (optional)

Mix all ingredients well. Store in an airtight glass container and label with an expiration date of one year.

WHOLE GRAINS POULTRY SEASONING

This is the perfect seasoning for classic meals such as Thanksgiving dinner.

YIELD: 1–2 cups

- ⅓ cup dried sage
- ¼ cup dried cutting celery (or substitute ⅛ cup celery seed)
- ¼ cup dried lemon peel
- ¼ cup dried marjoram
- ¼ cup dried parsley
- ¼ cup dried savory (either winter or summer savory)
- ¼ cup dried thyme
- ¼ cup dried rosemary (optional)

Combine all ingredients and blend well. Use a spice grinder or a blender to make a powder. Store in an airtight glass jar and label with an expiration date of one year.

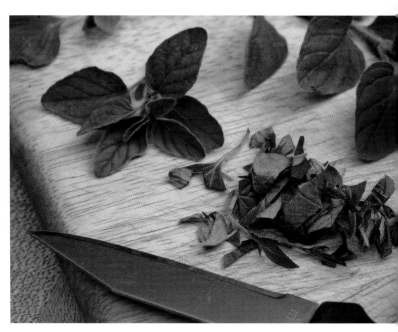

Freshly harvested Greek oregano is coarsely chopped and then added to pizza or pasta dishes. It is equally good used fresh or dried.

Culinary Herbal Vinegars

Culinary herbal vinegars are easy to prepare and make handsome gifts. You can choose from a wide variety of herbs according to what you like. Once your vinegars are made, use them to create vinegar and oil salad dressings, to top steamed vegetables and rice dishes, or to drizzle on breads for a simple appetizer.

I like red and white wine vinegars as my base. Don't use white distilled vinegar unless you're sure it is certified organic. Nonorganic white distilled vinegars are often processed with harsh and toxic chemicals that you certainly don't want to put into your body.

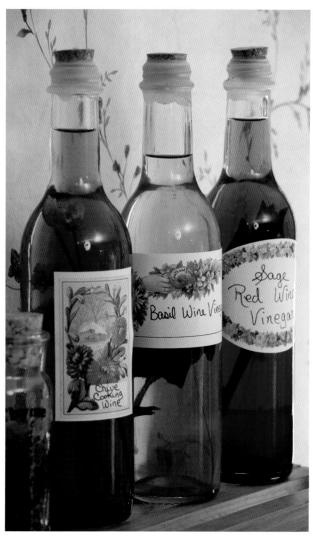

Culinary herbal vinegars are fantastic in homemade salad dressings. They also make wonderful gifts at holiday time or for a new bride stocking her kitchen.

For the first steps of vinegar preparation, you'll need four clean quart-size glass jars with tight-fitting lids. For the final step, you'll want clean, decorative bottles that can be tightly closed with lids or corks.

Warm the vinegar until it's hot (but not boiling). As it's heating, place two or three sprigs of fresh, rinsed herbs into each quart jar. Each sprig should be about 4 inches long. Pour the hot vinegar into each jar up to its neck so that the herbs are covered with the vinegar. Tightly cap, then label the jar with all the ingredients and the date you prepared it. Let it stand at room temperature for 10–14 days, and then strain out the herbs, retaining the vinegar as your final product. (You can compost the used herbs.)

Next, reheat the vinegar until it's very hot (but not boiling). Once it's hot enough, using a funnel, carefully pour it into decorative bottles. Fill each bottle to just below the neck and cap tightly with a lid or cork. Let the vinegar cool completely.

When it's cool, melt a small amount of beeswax in a small pan and carefully dip the lid or cork of each bottle into it to coat with a thin layer of wax. Now you've sealed the vinegar until you're ready to use it.

To each bottle, affix a beautiful label that includes all the ingredients, some ways to use the vinegar in the kitchen, and a one-year expiration date. Also include directions to shake well before using and to store in the refrigerator once opened. (Opened vinegar stored in the refrigerator is good for about a month.) Tie a ribbon around the top of each bottle and your culinary vinegar is finished. It will look lovely sitting on the countertop until you're ready to use it, or you can gift it to someone special in your life . . . maybe your mom or your grandma.

HERBS FOR INCREDIBLE CULINARY VINEGARS

> **Fennel leaf or seed** is great for pasta dishes.

> **Cayenne peppers** are very hot: use to add zing to salsas.

> **Dill weed or seed** makes excellent salad dressing.

> **Gingerroot** is nice drizzled over rice or steamed vegetables.

Herb Butters

Herb butters will make an ordinary meal seem extraordinary, and you can create them with very little effort. Sweet herbal butters are a treat on pancakes; savory herbal butters are delicious on breads and vegetables. Or substitute an herbal cream cheese for a different tasty treat.

But first, a word or two about the appropriateness of using real dairy butter and not a butter substitute, such as margarine. Good-quality organic butter from pasture-raised animals, be it from cows or goats, is a good wholesome food, and so delicious! So, enjoy your butter and put some herbs in it for a gourmet treat!

Sometimes I hold an herb butter–making event. This usually happens on a cold winter day while I'm working in the kitchen, the woodstove burning cheerfully. I've usually just prepared some bread and I'm waiting for it to rise. I often make several different kinds of herb butter from fresh herbs growing in the kitchen or in the greenhouse, and before you know it, I've gone through 2 pounds of organic butter. The beauty of this event is that I then have enough herb butter stored in the freezer, in packages just the right size to spread on a full loaf of

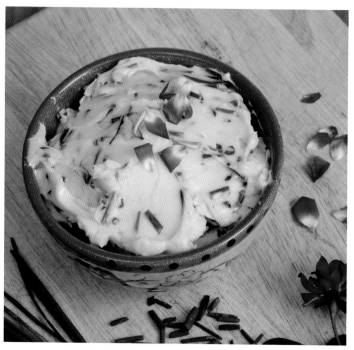

By making herbal butters a regular part of your meal preparation, you turn an ordinary meal into something special and beautiful. Chives with rose petals are always a hit at our house.

home-baked bread (about ½ cup of butter apiece), to last a month or so. I just pull out a package in the morning, and by the noon meal or suppertime the butter is thawed and ready to go.

SAVORY HERB BUTTERS

Butter is enhanced by any of the following herbs. Feel free to mix and match to create your own special blends. Add a few edible flowers, if you like, to make your butters as beautiful as they are delicious.

YIELD: approximately ½ cup

- ½ cup softened, lightly salted butter
- ¼ cup finely chopped fresh chives or garlic chives or
- ¼ cup finely chopped fresh parsley or fresh basil or
- ¼ cup finely chopped fresh thyme or oregano or
- 3 tablespoons finely chopped fresh tarragon or
- 2 tablespoons dill seeds

Blend the herb or herbs into the butter until they are well mixed. Store for up to three weeks in the refrigerator, or freeze for up to six months.
NOTE: If you want to substitute dried herbs for fresh in butters and cream cheese spreads, use just half the amount of herbs.

SWEET HERB BUTTERS

Any of the following herbs and spices, alone or in combination, make a delectable addition to butters. They're sure to be a big hit with family or friends.

YIELD: approximately ½ cup

- ½ cup softened, lightly salted butter
- 1 tablespoon orange juice and 1 tablespoon poppy seeds
- ¼ cup finely chopped fresh lemon balm and a pinch of ground cinnamon
- ¼ cup finely chopped fresh mint (spearmint, peppermint, orange mint)
- 3 tablespoons finely chopped walnuts
- 2 tablespoons honey
- 1 tablespoon ground cinnamon

Prepare the sweet herb butter as you would a Savory Herb Butter (see at left), then garnish with edible flowers or flower petals for an elegant touch.

Crystallized Herbs and Flowers

This is a delicious way to use therapeutic herbs. It's like having a sweet treat that's good for you. My favorites are honey-crystallized ginger and angelica roots. Flowers crystallized with sugar and egg whites are beautiful atop of a cake or on shortbread cookies.

There are two ways to prepare crystallized herbs and flowers. For honey-crystallized herbs: Prepare an herbal honey (see the directions on page 142). Once the honey is cooked, pour the mixture into a glass baking pan. Cover with plastic wrap and let sit for two to three days at room temperature.

Line a baking sheet with waxed paper. Strain out the herbs and place them in a single layer on the waxed paper. Cover loosely with another piece of waxed paper, to protect them from dust, making sure there's still good air circulation. Pour any excess honey into a jar and use for cooking or to sweeten beverages. Let the herbs sit for one week.

Dust the honey-covered herbs with table sugar — a light coating is all that's needed. Spread the herbs in a single layer on a piece of butcher paper or waxed paper and let them dry for one to two days. Store in a glass jar until ready to use. Crystallized herbs will usually keep for two to four weeks at room temperature or for several months in the refrigerator. Eat one or two pieces at a time.

To prepare sugar-crystallized flowers and leaves to decorate cakes and cookies, lightly but completely coat the flowers and leaves with lightly beaten egg whites; a pastry brush works well for this task. Sprinkle the flowers and leaves with very fine sugar until each is coated. Line a cookie sheet with waxed paper and transfer the finished flowers and leaves onto it to dry for a couple of days. (Drying time will vary depending on the humidity level.) Dried flowers will keep for a week or so, but don't wait too long to use them. Mints, along with violas and rose petals, are especially attractive as cake-top decorations.

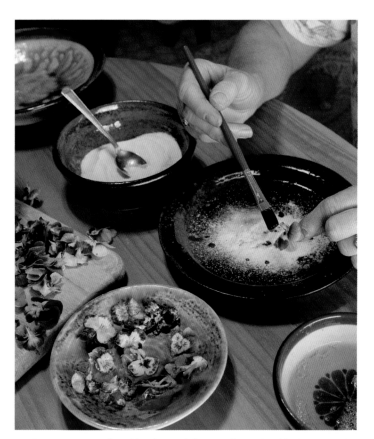

Prepare crystallized herbs and flowers from freshly harvested pansies, mint, and lemon balm leaves. Once dry, they're great for decorating cakes or frosted shortbread cookies.

DELICIOUS AND HEALTHY CRYSTALLIZED HERBS AND FLOWERS

> **Rosemary** flowers support healthy circulation.

> **Gingerroot** is great for digestive-tract health.

> **Violet** flowers enhance the skin and heart function.

> **Angelica** stalks are terrific for the respiratory and female reproductive systems.

> **Spearmint** leaves support the nervous system.

> **Borage** flowers promote skin health.

Simple Ways to Use Herbs

In my quest to cook with herbs, I have discovered many ways to incorporate them into meals. It is not unusual for recipes to call for a bit of this herb or that spice to make a dish more interesting. Now I challenge *you* to be as creative as you can be, using what you grow yourself, to make all your cooking delicious with the flavors of herbs. Do not limit yourself to what a recipe calls for. Recipes are wonderful guidelines and a good place to start, but be spontaneous. Add a bit of parsley to your everyday salad or sprinkle the breakfast yogurt with chopped spearmint or lemon balm. Consider all the wonderful possibilities!

As I have gotten older, I have also thought more about the concept of incorporating herbal medicines into my foods. I am forever questioning the patterns that my generation grew up with, particularly the belief that a pill can cure anything and everything. Pills certainly have a place in health care, but that place should be kept in perspective. It makes much more sense to me to use our daily whole foods and herbs not only for nutrition, but also to support our good health. While cooking with herbs, consider using medicinal herbs as part of your culinary approach. How wonderful to think of eating your medicines as a delicious part of a salad or spaghetti sauce.

All that is required is a stroll through the garden to harvest fresh ingredients or a look through the pantry of dried-herb stores to see what treasures are waiting for you to find them.

Enhance Your Salads

The addition of a few herbs can turn the usual salad into a gourmet event. Lettuces and other salad greens are quite easy to grow in a container garden or a traditional food garden with other vegetables such as green onions, cucumbers, summer squash, and, of course, carrots. Why not plant a generous variety of salad herbs like dill, basil, parsley, and cutting celery alongside your salad vegetables? And don't forget edible flowers. Now you'll have all the ingredients for a salad that is healthful and beautiful to the eye, and just wait till you taste it. Fabulous!

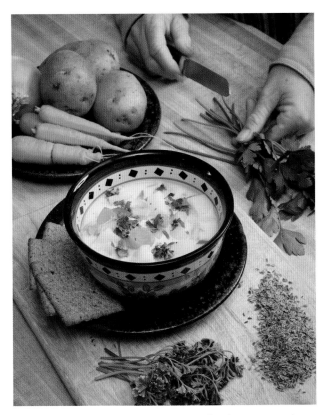

Dilly potato soup is a hearty soup that is very easy to prepare in a slow cooker. At serving time, garnish it with some freshly chopped parsley.

SUPER SALAD HERBS

Here are some good herbal salad ingredients and their supportive health benefits:

> **Basil, peppermint, spearmint, and parsley** promote good digestive function.

> **Borage, gotu kola, and violet leaves** are fantastic for skin concerns.

> **Catnip and sorrel** support the liver, gallbladder, and urinary tract.

> **Marsh mallow, hollyhock, and peppermint** are valuable for intestinal issues.

> **Garlic** supports cardiovascular health.

> **Sunflower seeds** are excellent for reproductive health and respiratory conditions.

GREEN HERB SALAD: A DAILY FAVORITE

The usual green salad goes with nearly every lunch or dinner meal plan. Make your normal green salad special by adding herbs to the mix.

SERVES 2

- 4 cups salad greens (lettuce, arugula, watercress, spinach)
- ¼ cup dill leaves, torn
- ¼ cup fennel leaves, torn
- 2 large leaves cutting celery, finely chopped
- 1 tablespoon chives or garlic chives, stems chopped
- ¼ cup edible flowers of your choice (see the Edible Flowers at a Glance chart, page 160)
  Freshly squeezed lemon juice or balsamic vinegar and oil dressing

Mix all ingredients, except edible flowers, in a salad bowl and toss gently using two wooden spoons. Just before serving, dress with the lemon juice or balsamic vinegar and oil, and sprinkle the flowers on top.

WAYS TO USE UNIQUE HERBS FOR A CULINARY PLEASURE

Say you've got some vegetables or perhaps a side dish or appetizer that needs a little something extra. Is there a way to incorporate lesser-known herbs into these dishes? Here are a few easy ideas:

Epazote is a traditional Mexican medicinal herb used in food preparation. Add it conservatively to bean dishes during the long cooking time. It has an unusual flavor that really enhances beans and gives a new flavor to burritos.

Prickly pear has been studied as a medicinal food for people with diabetes because it is so helpful in balancing blood sugar levels. Native American peoples of the Southwest and Latin America have been cooking it as a vegetable for years. I find it delicious when prepared with onions, garlic, peppers, and potatoes.

Nettles are quite popular in other parts of the world as a vegetable in soups and lasagnas. They're considered a whole-body tonic herb because they're so nutritious. Substitute freshly harvested nettles (remember to wear gloves when handling them) for the spinach portion of soups and casserole dishes.

Catnip pesto is a wonderful way to calm down and relax. Simply substitute catnip for half the basil in your favorite pesto recipe.

COTTAGE CHEESE AND GOTU KOLA LUNCH SALAD

This is an easy salad to take along as a brown-bag lunch.

SERVES 1

- ½ cup cottage cheese
- ½ teaspoon dill seeds
- 4–6 gotu kola leaves
- 2 sprigs lemon thyme

Stir together the cottage cheese and dill seeds in a bowl. Let the mixture sit for 15 to 30 minutes; the cheese will soften the seeds, and the seeds will infuse the cheese with a delicious flavor.

Just before serving, top with the gotu kola and the lemon thyme. As a variation, substitute sorrel leaves for the gotu kola, garlic chives for the dill seeds, and fresh oregano for the lemon thyme.

AUNT DIANE'S GREEK TOMATO SALAD

This is a quick and easy salad to prepare on a hot summer day. Putting the salad together won't keep you away from your outdoor activities, and it's remarkably delicious!

SERVES 4 TO 6

- 2 cups cherry tomatoes, halved
- 2 cups mozzarella cheese (balls or cubes)
- ¼–½ cup fresh basil leaves, shredded
- 1 tablespoon fresh oregano or thyme, finely chopped
- ¼ teaspoon garlic salt, or to taste
  Drizzle extra-virgin olive oil

Gently mix the tomatoes, cheese, basil, and oregano in a large bowl and sprinkle lightly with the garlic salt. Drizzle with olive oil to lightly coat. Refrigerate up to two days.

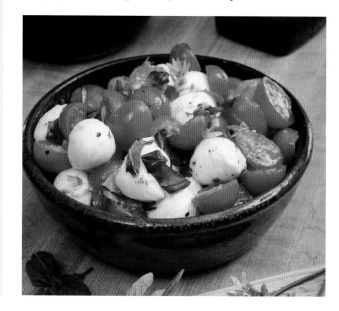

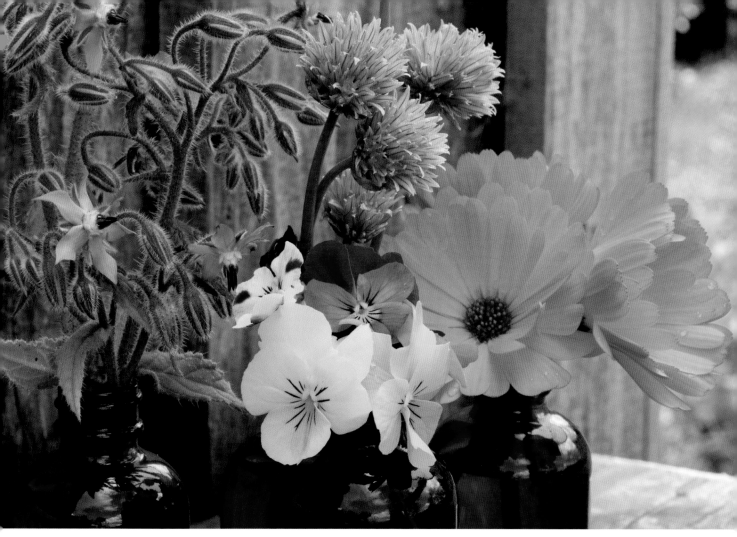

Don't Forget the Edible Flowers

The Japanese believe that color and presentation are as important to a meal as the taste of the food, and I agree with them. When it comes to adding color to meals, you can't do better than to grow a wide selection of edible flowers. It's a simple step to add those flowers to your dishes, and doing so, I guarantee, will change how you feel when you sit down to eat. Edible flowers take you to the next level, and suddenly their colors and forms are all it takes for you to be a "gourmet cook" in the eyes of family and friends. Privately, you can afford a little giggle, as you bask in their admiration, because all you did was sprinkle some petals in the salad, float some blossoms in the lemonade, and decorate the dessert with a few pretty flowers.

(Note: Always check with a reference guide to make sure the flowers you pick in the garden are safe to eat — not every flower is edible, and some are actually poisonous.)

} I love sprinkling borage flowers into a green salad, chopping chive flowers into herb butter, coloring my rice golden with calendula petals, and floating violas in my lemonade.

FLOWER POWER SALAD

Rich in antioxidants, this salad will benefit the circulatory system.

SERVES 2

- 2 tomatoes, sliced
- 1 green bell pepper, thinly sliced
- 4 fresh basil leaves
- 2 nasturtiums
- 2 strawberry flowers
- 2 violet flowers
- 1 tablespoon herbal vinegar

Lay the tomato slices on two salad plates. Spread the pepper slices on top of the tomatoes. On top of the peppers, place the basil leaves in the center of the plate in the form of a cross. Sprinkle the flowers on top, then dress with the herbal vinegar.

EDIBLE FLOWERS AT A GLANCE

COMMON NAME	LATIN BOTANICAL NAME	CULINARY USES
Agastache	*Agastache* species	Fruit and green salads, dessert decoration, beverages, honey, herb butter, and cream cheese spreads
Borage	*Borago officinalis*	Veggie salads, and pastas, dessert decoration, cream cheese spreads, sandwiches
Calendula	*Calendula officinalis*	Green salads, soups, pastas, and grains, dessert decoration
Catmint	*Nepeta × faassenii*	Fruit and green salads, dessert decoration, beverages, honey, herb butter and cream cheese spreads
Chamomile	*Matricaria recutita, Chamaemelum nobile*	Fruit and green salads, pastas, dessert decoration, beverages, honey, herb butter and cream cheese spreads
Chives, garlic chives	*Allium schoenoprasum, A. tuberosum*	Veggie salads and pastas, herb butter and cream cheese spreads, soups, sandwiches, grains
Cilantro	*Coriandrum sativum*	Green salads, pastas and grains, salsas, sandwiches
Dianthus, pinks	*Dianthus* species	Fruit and veggie salads, dessert decoration, beverages, honey, herb butter and cream cheese spreads, sandwiches
Dill	*Anethum graveolens*	Veggie salads and pastas, grains, herb butter and cream cheese spreads, soups, sandwiches, potatoes
Fennel	*Foeniculum vulgare*	Veggie salads and pasta, grains, sandwiches, herb butter and cream cheese spreads, honey, soups
Hollyhock and mallows	*Alcea* species, *Althaea* species, *Malva* species	Green salads, dessert decoration, herb butter and cream cheese spreads
Hyssop	*Hyssopus officinalis*	Green salads, dessert decoration, cream cheese spreads
Lavender	*Lavandula* species	Fruit and green salads, pastas and grains, dessert decoration, beverages, honey, cream cheese spreads
Lemon verbena	*Aloysia triphylla*	Fruit and green salads, herb butter and cream cheese spreads, dessert decoration, beverages, honey
Monarda	*Monarda* species	Veggie salads and pastas, soups, grains, dessert decoration, honey, herb butter and cream cheese spreads, sandwiches
Nasturtium	*Tropaeolum majus*	Fruit and veggie salads, soups and pastas, dessert decoration, beverages, honey, herb butter and cream cheese spreads, sandwiches, grains
Red clover	*Trifolium pratense*	Veggie salads, soups and pastas, honey, grains and hot cereals
Rosemary	*Rosmarinus* species	Fruit and veggie salads, pasta, soups, potatoes, dessert decoration, beverages, honey, herb butter and cream cheese spreads, sandwiches, grains
Roses	*Rosa* species	Fruit and veggie salads, dessert decoration, apple pie, beverages, honey, herb butter and cream cheese spreads, sandwiches
Sage	*Salvia officinalis*	Veggie salads, pasta and soups, honey, herb butter and cream cheese spreads, grains
Stevia	*Stevia rebaudiana*	Fruit salads, dessert decoration, beverages, honey, herb butter and cream cheese spreads, cereals
Thyme	*Thymus* species	Fruit and veggie salads, pastas, soups, potatoes, dessert decoration, beverages (lemon varieties), honey, herb butter and cream cheese spreads, sandwiches, grains
Violets, heartsease, pansies	*Viola* species	Fruit and veggie salads, pastas, dessert decoration, beverages, honey, herb butter and cream cheese spreads, sandwiches, grains

Savor the Main Dish

The main dish often centers around meat, but it's easy and nutritional to create a filling meal of grains and vegetables.

Whether you choose meat, vegetables, or grains, herbs play an active role in making the meal delicious. Parsley root, fresh garlic, rosemary, and hot chili peppers usually come to mind when I am planning a meal. Each imparts high flavor, and all are rich in antioxidants, good for digestion, and supportive to the urinary tract and the cardiovascular system.

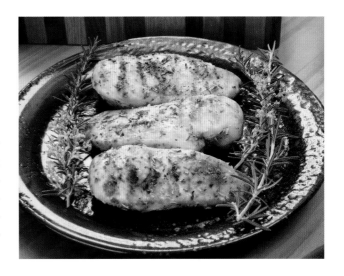

GINGER, RICE, AND EVERYTHING NICE

An autumn favorite at our house, this dish is delicious, warming, and filling, with a robust flavor. It contains herbs that are excellent to relieve the sinus congestion, coughs, and sore throats that accompany cold and flu season.

SERVES 2

- 3 cups water
- 1 cup uncooked brown rice
- 2 tablespoons powdered vegetable broth
- 2–3 tablespoons butter
- 4 cloves garlic, minced
- 3 mushrooms, sliced
- 1 celery stalk, thinly sliced
- 1 onion, quartered and sliced
- 1 red bell pepper, thinly sliced
- 1 tablespoon freshly grated ginger
- 2 tablespoons tamari or soy sauce

Bring the water, rice, and powdered vegetable broth to a boil in a 2-quart saucepan over medium heat. Reduce the temperature and continue to simmer gently until the rice is tender and most of the liquid is absorbed, about 30 to 45 minutes.

Meanwhile, during the last 10 to 15 minutes that the rice is cooking, heat the butter in a saucepan over medium heat. Sauté the garlic, mushrooms, celery, onion, and pepper until tender and translucent. This step takes only about 5 minutes or so.

Add the ginger and sauté for 3 to 5 minutes longer, then add the tamari and stir.

To serve, spoon the vegetables over the rice.

GRILLED ROSEMARY RED PEPPER CHICKEN

We love this chicken for a barbecue, but it does have a bite to it. If you want to tone it down, substitute thyme for the red pepper flakes. After you try this recipe, you may never want to eat plain grilled chicken again.

SERVES 4

- 2 teaspoons sea salt
- 1 tablespoon dried or 2 tablespoons fresh minced rosemary
- 1 teaspoon crushed red pepper flakes
- 2 teaspoons brown sugar
- 6 chicken thighs or boneless breasts, skin on
- 2 tablespoons olive oil, and more to coat the grill

Mix the salt, rosemary, red pepper, and brown sugar in a shallow bowl. Coat the chicken lightly with 2 tablespoons of the olive oil. With the back of a spoon, gently rub the spice mixture into the chicken. Let the chicken sit, covered, in the refrigerator for 30 to 60 minutes, but not longer or it will become too salty.

Coat the grill surface with an olive oil–soaked paper towel and heat the grill to medium high.

Grill the chicken for 3 to 5 minutes on each side to seal in the juices. Reduce the temperature to medium and slowly cook the chicken, turning often, until it is tender and done. This usually takes about 10 to 20 minutes more. On a gas grill, cover the chicken; on a charcoal grill, cook it uncovered. You can tell the chicken is ready if you insert a fork and it pulls back out easily.

Serve with rice or garlic-buttered noodles and a green salad.

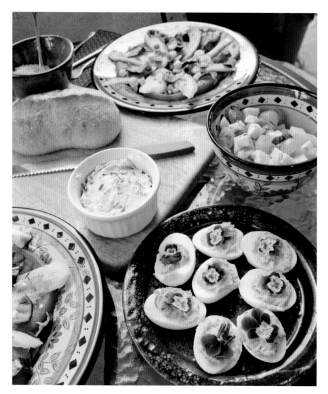

Garden-fresh tomato-cucumber salad is lovely served with pansy-topped deviled eggs and freshly baked bread with garlic chive herb butter.

Colorful, Nutritious Side Dishes

Side dishes are important because they balance the main part of the meal. They round out a meal nutritionally, and provide variation to your menus.

CATNIP PESTO WITH PASTA

This pesto is an easy side dish using fresh basil and catnip. It can also be frozen, so that during the winter you'll be able to enjoy this side made from the bounty of summer.

YIELD: approximately 1 cup

- 4 cups lightly packed fresh basil leaves
- 1 cup lightly packed fresh catnip leaves
- ½ cup walnut pieces, roasted or raw
- 1–2 fresh garlic cloves, to taste
  Extra-virgin olive oil
  Salt

Put the herbs, walnuts, and garlic into a food processor or blender and slowly purée, adding just enough olive oil to create a coarsely textured paste.

Add a heaping tablespoon of pesto to ½ pound of cooked, drained pasta, just before serving. Toss the pasta lightly with the pesto and salt to taste. Enjoy!

MASHED POTATOES, TURNIPS, AND PARSLEY

Most of us are familiar with common Italian or curled parsley leaves, but it's also great to cook with the roots of this same herb. They're delicious in this recipe, or added to vegetable soups.

SERVES 4–6

- 4 parsley roots
- 3 potatoes (any variety you have on hand will work)
- 1 turnip
- ½ stick butter (do not substitute margarine)
- ¼ teaspoon fresh garlic, minced
  Pinch of celery seed
- 1 cup sour cream
- ½ cup grated Parmesan cheese

Wash the vegetables. You can peel your potatoes and turnips if you like, but I usually just cut them up into quarters with the skins on. In a large saucepan, boil the parsley roots, potatoes, and turnip until tender. Pierce the potatoes with a fork to determine when they are tender; this will be about 20 minutes or so. Drain.

Mash the vegetables with a potato masher in a large bowl. Add the butter, freshly minced garlic, and celery seed. Stir in the sour cream and cheese and mix well.

To serve, top with your favorite sautéed vegetables (I like to use squash and carrots). Or serve as a side dish for a holiday dinner.

LENTIL AND RICE CASSEROLE

On cold days, this side dish really hits the spot; it is hearty and delicious! I also prepare it as a one-pot dish on camping and backpacking trips.

SERVES 4

- 4 cups chicken broth (chicken stock cubes for backpack version, and add 4 cups water at time of cooking)
- 1 cup brown basmati rice
- 1 cup lentils
- 1 onion, finely chopped (¼ cup dried minced onions for backpack version)
- 1 large tomato, coarsely chopped (1 cup dehydrated tomatoes for backpack version)
- 1 large clove fresh garlic, minced (¼ teaspoon dried minced garlic for backpack version)
- 1 teaspoon cumin seeds or rosemary, crushed
- ½ stick (4 tablespoons) salted butter (do not use margarine or a butter substitute)

Put all ingredients except butter in a large pot. Stir and bring to a boil. Lower heat, cover with a lid, and let mixture simmer gently for about 45 minutes, or until rice is tender. To serve, stir in the butter until it's melted.

If you're preparing the backpack version, place all dry ingredients into a large ziplock bag and pack the butter in a smaller bag. When it's time to cook, put the dry ingredients in a pan and add 4 cups of water. Then follow the recipe.

Glorious Soups and Stews

I am a big fan of soups and stews. Just chop the ingredients, simmer for the better part of a day, and serve hot with a loaf of homemade bread. That's a version of heaven! Soups and stews are also an easy way to incorporate medicinal herbs into your diet. A supportive soup for someone with a bladder infection might contain parsley, dandelion, nettles, and hollyhock. A person who is undergoing cancer treatments will surely appreciate a soothing soup prepared with Chinese astragalus and red clover to support and nourish the body during chemotherapy or radiation.

Soups and stews are extremely versatile. You can serve them in any season, and make them with a multitude of fresh-from-the-garden ingredients.

GINGER PUMPKIN SOUP

I love cooking this soup in fall or winter, when pumpkins and winter squash are abundant, harvested from my garden, and stored in large baskets in the kitchen. It's a perfect addition to Thanksgiving dinner, but really, we like this soup anytime. Any kind of winter squash may be substituted for the pumpkin.

SERVES 4–6

- 1 tablespoon butter
- 3–4 whole marsh mallow plants, chopped
- 1 tablespoon chopped gingerroot
- 4 cups vegetable or chicken broth
- 4–6 cups baked pumpkin
- ½ cup milk

Melt the butter in a skillet and sauté the marsh mallow and ginger until tender, about 5 minutes. Transfer to a large cooking pot, add the vegetable broth, and simmer gently for about 5 minutes, until the marsh mallow and ginger are softened.

Combine approximately 1 cup pumpkin, 1 cup broth mixture, and 2 tablespoons milk in a blender. Purée until smooth. Pour into another large cooking pot. Continue blending pumpkin, broth mixture, and milk in these ratios, until all the pumpkin has been puréed and poured into the large pot. Heat soup until just warmed through; do not boil.

DILLY POTATO SOUP

This is a good, nourishing soup, and is especially helpful for anyone recovering from illness, fatigue, or excessive stress. The dill supports digestion and decreases flatulence and belching.

SERVES 8–10

- 8–10 cups water
- 6 potatoes, peeled and cubed
- 2 carrots, sliced
- 1 cup fresh or frozen peas
- 1 onion, chopped
- 1 stalk celery, chopped
- 3–4 cloves garlic, minced
- 3 tablespoons dill seed
- 2 cups milk

In a large soup pot, boil the potatoes, carrots, celery, onion, peas, and garlic in the water until the vegetables are tender, about 30 minutes or so.

Mix in the dill seed. Pour the soup into a blender, add the milk, and purée. If necessary, warm the soup over low heat. Do not boil; it will easily scorch. Serve hot with salad or bread.

HEALTHY SOUP HERBS

For variety, try some of these supreme medicinal herbs in soups and stews:

> **Calendula** acts a broth-coloring agent and is also a good astringent herb for the intestinal tract.

> **Cilantro and lemongrass** are nice "coolers" for people who always feel overheated.

> **Dill** is a priority for digestive discomforts such as flatulence and belching.

> **Lovage** may be substituted for celery and is beneficial for a respiratory tract condition. It also aids digestion.

HEARTY VEGETABLE SLOW-COOKER SOUP

This soup is perfect for people with busy schedules and no time to stop and cook. Fill the slow cooker with the ingredients, plug it in, and forget about it until you're ready to eat. The aromas will entice you to the table.

SERVES 8–10

1	quart vegetable or chicken broth
4	cloves garlic, peeled and chopped
4-5	carrots, chopped
2	potatoes, chopped
1	onion, chopped
½	cup barley
½	cup French or red-veined sorrel, chopped
¼	cup fresh lovage root, chopped
¼	cup quinoa
6	calendula flowers, crushed
1	bay leaf, whole
½	teaspoon fresh rosemary or ¼ teaspoon dried rosemary
¼	teaspoon fresh or dried sage
¼	teaspoon fresh or dried thyme

Combine all ingredients in a slow cooker. Set the temperature on high for 30 minutes, then reduce to low. Let the soup cook all day, at least 6 to 8 hours.

Serve with fresh warm bread with whipped honey or herb butter.

HEARTY QUINOA-BEAN CHILI

Quinoa and beans are great sources of protein. The beans also support kidney health; the cumin, garlic, and chili powder improve digestion and circulation.

SERVES 6–8

1	cup dry pinto or adzuki beans
2	tablespoons olive oil
2	cloves garlic, minced
1	medium onion, chopped
1	red or green bell pepper, chopped
1	teaspoon cumin seeds
1	cup fresh or frozen corn
⅔	cup quinoa
1	(6-inch) piece of kelp
2-3	teaspoons chili powder
10	cups water
1-2	cups Colby or cheddar cheese, shredded

Put the beans in a bowl; cover with water and let soak 8 to 10 hours or overnight. Drain and rinse.

Warm the olive oil in a large soup pot over medium heat. Sauté the garlic, onion, pepper, and cumin seeds until the vegetables are tender, about 5 minutes.

Add the beans, corn, quinoa, kelp, chili powder, and 10 cups of water and mix well. Cook 1 to 2 hours, or until beans are tender.

To serve, remove the kelp. Top with a sprinkling of cheese, if desired. Accompany with freshly baked cornbread or tortillas.

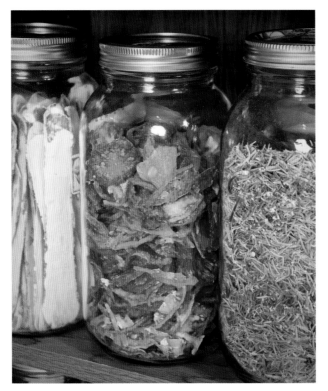

Keeping a well-stocked pantry of dried herbs and spices, fruits and vegetables, and many types of grains translates into creative meals that are nothing short of delicious.

BEANS AND HERBS — A HEALTHY, DELICIOUS COMBO!

People in South America often make beans and rice a core part of their meals. They also create amazing sauces to accompany them. Tomatoes, cilantro, epazote, and onions are all common ingredients in their cuisine. I happen to love beans and rice and these are super foods for kidney health: healthy, healing, and yummy! We use cooked beans and rice as filling for tacos and burritos, to make into chili, or just piled onto a plate, topped with salsa, and a flour tortilla on the side.

Home-Baked Bread: The Food of Life

Despite the preparation time, breads are easier to make than most people imagine. Few things taste better, and really . . . how can you eat homemade soup without fresh bread on the side?

M'LISSA'S FAIRY BREAD

This is one of my daughter M'lissa's favorite bread recipes.

YIELD: 1 loaf

- 2 cups flour
- ⅓ cup sugar
- 3 teaspoons baking powder
- ½ teaspoon salt
- 1 heaping teaspoon cinnamon powder
- ⅛ teaspoon clove powder
- 1 egg
- 1 cup milk
- ¼ cup melted butter
- 1 cup freshly harvested currants, raspberries, mulberries or blueberries . . . your choice, but only one kind of berry, please
- 1 tablespoon dried coarsely chopped lemon balm or chocolate peppermint
- ¼ cup semisweet chocolate chips

Preheat oven to 375°F. Grease and flour an 8-by-12-inch cake pan. Sift dry ingredients and spices together in a large mixing bowl. In a smaller bowl, beat together milk and egg; stir in butter. Beat all these ingredients together just until everything is moistened. Gently fold in berries, lemon balm or chocolate peppermint, and chocolate chips. Pour the batter into the cake pan and bake for 25 to 40 minutes, or until a knife inserted into the middle pulls out clean. Remove from oven and cool on rack.

BREAD WINNERS FOR HEALTH

Enhance whole grains and homemade breads with these herbs:

> **Dill and fennel** are delicious, promote good digestion, and relieve the discomfort associated with heartburn.

> **Lovage** is fantastic with rice and lentil dishes, and just the ticket for someone recovering from a respiratory infection.

> **Blueberries** contribute to good vision and are a sweet addition to cereals as well.

> **Cinnamon,** a delicious spice, improves digestion and circulation.

HOME-BAKED ROSEMARY BREAD

This is one of my favorite bread recipes. It is simple to make and you can vary it with different herbs and spices, according to your whim.

YIELD: 1 loaf

- 1 package baking yeast
- 1¼ cups warm water
- 3 cups flour, divided
- 2 tablespoons extra-virgin olive oil
- 2 tablespoons sugar
- 2 teaspoons salt
- 1–2 teaspoons dried rosemary, to taste

Sprinkle the yeast on the warm water in a large mixing bowl. Stir in 1½ cups of the flour and the oil, sugar, salt, and rosemary. Beat for approximately 2 minutes with an electric mixer. Stir in the remaining 1½ cups of flour. Cover the bowl with plastic wrap and let rise in a warm place until doubled (approximately 45 minutes).

Grease and flour a 9-by-5-inch loaf pan. Punch down the dough and beat again with electric mixer for 2 minutes or so. Pour into the loaf pan and let rise again for another 40 minutes.

Preheat the oven to 375°F.

Bake the bread for 45 to 50 minutes, or until the top of the loaf is golden brown.

Cool slightly on a baking rack, but serve while still warm for that fresh-from-the-oven goodness.

BASIL GRILLED CHEESE

We often eat these sandwiches for lunch, but they're also great as take-along snacks on hikes or bicycle rides.

SERVES 2

- 4 slices of hearty bread, each buttered on one side
- 2 slices of Colby or jack cheese
- 4 large basil leaves

Place a slice of bread, buttered side down, in an electric skillet set at 350°F or in a hot skillet on top of the stove, set on medium. Top with a slice of cheese and two basil leaves, then top with another slice of bread, buttered side up. Cook until golden brown on the first side. Using a spatula, turn the sandwich to cook the second side golden brown. Repeat to make a second sandwich. Delicious!

Breakfast Food

Breakfast is considered the most important meal of the day, yet it's the one everyone seems to skimp on. Whole grains and cereals nourish and support the nervous and immune systems. Nurture yourself with these foods — you deserve it!

Whole-Grain Oats

Oats are one of nature's most nutritious foods. They're certainly one of my favorite grains, and daily consumption is absolutely necessary. High in calcium and protein, oats nourish the nervous system and the skin and support good bone health. They relieve itchy skin, keep stress levels in check, and act as an excellent reproductive-organ tonic. Eat your oatmeal: That's my advice to every person on the planet!

OATMEAL CHERRY CRISP

This recipe is adapted from Aunt Sherry's oatmeal apple crisp. It's always a big hit for breakfast, and our farm crew like it for a nutritious snack at morning break. Sometimes I double the dry ingredients and the butter to make an extra thick layer of oatmeal topping because it's so yummy!

SERVES 4–6

- 4 cups sour pie cherries, pitted (fresh, frozen, or canned)
- 1 tablespoon lemon juice
- 1 cup rolled oats
- ⅓ cup flour
- ½ cup brown sugar
- 1 teaspoon cinnamon
- ½ teaspoon salt (optional)
- ⅓ cup melted butter (do not use margarine)
  Whole-milk vanilla yogurt (optional)

Put the cherries in a baking dish and sprinkle with the lemon juice. In a large mixing bowl, combine the oats, flour, brown sugar, cinnamon, and salt, until well mixed. Add the butter and again mix well until mixture is crumbly.

Preheat the oven to 375°F.

Sprinkle the topping mix over the cherries and bake for about 30 minutes, or until topping just begins to turn golden. Serve topped with whole-milk vanilla yogurt for extra taste and nutrition. **NOTE:** You can substitute other types of fruit for the cherries, like apples, peaches, or plums.

BLUEBERRY-CINNAMON MUFFINS

These muffins are terrific for breakfast or snacking; you may want to make a double batch and freeze half for another time.

YIELD: 12 muffins

- 2½ cups whole wheat flour
- 3 teaspoons baking powder
- 1 teaspoon sea salt (optional)
- 1½ teaspoons ground cinnamon
- ⅓ cup honey
- ¼ cup milk
- 1 egg
- ¼ cup melted butter
- 1 cup fresh or frozen blueberries

Grease or line a dozen muffin cups. Preheat the oven to 400°F. In a mixing bowl, sift together the flour, baking powder, cinnamon, and sea salt, if using.

Beat together the honey, egg, and milk in a separate bowl. Stir in the butter and the flour mixture and beat just until moistened.

Fill muffin cups two-thirds of the way and bake for 20 to 25 minutes, or until a toothpick inserted into the middle of one muffin comes out clean. Serve with honey or enjoy them just as they are.

LICORICE AND BANANA OATMEAL

Try this for a new take on traditional oatmeal. The licorice makes the cereal sweet; the bananas are just delicious.

SERVES 2

- 1 ripe banana, mashed well
- 2 pinches of powdered licorice root
- 2 bowls of well-cooked oatmeal (use regular or organic uncooked oats, not the quick-cooking or precooked variety)
  Organic milk (optional)

Blend the banana and licorice into the bowls of oatmeal. Add a little organic milk, if desired, and start your day in style.

Purslane

Portulaca oleracea

In midsummer, when the weather gets hot, purslane emerges in the garden in abundance. This succulent plant is easy to spot, as it rambles close to the ground. For several weeks, there's enough purslane to serve it daily as part of our meals.

Purslane is a rich source of essential fatty acids and vitamin C, making it excellent for healthy skin and women's reproductive systems. It tastes slightly tangy, with a bit of a lemony flavor. Add it fresh to salads and dice into salsas. Chop it up and fry it with potatoes, onions, garlic, and sweet frying peppers for a fantastic skillet dinner. You can even boil it up like pasta and serve it topped with spaghetti sauce and Parmesan cheese.

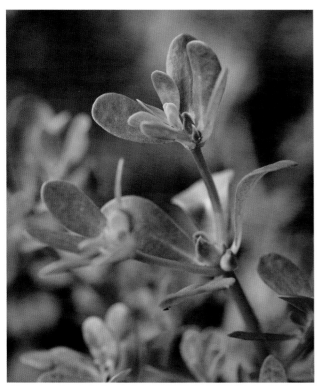

The zingy flavor of purslane in the heat of the summer season is refreshing and delicious, not to mention highly nutritious.

PURSLANE SKILLET DINNER

This is a simple but flavorful dish that's quick to prepare. Serve it for breakfast as a robust start to the day, or serve with salad.

SERVES 2

4–6	tablespoons butter (do not use margarine)
4–6	large potatoes, chopped or grated
1–2	cups purslane, coarsely chopped
2–3	cloves garlic, peeled and minced
2	sweet frying peppers, sliced thin
1	large onion, sliced thin
4	eggs
	Cheddar cheese, grated
1	large tomato, chopped
2–3	green onions, chopped
	Hot sauce (optional)

Put the butter, potatoes, purslane, garlic, peppers, and sliced onion in a large skillet (or an electric skillet). On medium high (350°F), fry gently until the potatoes are golden brown, stirring frequently to prevent burning. Turn out onto two platters and cover to keep warm.

In the same skillet, fry the eggs. Put two eggs on top of each platter of potato. Sprinkle generously with grated cheese and top with the tomato and green onions. Flavor with hot sauce, if desired.

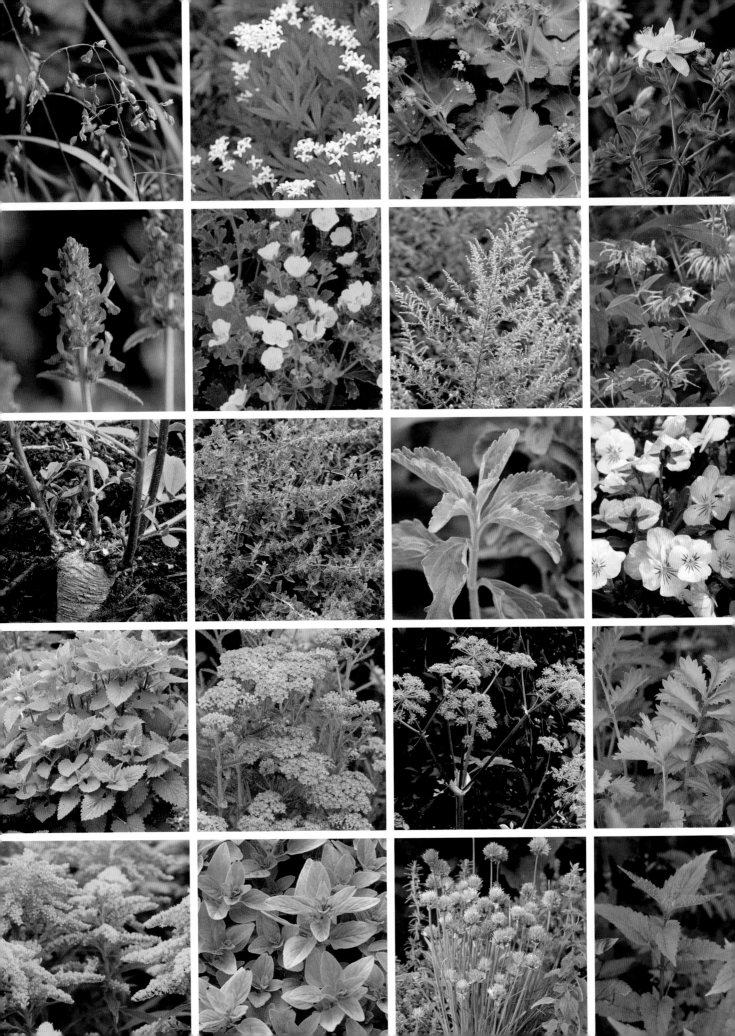

CHAPTER TEN

Herb Personalities

A Closer Look at Each Plant

In this chapter you will become better acquainted with the individual herbs and how they exist in their natural habitat. Understanding a plant's personality traits will help you design a garden that is appropriate for your site, climate, and personal needs. You'll also get to know the best ways to use each plant for cooking, to support your health, and in your home. Remember to consult a reliable reference book for more detailed information on medicinal usage, dosages, and cautions (see Recommended Reading, page 246).

This is also where you will become familiar with the growing and propagation requirements of your herbs. I present here information gleaned from my experiences and from other growers. Do keep in mind that plants often have a will of their own, and each time you grow them you're bound to learn something new about them. A respectful approach to growing them will yield success.

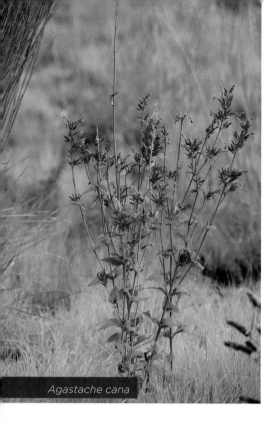

Agastache cana

Agastache

Agastache species

The many species of Agastache *have several things in common: They're beautiful, they attract pollinators like hummingbirds and sphinx moths, they're good digestive herbs, and they taste great!*

COMMON SPECIES OF AGASTACHE: Sunset hyssop (*A. rupestris*), double bubblegum mint (*A. cana*), coronado mint (*A. aurantiaca*)

PERSONALITY: Perennial; herbaceous (Zones 5–9)

HEIGHT: 1 to 3 feet (30 cm–0.9 m)

BLOOM TRAITS: Spikes of bright flowers in shades of purple, pink, and orange in midsummer through late fall

LIKES/DISLIKES: Agastaches are typically sun-tolerant and prefer open areas. They also perform nicely at lower mountain elevations.

PROPAGATION/MAINTENANCE: Most agastaches are easy to grow from seed. Sow in late winter in a greenhouse or direct-sow them into the garden in late fall for spring emergence. Expect 40–75 percent germination, depending on the species, in 2 to 3 weeks. Agastaches grow in clumps and should be spaced about 12 to 15 inches (30–38 cm) apart. They use low to moderate water.

SUN/SOIL: Full sun preferred; grows well in poorer soils like clay, gravel, and sand.

COMPANION/COMPLEMENTARY PLANTING: Grow in community with southernwood, winter savory, and lavenders.

HARVESTING: Harvest the upper third of the plant, preferably when in flower, using a pair of snips or scissors.

CULINARY USE: The leaves and flowers vary in flavor from minty root beer and licorice mint to the taste and smell of bubblegum (hence the name). The leaves and flowers are nice made into herbal honey and cream cheese spreads, or sprinkled into fruit salad and over ice cream.

MEDICINAL BENEFITS: All the agastaches support digestion and help to lower fevers. A tea from these plants makes a soothing sore throat gargle.

PARTS USED: Aerial parts with or without flowers, fresh or dried

HOME PHARMACY USES: Infusion, traditional tincture, syrup, elixir, bath herb, honey

EDIBLE FLOWERS: Add brightly colored flowers to fruit salads or pasta salad for a zippy taste, add to cream cheese spread or herb butter, or float in lemonade. The flowers are also quite beautiful as cake decorations.

Angelica

Angelica archangelica

Angelica is gaining recognition as a substitute herb for the environmentally at-risk osha plant (Ligusticum porteri). *Angelica is often combined with rosemary and yerba mansa for optimum benefit.*

PERSONALITY: Biennial or monocarpic perennial (once angelica flowers and seeds, it dies, usually in 2 years, occasionally in 3 years); herbaceous (Zones 5–9)

HEIGHT: 4 to 6 feet (1.2–1.8 m)

BLOOM TRAITS: Umbels have clusters of yellowish green flowers.

LIKES/DISLIKES: Angelica grows in moist soil and full to partial shade, usually near streams in sandy/loamy soil.

PROPAGATION/MAINTENANCE: Sow seeds immediately upon ripening or store in the freezer until ready to sow. Expect between 30 and 50 percent germination, depending on seed freshness. Sprouting usually occurs in 3 to 4 weeks. Transplant outdoors 1 to 2 weeks before the last frost. Space plants 15 inches (38 cm) apart. Angelica grows in clumps with a large taproot system. It needs moderate to heavy watering.

SUN/SOIL: Shade, partial shade, full sun; prefers a richer loam soil, but is tolerant of clay or sandy soils that are rich in organic matter.

HARVESTING: Harvest first-year roots in late fall; dig second-year roots in early spring; use a needle-nose spade or fork. Harvest stalks with snips any time during the growing season.

Calendula

Calendula officinalis

Calendula may be used as an herbal food coloring for broth, rice, and even frosting, to which it imparts a rich golden color. King Henry VIII of England reputedly liked his food highly seasoned and brightly colored, and his cooks relied heavily on calendula to meet his demands. The plant is often called pot marigold or French pot marigold, a tribute to its early culinary uses.

COMMON VARIETIES OF CALENDULA: 'Alpha', 'Radio Heirloom', 'Déjà vu', 'Resina', 'Indian Prince'

ETHNIC AND OTHER NAMES: French pot marigold

PERSONALITY: Annual; herbaceous

HEIGHT: 12 to 15 inches (30–38 cm)

BLOOM TRAITS: Bright yellow and orange flowers bloom from early summer until a killing frost. They close up at night and reopen in early to mid-morning.

LIKES/DISLIKES: Calendula is now considered a garden plant only. Its origin is not known, but it is a common choice for nearly all types of gardens.

PROPAGATION/MAINTENANCE: Propagate calendula from seeds. They are easy and require no pretreatment. They are best sown directly into the ground, but you can start them indoors and transplant them later. Germination is normally very reliable, around 80 percent. Seeds take 1 to 2 weeks to sprout. This plant, which grows in clumps, does not spread by roots or runners, but it does self-sow vigorously. Space 10 inches (25 cm) apart and provide light to moderate amounts

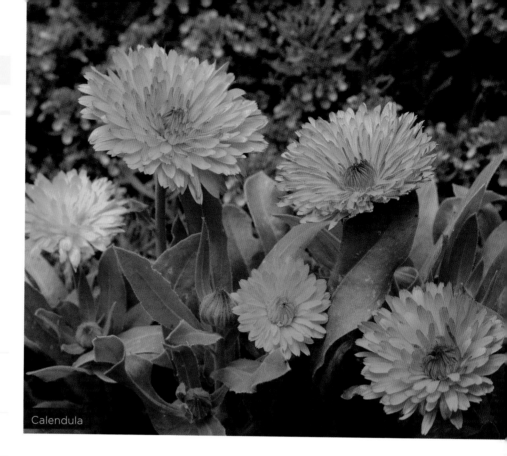
Calendula

of water. Deadheading the flowers regularly will result in nonstop blooming throughout the summer until a killing frost in the fall.

SUN/SOIL: Full sun; will grow in nearly every type of soil, as long as it isn't overly moist.

COMPANION/COMPLEMENTARY PLANTING: Calendulas tend to attract aphids, whiteflies, and thrips. Use them as a magnet plant: Set them in around other plants that are troubled by those pests.

HARVESTING: Only the flowers of calendula are harvested; pick by hand when they are just fully opened. Don't pick flowers that have already begun to form seed; these will not be as medicinally active. Remove spent blossoms to promote blooming throughout the summer and early fall. Once all the flowers go to seed, calendula will die.

MEDICINAL BENEFITS: Excellent for skin health, but also appropriate for gastrointestinal tract concerns

PARTS USED: Flowers, fresh or dried

HOME PHARMACY USES: Infusion, traditional tincture, ointment, salve, cream, foot soak, bath herb, infused oil, liniment, insect repellent, sunburn relief spray

EDIBLE FLOWERS: Calendula flowers are known in the herbal world as a food coloring. Add ½ cup or so to the soup kettle and the broth will taste great and have a golden glow. Remove the petals from the center portion of the flower and sprinkle them into green salads, or add them to a cream cheese spread for a beautiful touch.

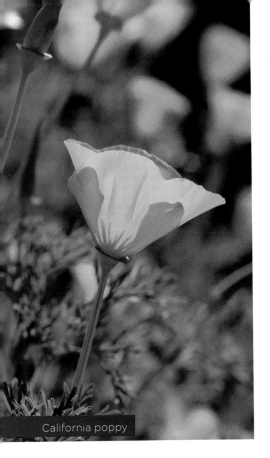

California poppy

California Poppy

Eschscholzia californica

Few plants look as stunning as a mass planting of California poppies. Their grayish green, feathery foliage and dramatic orange flowers never fail to stop people in their tracks. Use the edible flowers to decorate a cake or create a confetti effect in a cream cheese spread.

COMMON VARIETIES: 'Misson Bells', 'Thai Silk'

PERSONALITY: Annual; herbaceous

HEIGHT: 12 inches (30 cm)

BLOOM TRAITS: Vibrant, bright orange flowers bloom from late spring until a killing frost.

LIKES/DISLIKES: These plants prefer to grow in wide-open, grassy areas, where they happily intermix with native grasses and other wildflowers. They are native to the California Sierras.

PROPAGATION/MAINTENANCE: Stratify seeds for a week or so and then sow them directly into the garden soil, or start them early indoors and transplant outdoors in late spring. Space 10 to 12 inches (25–30 cm) apart and provide light to moderate amounts of water. Germination is usually around 70 percent and occurs in 7 to 14 days. Although individual plants do not spread, California poppies are vigorous self-sowers and can easily fill in a given space within 2 years.

SUN/SOIL: Sun, partial shade; no special soil needs

HARVESTING: The entire plant is harvested when the poppies are in bloom. At this stage you will have present both poppy flowers and the seedpods. Pull up the entire plant or use a garden fork if the ground is not moist enough to extract them. They have a large orange taproot that is usually easy enough to pull out by hand.

MEDICINAL BENEFITS: A wonderful nervine that is excellent for relieving stress and anxiety, it also offers pain relief and acts as a sleep aid.

PARTS USED: Whole plant in flower, fresh or dried

HOME PHARMACY USES: Infusion, traditional tincture, syrup, elixir, ointment, salve, cream, foot soak, bath herb, infused oil, honey, liniment

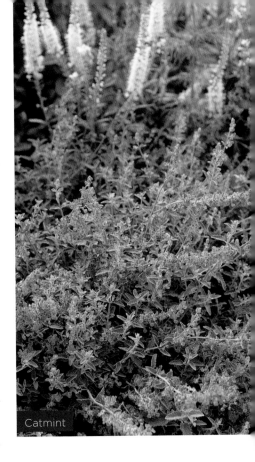

Catmint

Catmint

Nepeta × faassenii

An attractive spicy member of the mint family, catmint grows very well in a dryland garden. Cats will pay attention to catmint when it is bruised, but otherwise seem to ignore its intense fragrance and bright blue flowers, preferring traditional catnip.

COMMON VARIETIES: 'Blue Hill', 'Six Hills Giant', 'Walker's Low'

PERSONALITY: Perennial; herbaceous (Zones 4–9)

HEIGHT: 12 to 15 inches (30–38 cm)

BLOOM TRAITS: Bright blue flowers start in late spring and continue off and on throughout summer and early fall.

LIKES/DISLIKES: Catmint prefers an open sunny area that is moderately moist to somewhat arid. It is well suited to Southwestern xeric gardens. In this type of dryland garden, there is often spring moisture available to the garden in the form of melting snow and rain, but summer and autumn are quite dry and hot, with a short monsoon season in midsummer.

PROPAGATION/MAINTENANCE: The true species of catmint is easily grown from seed. Seeds do not require any special treatment prior to sowing. Sow indoors in late winter or early spring. Germination occurs at about 80 percent in 2 to 3 weeks. Many of the varieties, such as 'Walker's Low', will not grow true from seed, so tip cuttings must be used to propagate them. Dip cuttings in liquid or powder rooting hormone and stick each cutting into evenly moist soil. Keep in a warm location during the rooting process; keep the soil moist but not soggy. Transplant rooted cuttings or seedlings outdoors in mid- to late spring, and space about 15 inches (38 cm) apart. Lightly water plants once they are established. *Tip:* Once flowers fade, cut back the plant to 4 inches (10 cm) above the ground and in a few weeks the plant will be lush and blooming again.

SUN/SOIL: Full sun to partial shade; prefers well-drained soil

COMPANION/COMPLEMENTARY PLANTING: Grow in community with rue, lavender, santolina, and California poppy.

HARVESTING: Harvest the upper-third part of the plant, preferably while in flower. Use snips or scissors for the task.

TEA: The flowering aerial parts make a nice-tasting beverage tea.

EDIBLE FLOWERS: The flowers lend a pleasantly spicy flavor to green leafy and fruit salads. They are also nice for decorating cakes, and look lovely floating in a pitcher of lemonade.

Catnip

Nepeta cataria

Most people are familiar with catnip only for its intoxicating effect on cats, but it is a great herb for humans, too. Interestingly, catnip acts as a stimulant on cats but as a sedative on people.

ETHNIC AND OTHER NAMES: *Nebada* (Spanish)

PERSONALITY: Perennial; herbaceous (Zones 3–7)

HEIGHT: 15 to 24 inches (38–60 cm)

BLOOM TRAITS: Spikes of small, white, purple-spotted, not especially showy flowers bloom on and off from summer to fall.

LIKES/DISLIKES: Catnip is found in many types of environments. It is likely to be discovered in disturbed areas, such as alongside streams, ponds, lakes, roadsides, and waste ground.

PROPAGATION/MAINTENANCE: Seeds will germinate at a higher percentage if you stratify them for a couple of weeks before sowing. Then sow directly outdoors into the garden in early to mid-spring, or start early indoors and transplant outside in mid- to late spring. Germination is normally about 50 percent. Space plants 12 inches (30 cm) apart and provide low to moderate amounts of water. Catnip reseeds itself readily.

SUN/SOIL: Full sun, partial shade, shade; no special soil needs

COMPANION/COMPLEMENTARY PLANTING: French or red-veined sorrel, nasturtium, shiso, and sage make good neighbors for catnip.

HARVESTING: All of the aerial parts can be harvested at any time during the growing season. Use scissors or snips to cut the plant back to 3 to 4 inches (7.5–10 cm) above

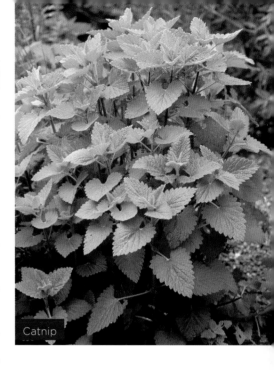

Catnip

the ground. The plant will grow back within only a couple of weeks. Plants provide several harvests throughout the season.

CULINARY USE: Substitute traditional or lemon catnip for one-quarter of the sweet basil when making pesto to give a new twist to an old-time favorite sauce.

MEDICINAL BENEFITS: Catnip has many medicinal uses, including nervous system support, pain relief, and stress relief. It is also recommended for the digestive tract, cold and flu symptoms, and children's health concerns.

PARTS USED: Aerial parts, fresh or dried

HOME PHARMACY USES: Infusion, traditional tincture, cider vinegar tincture, syrup, elixir, ointment, salve, cream, foot soak, bath herb, infused oil, honey, liniment, sleep pillow

CRAFTING: Kitty toys are fun and easy to make. Sew small pillows, approximately 4 inches square, from cute cat fabric, but leave one side unsewn. Fill the pillow as full as possible with crushed dried catnip and then stitch the pillow securely closed. Our three cats *love* these homemade treats!

Cayenne

Capsicum species

Cayenne is a member of the Solanaceae, the nightshade family, which includes potatoes, eggplant, and bell peppers. Never eat the leaves, stems, or flowers of the cayenne pepper plant; they can be toxic. The fruits, however, are perfectly safe. Be conservative in how much cayenne you add to your recipes or remedies; these peppers are hot!

ETHNIC AND OTHER NAMES: *Poivre de Cayenne* (French), *peperone* (Italian), *pimiento, chile* (Spanish), *Cayennepfeffer* (German), *kajennpeppar* (Swedish)

PERSONALITY: Annual; herbaceous

HEIGHT: To 24 inches (60 cm)

BLOOM TRAITS: White and somewhat star-shaped flowers bloom in early to midsummer, followed by the formation of green fruits. The fruits will turn bright red upon maturity.

LIKES/DISLIKES: Cayennes are probably native to South America. They are only a cultivated plant at this time, although there are some types of chilies, like chiltepines, that can still be found growing in the wilds of North and Central America. Cayennes prefer hot and somewhat dry areas, where there are long summers and bright sunny days.

PROPAGATION/MAINTENANCE: Start cayenne in late winter or early spring indoors in a bright, sunny, warm location. Seeds require no special treatment, but seedlings appreciate very warm temperatures. Expect good germination in about 1 week. We reliably get 80 to 90

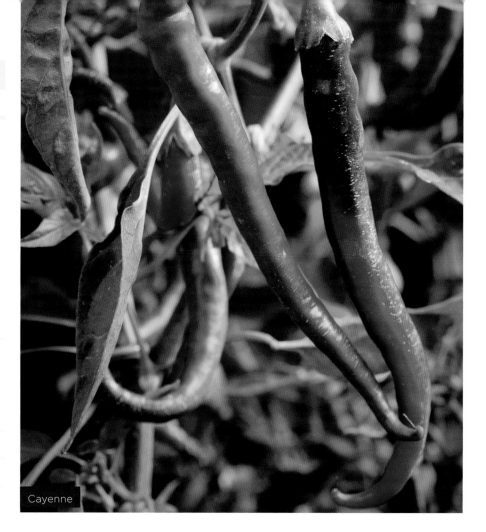

Cayenne

percent germination if all growing conditions are right. Transplant cayenne outdoors, 12 inches (30 cm) apart, after all danger of frost has passed. The plant grows in clumps and requires little watering.

SUN/SOIL: Full sun; prefers dryish soil, but is tolerant of others

COMPANION/COMPLEMENTARY PLANTING: Grow near basil and cilantro to enhance each herb's flavor. Any of these hot chilies are perfect additions to the veggie garden or the container gardens.

HARVESTING: Pick the bright red fruits (chilies) in late summer or even in early fall before the frost hits. The chilies are handpicked and gloves are recommended; capsicum resin on the skin can cause burning, especially for people who have fair or sensitive skin.

CULINARY USE: Add some zip to your cooking by incorporating a bit of dried crushed cayenne. It is good sprinkled over pizza, or try it combined with rosemary for an amazing grilled chicken dish. Hot pepper substitutes for cayenne include: habañero, serrano, jalapeño, Scotch bonnet, and chiltepine.

MEDICINAL BENEFITS: An excellent herb for heart and circulatory health, cayenne is also used in topical remedies for pain relief, especially of the joints and muscles.

PART USED: Fruit, fresh or dried

HOME PHARMACY USES: Traditional tincture, cider vinegar tincture, ointment, salve, cream, foot soak, infused oil

Chamomile

Matricaria recutita,
  Chamaemelum nobile

Chamomile flowers are cheerful and delicate but labor-intensive to pick. In many cases the leafy flowering tops can be used instead of just the flowers, and they are much easier to harvest.

ETHNIC AND OTHER NAMES:
Manzanilla (Spanish)

PERSONALITY: German chamomile (*Matricaria recutita*), annual; Roman chamomile (*Chamaemelum nobile*), perennial; herbaceous (Zones 4–9)

HEIGHT: German, to 24 inches (60 cm); Roman, 8 to 10 inches (20–25 cm)

BLOOM TRAITS: White, daisylike flowers bloom from June through frost.

LIKES/DISLIKES: Both genera are considered garden dwellers.

PROPAGATION/MAINTENANCE: German chamomile is easy to grow from seed, and can be direct-sown in garden or field. Keeping the tiny seeds moist for germination can be difficult, so try starting plants indoors and transplanting after frost danger has passed. Allow 3 to 5 weeks before transplanting outdoors. Space 10 inches (25 cm) apart. Seeds consistently germinate at 50 to 70 percent in about 2 weeks. This genus grows as a single plant and needs light to moderate watering.

Roman chamomile is also easy from seed, but the germination rate is just 40 to 60 percent. Instead, propagate by divisions. Roman chamomile spreads by rhizomatous roots. Space the plants 8 inches (20 cm) apart, which enables plants to fill in as a ground cover. Provide light to moderate amounts of water.

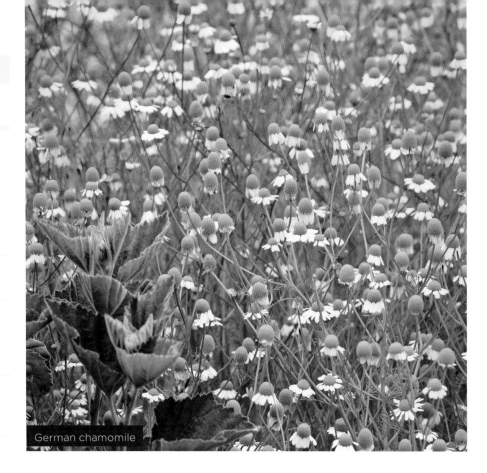

German chamomile

SUN/SOIL: Full sun, partial shade; grows best in well-drained soil

COMPANION/COMPLEMENTARY PLANTING: German chamomile is great planted with lavender, rosemary, and hyssop. It is very happy growing in a container, too. Roman chamomile is perfect planted among stepping-stones to create garden pathways. You may also grow it to cover an earthen bench — it will be wonderfully fragrant to sit upon.

HARVESTING: Harvest during the blooming season. If only flowers are used, pick by hand or with the help of a chamomile rake (a special tool designed for the purpose). If you want to harvest the flowers with 2 to 3 inches (5–7.5 cm) of stems attached, use a pair of snips.

MEDICINAL BENEFITS: A sedative and nervine herb, chamomile has calming, soothing, and anti-inflammatory actions. It is an excellent digestive herb, sleep aid, children's herb, and skin aid.

PARTS USED: Flowers and flowering tops, fresh or dried

HOME PHARMACY USES: Infusion, cider vinegar tincture, traditional tincture, syrup, elixir, ointment, salve, cream, foot soak, bath herb, sleep pillow, infused oil, honey, liniment

EDIBLE FLOWERS: Both German and Roman chamomile flowers are used to decorate cakes, as an addition to green and fruit salads, or as pretty floats in a party punch bowl. They make a delicious tea, especially combined with spearmint, served iced or hot.

CRAFTING: Chamomile flowers smell a bit like apples and are often an ingredient of potpourri.

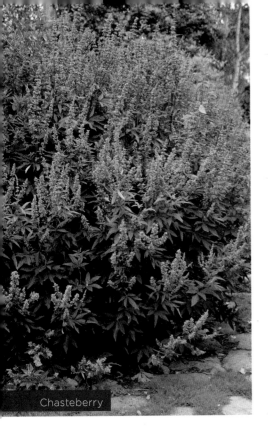

Chasteberry

Chasteberry

Vitex agnus-castus

In the Middle Ages, chasteberry was called monk's pepper. Monks ground the herb and used it as a substitute for the similar-tasting black pepper. These clergymen believed the plant would suppress the libido, but in fact it does not.

ETHNIC AND OTHER NAMES: Vitex, *palo santo* (Spanish)

PERSONALITY: Perennial; woody (Zones 6–9)

HEIGHT: 2 to 10 feet (0.6–3.0 m)

BLOOM TRAITS: Gorgeous lavender-colored spikes of flowers bloom in mid- to late summer beginning in the second year. In the colder parts of its range, chasteberry may not flower or form fruit.

LIKES/DISLIKES: Chasteberry is from the Mediterranean region. It likes hot temperatures and appreciates some humidity. In cooler climates, chasteberry dies back in winter and is quite late coming up again in spring . . . be patient.

PROPAGATION/MAINTENANCE: Stratify seeds for 3 to 4 weeks, then scarify them and soak them in warm water for 30 minutes before sowing immediately indoors. Seeds may take up to 4 weeks to germinate. The germination rate is 50 to 60 percent, although I occasionally get better results. Transplant outdoors, 12 to 24 inches (30–60 cm) apart, in late spring when the weather is well settled. This herb grows in clumps and requires moderate watering.

SUN/SOIL: Full sun, partial shade; well-drained soil

HARVESTING: The leaves and tender stem growth of the upper 4 inches (10 cm), along with the flowers and ripening seeds, may be harvested for medicinal purposes. (Most buyers prefer only the ripened berries, without the leafy and flowering portions.) Use snips to harvest leafy parts; if only berries are desired, gently rub them loose from the stems, then screen them out of the leafy and flowering parts. I make my remedies with the leafy, flowering portions along with the berries.

MEDICINAL BENEFITS: Considered a tonic herb for both the male and female reproductive systems

PARTS USED: Leaves, flowers, and berries, fresh or dried

HOME PHARMACY USES: Decoction, traditional tincture, cider vinegar tincture, syrup, elixir

Chives

Chives

Allium schoenoprasum

Growing chives in the garden or on the windowsill is one way to keep a fresh supply available. Nothing compares to their taste in scrambled eggs or on a grilled cheese sandwich. Dried chives just aren't the same.

ETHNIC AND OTHER NAMES: *Ciboulette* (French), *cipollina* (Italian), *cebolleta* (Spanish)

PERSONALITY: Perennial; herbaceous (Zones 4–9)

HEIGHT: 12 inches (30 cm)

BLOOM TRAITS: Big pink flowers from mid-spring on and off throughout summer and early fall

LIKES/DISLIKES: Primarily a garden herb, chives prefer to grow in open, sunny areas, but are quite flexible, making themselves at home throughout the garden.

PROPAGATION/MAINTENANCE: Chives are easiest to grow from seed and require no special treatment. Sow them directly into the garden soil in early spring, or start them indoors for transplanting into the garden later in spring or early summer. Germination is about 80 percent and sprouting occurs in about 2 weeks. Chives can also be propagated by root divisions in early spring or fall. Plants grow in clumps, so space them 12 inches (30 cm) apart and water moderately.

SUN/SOIL: Full sun to full shade; adaptable to different soil types, but prefers a well-drained location

COMPANION/COMPLEMENTARY PLANTING: Grow with heartsease, summer savory, and red shiso. Chives are wonderful in food gardens or as a windowsill or countertop herb.

HARVESTING: Cut the aerial parts. Do not pull chives up from the ground, as this will kill them outright. Flowers may be picked, too. Snips or scissors are the perfect tool.

CULINARY USE: The green leafy parts are delicious added to egg dishes or sprinkled into vegetables or pasta salads. They are a perfect garnish for onion and potato soups. Chives taste best fresh. For when you don't have fresh chives, freeze them and add them later to cooked dishes as an acceptable alternative. Dried chives taste a bit like sawdust, in my opinion, and I don't go to the trouble of drying them. In winter I keep a pot of chives growing indoors so I always have a ready supply.

EDIBLE FLOWERS: The pink flowers lend a mild onion flavor to green salads, herb butter, and cream cheese spreads for bagels or steamed vegetables.

Cilantro, Coriander

Coriandrum sativum

The leafy parts of this herb are known as cilantro; the seeds are called coriander. Both are recognized in cooking circles, but few people think of this plant as a medicinal herb. Restaurants and farmers' markets are good outlets for fresh cilantro, and coriander is sold as a spice.

ETHNIC AND OTHER NAMES: *Coriandre* (French), *coriandolo* (Italian), *Koriander* (German)

PERSONALITY: Annual; herbaceous

HEIGHT: 10 to 12 inches (25–30 cm)

BLOOM TRAITS: Small, delicate white flowers appear as temperatures warm and the plant bolts to seed.

LIKES/DISLIKES: Considered a garden herb, cilantro grows in moist gardens from tropical to temperate climates during the cooler parts of the growing season. It does not tolerate hot temperatures and will rapidly bolt.

PROPAGATION/MAINTENANCE: Sow untreated seeds outdoors in early to mid-spring or start indoors and transplant outdoors in mid- to late spring. Seeds do not germinate well in the heat of summer. You can also sow in late summer or very early fall for a fresh supply before frosts. Space plants 8 to 10 inches (20–25 cm) apart, and provide moderate to high amounts of water. This herb grows in clumps.

SUN/SOIL: Full sun, partial shade, shade; no special soil needs. Growing cilantro in more shade helps slow the inevitable bolting that is triggered by intense full sun and very hot temperatures.

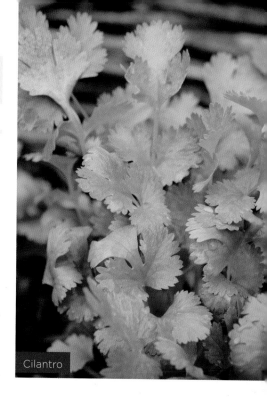
Cilantro

COMPANION/COMPLEMENTARY PLANTING: Cilantro will be happy planted with garlic chives and salad burnet, or in a shady part of a food garden.

HARVESTING: Harvest aerial parts with snips or scissors before the plant goes to flower. Handpick seed clusters and gently rub the golden brown seeds from the stems.

CULINARY USES: My favorite way to use cilantro is to chop fresh leaves with tomatoes, some green onions, and a bit of minced fresh garlic. We top all types of Mexican dishes with it, or add it to sandwiches for a zippy flavor. Coriander seed is great in home-baked bread.

MEDICINAL BENEFIT: Good for digestive health

PARTS USED: Fresh aerial parts and dried seeds

HOME PHARMACY USES: Cider vinegar tincture, traditional tincture, honey

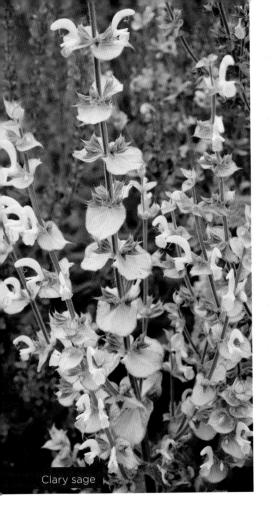

Clary sage

LIKES/DISLIKES: Clary sage is a Mediterranean plant that prefers a hot and dry climate.

PROPAGATION/MAINTENANCE: Sow seeds indoors for transplanting outside in late spring, or sow directly outdoors in mid-spring. No special treatment is required. Expect 60 to 70 percent germination about 2 weeks after sowing. Clary sage gets quite large in circumference, so space plants 24 inches (60 cm) apart. Water moderately.

SUN/SOIL: Full sun; prefers well-drained soil

HARVESTING: Harvest aerial parts when in flower; snips work well. I wear gloves because the oil of clary sage penetrates my skin and the fragrance stays with me for hours. Some people really like the smell, but I am not that fond of it.

MEDICINAL BENEFITS: Clary sage is used a great deal for women's health concerns. It is also popular as a fragrance fixative, and is often a relaxing component in massage oils.

PARTS USED: Aerial parts in flower, fresh or dried

HOME PHARMACY USES: Traditional tincture, ointment, salve, cream, foot soak, bath herb, sleep pillow, infused oil, honey, liniment

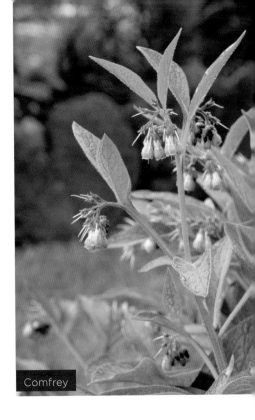

Comfrey

Clary Sage

Salvia sclarea

Clary sage is known primarily as an esteemed essential oil. It also contributes wonderful healing properties to women's health formulas.

PERSONALITY: Biennial or perennial; herbaceous (Zones 5–9)

HEIGHT: 3 feet (0.9 m)

BLOOM TRAITS: Beautiful lavender, pink, or white flowers bloom from midsummer through late summer.

Comfrey

Symphytum × uplandicum

Much of the comfrey used in herbal products has been mislabeled as Symphytum officinale, *but is in fact* S. × uplandicum. *This is important because the research that has made everyone skeptical about comfrey's safety was apparently conducted using* S. officinale. Symphytum × uplandicum *has considerably lower levels of pyrrolizidine alkaloid, a substance that can be toxic to the liver. Comfrey is a fantastic herb for the muscular and skeletal systems and promotes skin health.*

PERSONALITY: Perennial; herbaceous (Zones 3–9)

HEIGHT: 3 to 4 feet (0.9–1.2 m)

BLOOM TRAITS: Lilac-rose flowers fade to purple, violet, or blue (*S. officinale* has white, cream, mauve, or pink flowers).

LIKES/DISLIKES: Comfrey prefers moist soil near streams and ponds. It likes dappled sunlight.

PROPAGATION/MAINTENANCE: Comfrey is a sterile plant and must be propagated by root divisions. These will do best if divided outdoors in mid- to late spring. Space plants 24 inches (60 cm) apart. Comfrey will spread only if the root is dug up and divided or accidentally chopped up and dispersed in the soil (as might occur with a tiller or plow). Water moderately.

SUN/SOIL: Full sun, partial shade; prefers rich, loamy or sandy soil but will grow in most soils.

COMPANION/COMPLEMENTARY PLANTING: Grow with costmary, French sorrel, and horseradish.

HARVESTING: Historically, both roots and leaves of comfrey have been used. The leaves are just as good medicinally as the roots, though, and if you never dig the roots, you will never have to worry about comfrey spreading to parts of the garden where it is not welcome. Harvest the leaves with snips or handpick them any time during the growing season. For 14 years I have been harvesting the same comfrey plant (leaves only) and I still have only that single plant. If you feel you must harvest roots, do so in the spring or fall, using a needle-nose spade or a garden fork.

MEDICINAL BENEFITS: Well known for its support of muscles and bones, comfrey is also excellent for healing topical wounds.

PARTS USED: Leaves, fresh or dried. Roots may also be used fresh or dried.

HOME PHARMACY USES: Ointment, salve, cream, foot soak, bath herb, infused oil, liniment

Costmary

Tanacetum balsamita

Costmary was an important herb in the Middle Ages for medicine, for brewing ale, and as a flavorful salad herb. Today it is not as commonly known, but its wonderful, spearmintlike flavor and pretty nature make it a welcome addition to the garden.

ETHNIC AND OTHER NAMES: Balsamita, *menthe-coq*, *grande balsamite* (French)

PERSONALITY: Perennial; herbaceous (Zones 4–8)

HEIGHT: 12 to 24 inches (30–60 cm)

BLOOM TRAITS: White flowers from early summer to fall

LIKES/DISLIKES: Costmary thrives in nearly every growing situation aside from tropical conditions. A native of Asia, it is naturalized or grown as a garden plant throughout the temperate world.

PROPAGATION/MAINTENANCE: Costmary seed is tiny and should not be planted too deep, however, it germinates easily in 2 to 3 weeks at around 80 percent. Start plants indoors and transplant to the garden in mid- to late spring. Space plants 2 to 3 feet (0.6–0.9 m) apart. Costmary will thrive in dry conditions, but I find that moderate watering works best for the plants in my garden, where they grow in hot afternoon sun. Here is a useful hint: Once costmary produces flowers, the plant has a tendency to flop. When this happens, cut it back to 3 to 4 inches (8–10 cm) above the ground. It will fill out in a couple of weeks and will soon be flowering again.

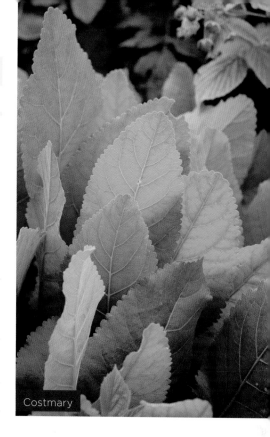

Costmary

SUN/SOIL: Full sun to partial shade; adaptable to different types of well-drained soil

HARVESTING: Harvest the aerial parts with snips or sturdy scissors.

CULINARY USE: Add young leaves to a leafy green salad. They have a spicy, balsamic-type taste, so just a few leaves will do; you don't want them to overwhelm the salad's flavor.

MEDICINAL BENEFITS: Good astringent for toning the skin

PARTS USED: Leaves, fresh or dried

HOME PHARMACY USES: Skin wash, liniment, ointment, cream, bath herb, foot soak

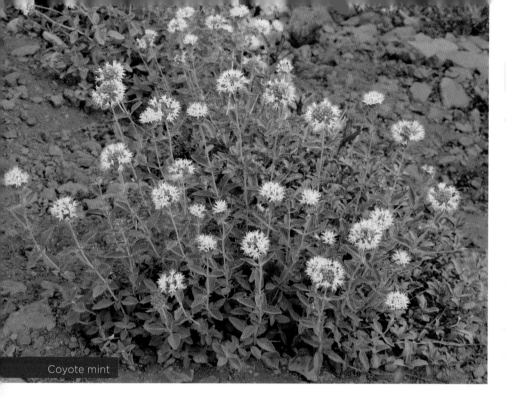
Coyote mint

Coyote Mint

Monardella odoratissima

Coyote mint is a spunky little plant that looks a bit like a miniature monarda. They are distant cousins within the mint family.

PERSONALITY: Perennial; herbaceous (Zones 6–9)

HEIGHT: 10 to 12 inches (25–30 cm)

BLOOM TRAITS: Pale lavender flowers bloom from early to midsummer.

LIKES/DISLIKES: Coyote mint is native to the dry, high mountain desert areas of the Southwestern states.

PROPAGATION/MAINTENANCE: When propagating from cuttings, use liquid rooting hormone and do not overwater. I prefer to grow this plant from seed. Stratify the seeds for 3 months before sowing and then expect a 3- to 4-week germination period. Germination varies greatly, but a good rate is 50 percent. These plants will spread, so

space them 12 to 15 inches (30–38 cm) apart. Water lightly.

SUN/SOIL: Full sun; soil that isn't too rich or moist

COMPANION/COMPLEMENTARY PLANTING: Hyssop, horehound, and southernwood are good companions.

HARVESTING: Cut aerial parts with scissors or snips in mid- to late summer.

CULINARY USE: Coyote mint honey is delicious. Drizzle some over toast for breakfast or onto a simple custard dessert.

MEDICINAL BENEFITS: Excellent for symptoms of winter illnesses, especially those of the throat; also used for respiratory tract and digestive conditions.

PARTS USED: Aerial parts (preferably in flower), fresh or dried

HOME PHARMACY USES: Infusion, traditional tincture, cider vinegar tincture, syrup, elixir, foot soak, sleep pillow, bath herb, infused oil, honey, liniment

Cutting Celery

Apium graveolens

Cutting celery is all about the leafy tops. It's a true celery, with all that great flavor, but you use the cut leaves, as you would parsley, instead of the stalks. This is an excellent seasoning herb and a must-grow plant for every windowsill herb gardener.

PERSONALITY: Biennial; herbaceous (Zones 5–9)

HEIGHT: 12 to 15 inches (30–38 cm)

BLOOM TRAITS: Clusters of white flowers in the second year during mid- to late summer

LIKES/DISLIKES: Cutting celery likes moist soil and partial shade, preferring a streamside home and moderately rich soil.

PROPAGATION/MAINTENANCE: Easily grown from seed; sow in early spring outdoors or start indoors for transplanting into the garden in late spring. Expect 80 to 90 percent germination, in about 2 weeks. Cutting celery grows in a clump. Provide moderate water, and space plants 12 inches (30 cm) apart.

SUN/SOIL: Partial to full shade; adaptable to various soil types but prefers a moderately rich soil.

COMPANION/COMPLEMENTARY PLANTING: Sorrel, watercress, and horseradish; cutting celery is a nice addition to food gardens and does well as a container herb indoors or on the patio.

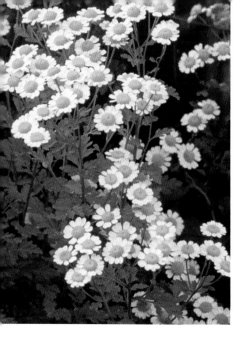

in mid-spring. Typically, feverfew germinates at a 65 to 70 percent rate and takes approximately 2 weeks to sprout. It is a vigorous, self-sowing herb, so space plants 12 inches (30 cm) apart. Water moderately.

SUN/SOIL: Full sun, partial shade; prefers a richer loamy soil, but is tolerant of most soils

COMPANION/COMPLEMENTARY PLANTING: Plant in community with anise hyssop, licorice, and monarda. It also seems to deter insects from the garden.

HARVESTING: Harvesting can include leaves only or flowering aerial parts, depending on your preference. Herbalists tend to go back and forth between the two. Most of the research was done on feverfew leaf, so I like to use the leafy parts. Scissors or snips work nicely to gather what you need.

MEDICINAL BENEFITS: Feverfew is used mainly to treat headaches, especially migraines.

PARTS USED: Leaves and flowering aerial parts, fresh or dried

HOME PHARMACY USES: Infusion, traditional tincture, cider vinegar tincture, syrup, medicinal food

Garlic

Allium sativum

One of the earliest cultivated plants, garlic has traveled the world, from Asia to the Middle East to the Americas and beyond, as one of our most important medicinal herbs and culinary seasonings.

ETHNIC AND OTHER NAMES: *Ajo* (Spanish), *Knoblauch* (German), *aglio* (Italian), *ail* (French)

PERSONALITY: Perennial or biennial; bulb (Zones 4–11)

HEIGHT: 15 to 24 inches (38–60 cm)

BLOOM TRAITS: Garlic doesn't produce the usual flowers. Instead, "scapes" make a coil and a bulbil (a cluster of mini cloves) at the top of the stalk.

LIKES/DISLIKES: Native to the steppes or grassy plains of central Asia, garlic prefers open, sunny areas.

PROPAGATION/MAINTENANCE: Plant garlic starting in early fall through the last hard frost. Break apart the individual cloves in a healthy organic bulb. Cloves are teardrop-shaped and should be planted about 4 inches apart and 1.5 to 2 inches deep in well-worked and well-drained soil. Cover with soil, then mulch the entire garlic area with 3 inches or so of fresh barley straw. Garlic is winter-hardy, if it is mulched well, and will send up tops that resemble a green onion. Water periodically throughout the winter months, if your winter is dry with periodic warm-ups. In spring, garlic will really begin to grow. Keep it well weeded for best bulb formation. Garlic stays in a clump and prefers a sunny location with moderate water.

SUN/SOIL: Full sun to partial shade; tolerant of different soil types provided they are well drained and high in organic matter

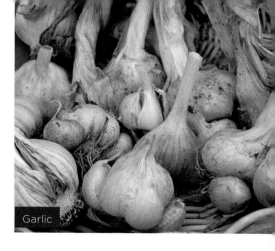

Garlic

COMPANION/COMPLEMENTARY PLANTING: Grow garlic in food gardens with costmary, winter savory, or hyssop. Aphids dislike garlic, making it a useful companion to herbs such as chamomile.

HARVESTING: Green stalks can be harvested and used fresh in cooking. Harvest bulbs in summer when the stalks have five leaves or have become yellowed. Lift the garlic from the soil, using a digging fork. Shake off excess soil gently, but do not wash the garlic. Group into bunches of four or five stems; tie with a slip-knotted string; and hang in a dry, dark, and airy location. You can also dry bulbs by laying them loosely on a screen. Garlic skins become papery and the flavor stronger as the bulbs dry. Once dry, gently rub off any lingering loose soil. Store garlic in a cool location, but protect from freezing and excess moisture. Garlic will hold approximately 6 months when properly stored.

CULINARY USE: Garlic is a must-have cooking herb. Add it to any savory dish, vegetables, and herb butter for home-baked bread.

MEDICINAL BENEFITS: Long recognized as an antimicrobial herb, garlic is also important to support heart and circulatory health.

PARTS USED: Bulb divided into individual cloves, fresh or dried

HOME PHARMACY USES: Traditional tincture, cider vinegar tincture

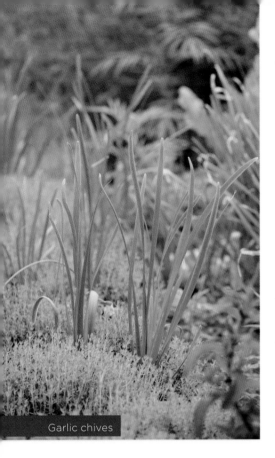

Garlic chives

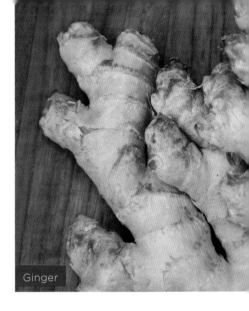

Ginger

Garlic Chives

Allium tuberosum

Stronger in flavor than typical chives, garlic or Chinese chives are a great choice for those who like a mild garlic flavor but do not want to experience a full-fledged garlic event.

ETHNIC OR OTHER NAMES: Chinese chives, *jiu-zi* (Chinese)

PERSONALITY: Perennial; herbaceous (Zones 4–9)

HEIGHT: 12 to 15 inches (30–38 cm)

BLOOM TRAITS: White star-shaped, lightly fragrant flowers in clusters. Flowering occurs any time from late spring through early fall.

LIKES/DISLIKES: Open meadow areas in temperate or subtropical climates

PROPAGATION/MAINTENANCE: Sow the seeds in spring or early summer, either directly in the garden or indoors for transplanting later. Seeds sprout in about 2 weeks and germination is high, 80 to 90 percent. Garlic chives grow in clumps spaced around 12 inches (30 cm) apart and require moderate water. Garlic chives can spread if they are growing in a moist climate, but here in Colorado, with more arid growing conditions, they seem to stay put.

SUN/SOIL: Full sun to partial shade; well-drained soil

COMPANION/COMPLEMENTARY PLANTING: Garlic chives are great windowsill or patio container herbs. They are nice in food gardens, grown with dill, sage, and parsley.

HARVESTING: Harvest the green stems or the unopened buds. Opened flower clusters may also be harvested. Cut with snips or scissors.

CULINARY USE: Garlic chives taste stronger than chives but are milder than true garlic. Use the fresh stems or unopened flower buds in stir-fries, soups, salads, and vegetable dishes. Like their chive cousins, garlic chives are used fresh or can be frozen. Dried chives are not as tasty.

EDIBLE FLOWERS: The white starry flowers are very pretty in green salads, or with tomato cucumber salad, lending a gentle garlic flavor that is delightful. Use the flowers in herb butter and spread on corn on the cob for a midsummer vegetable treat.

Ginger

Zingiber officinale

Ginger makes a nice houseplant or container herb on the patio in nontropical climates. In tropical gardens it should be planted as an understory plant, as it prefers partial to full shade.

ETHNIC AND OTHER NAMES: *Ajenjibre* (Mexican Spanish), *jengibre* (Spanish), *gingembre* (French), *Ingwer* (German), *zenzero* (Italian), *ingefära* (Swedish)

PERSONALITY: Perennial; herbaceous (Zones 9–11)

HEIGHT: 3 to 4 feet (0.9–1.2 m)

BLOOM TRAITS: Spikes are clad in waxy, yellowish green flowers with some purple on the lip. Ginger rarely flowers under cultivation.

LIKES/DISLIKES: A shade-loving plant, ginger grows in hot, moist, tropical regions.

PROPAGATION/MAINTENANCE: Propagate by planting the rhizomes. They grow in "sections" that can be broken apart easily at the joints. Look for buds, called eyes, on each section; plant a rhizome with the eyes facing up toward the soil surface. Plant rhizomes 1 to 2 inches

(2.5–5 cm) below the surface of the soil, about 15 inches (38 cm) apart. Ginger rarely produces seeds, and when seeds do form they are sterile. Ginger grows mainly in a clump and spreads slowly by rhizomes. It requires a great amount of water.

SUN/SOIL: Shade to partial shade; prefers a rich, loamy, and well-worked soil that is kept evenly moist

COMPANION/COMPLEMENTARY PLANTING: Ginger is an excellent container herb indoors in indirect light. It will also do nicely on a protected shaded patio. Grow in a shady container garden with turmeric, gotu kola, and nasturtium.

HARVESTING: A garden fork is ideal. Harvesting times depend on how the ginger will be used. For fresh preparations, harvest rhizomes between 4 and 7 months of age. The older (7 to 9 months), more pungent, and less fleshy rhizomes are harvested for dried preparations.

CULINARY USE: Fresh ginger is tasty when finely grated over steamed vegetables and rice. Dried ginger can be finely or coarsely ground in a spice grinder and then used in cookie recipes like gingersnaps and oatmeal cookies. Add 1 tablespoon of ground dried ginger to 2 cups of dry beans in the overnight presoak water to help prevent flatulence.

MEDICINAL BENEFITS: Ginger is a warming herb, often used for the circulatory and digestive systems. It is a well-known antioxidant and has anti-inflammatory properties. Ginger is used for fevers, nausea, dizziness, and headaches; as a heart tonic; and to support the male and female reproductive systems.

PARTS USED: Rhizome, fresh or dried

HOME PHARMACY USES: Infusion, traditional tincture, cider vinegar tincture, syrup, elixir, ointment, salve, cream, foot soak, bath herb, infused oil, honey, butter, liniment

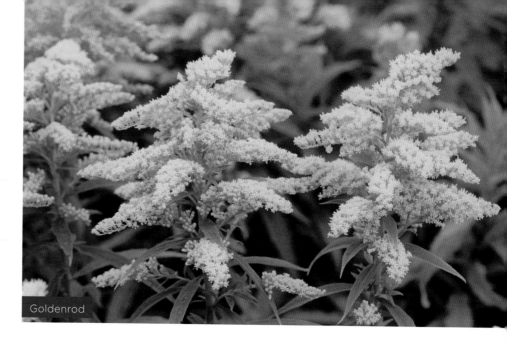
Goldenrod

Goldenrod

Solidago species

The flowers and young shoots of this stunning herb are used to create beautiful yellow dyes for cotton and wool. Goldenrod is a late-summer flower that always signals the garden's transition to the next season.

PERSONALITY: Perennial; herbaceous (Zones 4–9)

HEIGHT: 2 to 4 feet (0.6–0.9 m)

BLOOM TRAITS: Large fans of golden yellow flowers bloom in the later months of summer.

LIKES/DISLIKES: Found in a variety of habitats, goldenrod grows on prairies as well as mountains. It is commonly found near streams and lakes. It seems to prefer open spaces, and I often see it along roadsides.

PROPAGATION/MAINTENANCE: Stratify seeds in moist peat moss or sand in the refrigerator for 7 to 10 days. This method will give you reliable germination, 90 percent or better. Sow indoors and transplant outside in mid- to late spring, or sow seeds directly in the garden in early spring. Goldenrod grows in clumps and should be spaced 12 inches (30 cm) apart. Water lightly or moderately.

SUN/SOIL: Full sun; no special soil needs

COMPANION/COMPLEMENTARY PLANTING: Grow in community with red clover, catnip, and potentilla

HARVESTING: Aerial parts, while in flower, are harvested in late summer with snips or scissors.

MEDICINAL BENEFITS: Goldenrod is used primarily for conditions of the urinary and respiratory tracts. Traditionally, Native Americans have used this plant for toothache, fever, and coughs.

PARTS USED: Aerial parts in flower, fresh or dried

HOME PHARMACY USES: Infusion, traditional tincture, syrup, foot soak, bath herb, honey

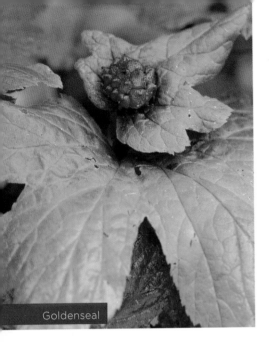

Goldenseal

Goldenseal

Hydrastis canadensis

In the United States, goldenseal is classified as an at-risk plant by the Convention on International Trade of Endangered Species (CITES). Its wild harvesting is strictly governed for export sales, but goldenseal needs more help! Many of the wild rhizomes are harvested for domestic use in the United States, and that is not nearly so closely controlled. Groups like United Plant Savers are working hard to help protect this medicinal plant from extinction in the wild. Cultivation is greatly encouraged, especially if you garden in the upper Midwest or the northeastern parts of North America.

PERSONALITY: Perennial; herbaceous (Zones 3–9)

HEIGHT: 10 to 15 inches (25–38 cm)

BLOOM TRAITS: Greenish white flowers appear in spring. Bright red berries form from the flowering parts later in the summer.

LIKES/DISLIKES: Goldenseal is a woodland plant that grows in fairly dense shade and moist, humusy soil.

PROPAGATION/MAINTENANCE: Goldenseal is often propagated by root divisions in the fall. You can also grow it from seeds, although this is more difficult. Buy seeds from a reliable source, and when they arrive, stratify them in moist sand in the refrigerator for a couple to several weeks, until the seeds sprout. Once sprouted, handle the seeds gently to avoid breaking off the tiny sprout, and plant the seeds immediately. Sow seeds in late fall or very early in spring, in a seedbed that is well shaded and not too hot. Let seedlings grow in the seedbed until the following year, then transplant them, 8 to 10 inches (20–25 cm) apart, into their permanent garden home. Goldenseal grows in clumps, and requires moderate watering.

SUN/SOIL: Shade, partial shade; prefers a humusy soil that is rich in composting hardwood tree leaves; is remarkably adaptable to a variety of soils

HARVESTING: Rhizomes are usually harvested between 4 and 6 years of age. With a garden fork, dig rhizomes in the fall rather than in the spring, so the plant has a chance to propagate itself from seed first.

MEDICINAL BENEFITS: Goldenseal is used for the acute stages of winter illnesses and respiratory conditions. It is also helpful for some skin conditions. It has been improperly used for many years as a tonic and detoxification herb, and that has seriously contributed to its threatened extinction.

PARTS USED: Rhizome, fresh or dried

HOME PHARMACY USES: Decoction, traditional tincture, syrup, elixir, ointment, salve, cream, foot soak, bath herb, infused oil, butter, liniment

Gotu Kola

Centella asiatica

Have you ever heard that elephants have an incredibly long and sharp memory? Is it a coincidence, then, that elephants often favor the memory- and brain-enhancing gotu kola?

PERSONALITY: Annual in North America, perennial in tropical climates; herbaceous (Zones 8–11)

HEIGHT: 6 to 8 inches (15–20 cm)

BLOOM TRAITS: Greenish flowers that sit underneath the leaves are barely visible. They bloom in early spring.

LIKES/DISLIKES: Grown as a garden plant in temperate climates. In tropical climates or where it grows wild, it is found along open ditches with good exposure to moisture.

PROPAGATION/MAINTENANCE: Gotu kola is difficult to grow from seed; greater success is had when it is grown from layerings or root divisions. I find that root divisions are the easiest method, and the most successful, but layering also works well. When doing root divisions, simply separate the parent into several divisions and plant those into individual pots. The newly divided tiny plants must be kept moist but not overly wet. Night temperatures should be near 70°F (21°C), with daytime temperatures 80 to 90°F (26–36°C).

Gotu kola also grows very nicely as a hanging houseplant. This herb is sprawling, and it roots wherever its stems make contact with soil. Space 10 inches (25 cm) apart and water well and often.

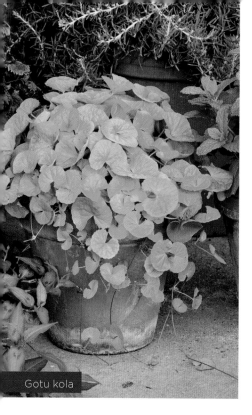

Gotu kola

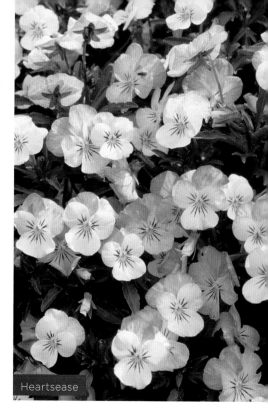

Heartsease

Viola tricolor, V. cornuta

This charming herb just makes you feel happy. Hundreds of years ago, in Europe, it was considered a symbolic romantic herb for couples.

COMMON VARIETIES: 'Arkwright Ruby', 'Bowles' Black', 'King Henry', 'Helen Mount', 'Azurella'

ETHNIC AND OTHER NAMES: Johnny-jump-up, wild pansy

PERSONALITY: Annual, short-lived perennial (Zones 4–9)

HEIGHT: 4 to 8 inches (10–20 cm)

BLOOM TRAITS: Flowers range in color from blues and purples, whites and creams, to yellows, pinks, maroons, deep violet, and bicolor/tricolor versions. Plants bloom throughout the year in mild winter conditions, though flowering does slow during the very hottest part of the summer months.

LIKES/DISLIKES: This little plant is not at all fussy. It will grow in open, sunny areas that are not too hot, or in shady treed places. Because of its self-sowing nature, it readily naturalizes.

PROPAGATION/MAINTENANCE: Sow seeds at any time of the year, when temperatures are warm to mildly cool. Germination takes between 1 and 2 weeks and is around 80 percent. Seeds do not germinate as well at very hot temperatures. Either direct-sow the seeds in the garden or transplant young plants into the garden in early spring through early summer or again in fall. Heartsease easily reseeds. Space plants about 8 inches (20 cm) apart. Provide moderate to heavy water.

Heartsease

SUN/SOIL: Partial shade to full sun; prefers a rich garden loam, but will grow in almost any well-worked soil

HARVESTING: Harvest at any time during the hot growing season for outdoor plants. If you are growing plants indoors or in a greenhouse, you can harvest year-round. Use small snips or scissors to harvest the aerial parts.

CULINARY USE: Fresh gotu kola leaves can be used like any leafy green in salad or as a lettuce substitute on sandwiches or in tacos.

MEDICINAL BENEFITS: Traditionally used as a tonic herb that supports skin health and brain health by promoting good memory and concentration, gotu kola is also being researched for its anticancer properties for the skin.

PARTS USED: Aerial parts, fresh or dried

HOME PHARMACY USES: Infusion, traditional tincture, cider vinegar tincture, syrup, elixir, ointment, salve, cream, foot soak, bath herb, infused oil, honey

SUN/SOIL: Partial shade preferred, but will tolerate both full sun and full shade; no special soil needs

HARVESTING: Flowers and leaves, gently hand-picked

MEDICINAL BENEFITS: Supportive for skin conditions, anti-inflammatory benefits, and as a soothing sore throat gargle

PARTS USED: Leaves, fresh or dried

HOME PHARMACY USES: Infusion, traditional tincture, skin wash, throat gargle, syrup, ointment, salve, cream, foot soak, bath herb, honey, liniment

EDIBLE FLOWERS: The flowers are beautiful in green or fruit salads, cream cheese spreads and herb butter, and crystallized. Float them in lemonade and iced tea; use them to decorate cakes, too.

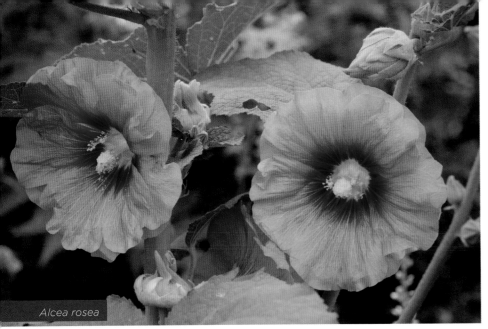
Alcea rosea

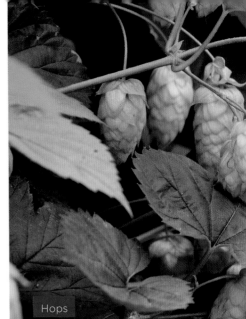
Hops

Hollyhock

Alcea rosea, A. rosea var. *nigra,*
  A. rugosa

Many people grow hollyhock in their gardens, but not many folks realize that this plant has edible flowers as well as medicinal properties in its flowers, leaves, and roots. Enjoy both its beauty and its health benefits.

COMMON VARIETIES OF HOLLYHOCK: 'Old Fashioned Pink', 'Chaters', 'Black Heirloom', 'Outhouse Classic'

PERSONALITY: Biennial; herbaceous (Zones 3–9). Yellow hollyhock (*Alcea rugosa*) is the only perennial kind.

HEIGHT: 6 to 8 feet (1.8–2.4 m)

BLOOM TRAITS: Flowers mainly in pinks, reds, whites, and yellows, but also a black-flowered form originally grown by Thomas Jefferson. Blooming begins in midsummer and often continues until early fall.

LIKES/DISLIKES: Hollyhocks are grown throughout the temperate parts of the world.

PROPAGATION/MAINTENANCE: You'll get more consistent results if you stratify seeds for a few weeks and then sow indoors. Germination is about 70 percent, and sprouting takes place in about 2 weeks. Transplant outside after danger of frost is past. I germinate them at a nighttime temperature of 70°F (21°C). Space 15 inches (38 cm) apart; plants will grow in clumps. Water moderately.

SUN/SOIL: Prefers full sun and loamy soil; adaptable

COMPANION/COMPLEMENTARY PLANTING: Grow with licorice, lemon balm, and feverfew.

HARVESTING: Leaves are hand-picked or snipped at any time during the growing season. Hand-pick flowers when in bloom. Dig up roots with a needle-nose spade in late summer or early fall.

MEDICINAL BENEFITS: Used for the gastrointestinal tract and as a soothing herb for throat conditions

PARTS USED: Leaves, flowers, and roots, fresh or dried

HOME PHARMACY USES: Decoction, traditional tincture, ointment, salve, cream

EDIBLE FLOWERS: Hollyhock flowers are beautiful added to green leafy or fruit salads. Use the flowers whole or pull off the petals and scatter them in a dish. You can also decorate cakes with them.

Hops

Humulus lupulus

Resins in hops are strong after a morning of picking; enough of them may be absorbed through the skin to make you feel very relaxed, perhaps even ready for a nap. High-quality, insect-free, certified organic hops are difficult to find. Give this herb a sturdy fence, trellis, or building to climb in the garden and it will make itself at home.

ETHNIC AND OTHER NAMES: *Hopfen* (German), *luppolo* (Italian), *houblon* (French), *lúpulo* (Spanish)

PERSONALITY: Perennial; herbaceous, vining (Zones 4–8)

HEIGHT: 8 feet (2.39 m) and taller

BLOOM TRAITS: Green strobiles, which are the hops' flowers and look a bit like a papery green pine cone, are abundant by late summer.

LIKES/DISLIKES: Hops grow in disturbed soil, vining onto structures, trees, and fences.

PROPAGATION/MAINTENANCE: Root divisions are best. Seed germinates very poorly and sporadically over

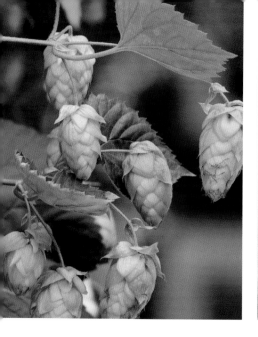

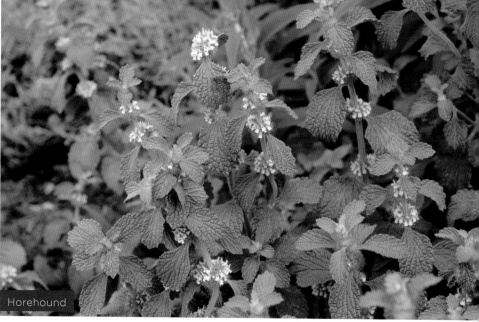

Horehound

6 to 8 weeks, often with only a 5 to 10 percent success rate. Stratifying seeds for 3 to 6 months and then soaking them overnight in warm water before sowing may help. Hops can also be propagated by cuttings or by layering; tip cuttings are less successful than layering. Hops spread easily by root runners, and stems root every place they make contact with the soil. Space plants 6 to 8 feet (1.8–2.4 m) apart; a strong trellis system will be required. Do not plant with less vigorous herbs. Water moderately to heavily.

SUN/SOIL: Sun, partial shade; prefers normal to rich garden soil, but will tolerate poorer soils

HARVESTING: Handpick strobiles (flowers) when they are fully developed but still goldish green (not tan).

MEDICINAL BENEFITS: Used as a sleep aid and to relive pain, hops are strong, so use them carefully.

PARTS USED: Strobiles, fresh or dried

HOME PHARMACY USES: Infusion, traditional tincture, sleep pillow, bath herb, foot soak

Horehound

Marrubium vulgare

This plant, often an ingredient in old-fashioned cough syrups and cough drops, is excellent bee fodder, especially in high mountain desert climates. Of course, bees are welcome creatures because they are essential garden pollinators.

ETHNIC AND OTHER NAMES: *Marrubio* (Spanish)

PERSONALITY: Perennial; herbaceous (Zones 3–8)

HEIGHT: 12 to 24 inches (30–60 cm)

BLOOM TRAITS: Blooms from July till frost, with small white flowers

LIKES/DISLIKES: Commonly found in grasslands, prairies, pastures, and meadows, horehound grows in dry, sandy wash areas, in rocky soil, and in juniper forests.

PROPAGATION/MAINTENANCE: Horehound is easily propagated from seed. No special treatment is required and seeds germinate in 2 to 3 weeks, consistently at 70 to 80 percent. Transplant outdoors in mid- to late spring. Tip cuttings and root divisions (see chapter 4)

are also methods to propagate horehound. Horehound will not grow well if overwatered. It grows in clumps and readily reseeds. To prevent too many volunteer seedlings, cut back horehound to 3 inches above the ground once flowering is finished and before seeds mature and drop. Space plants 12 inches (30 cm) apart.

SUN/SOIL: Full sun; poorer soil is preferred.

COMPANION/COMPLEMENTARY PLANTING: Horehound grows nicely with thyme, rosemary, and feverfew.

HARVESTING: Harvest anytime during the growing season. Aerial parts are harvested with snips.

MEDICINAL BENEFITS: This herb is used to relieve symptoms of winter illnesses, especially coughing.

PARTS USED: Aerial parts, fresh or dried

HOME PHARMACY USES: Traditional tincture, syrup, infusion, honey, elixir

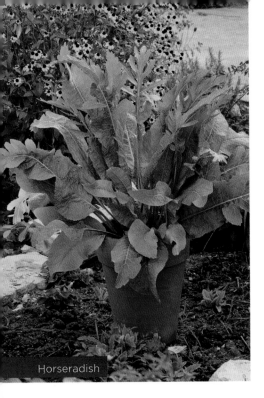

Horseradish

Horseradish

Armoracia rusticana

Horseradish has been cultivated for hundreds of years — so long, in fact, that no one seems to know for sure what part of the world it is indigenous to.

ETHNIC OR OTHER NAMES: *Raifort* (French), *Meerrettich* or *Kren* (German), *rafano* (Italian), *rabano picante* (Spanish), *pepparrot* (Swedish)

PERSONALITY: Perennial; herbaceous (Zones 4–9)

HEIGHT: 2 to 3 feet (0.6–0.9 m)

BLOOM TRAITS: It is rare to see horseradish in bloom, but when it is, it produces white flowers.

LIKES/DISLIKES: Horseradish prefers an open sunny area that is not too dry. Found in the wild, it would most likely choose a moist, open meadow.

PROPAGATION/MAINTENANCE: The best way to propagate horseradish is by root divisions; the plant does not produce seed. Dig a portion of root and remove the loose soil. Cut the root into pieces, 1 to 2 inches in length, and set about 1 inch deep in moist soil, either directly in the garden or in pots. Nearly every piece of root will sprout into a new plant within 4 weeks. A word of caution: Each sliver of root will potentially take, so don't carelessly spread bits of root around in the garden or you'll end up with a horseradish forest! Horseradish grows in a large clump, so space plants about 3 feet (0.9 m) apart. Provide moderate to high water.

SUN/SOIL: Full sun preferred but will tolerate dappled shade; adaptable to different soil types

COMPANION/COMPLEMENTARY PLANTING: Horseradish is perfect as a permanent occupant of food gardens. It can easily be grown in a container that is 15 to 24 inches (38–60 cm) deep by patio gardeners and those not wanting to risk it spreading in the garden. Grow in the herb garden with garlic, sorrel, and red clover.

HARVESTING: Harvest roots any time ground can be worked. The roots are large and deep, so use a needle-nose spade or a garden fork.

CULINARY USE: The roots are spicy-hot and delicious made into a sauce and served with roast beef or pork. A small amount of grated fresh horseradish root is also tasty on steamed vegetables or sprinkled on a baked potato with sour cream.

MEDICINAL BENEFITS: The root is excellent for the upper respiratory tract and winter illness and flu symptoms.

PART USED: Root, fresh only

HOME PHARMACY USES: Traditional tincture, cider vinegar tincture, foot soak, honey

Hyssop

Hyssopus officinalis

Many herbs carry the common name hyssop, but most of them are actually members of the genus Agastache. They should not be confused with this true hyssop, which is a beautiful herb useful both medicinally and as a tasty tea.

COMMON VARIETIES: 'Nector Pink', 'Nector White'

PERSONALITY: Perennial; woody (Zones 4–9)

HEIGHT: 12 to 15 inches (30–38 cm)

BLOOM TRAITS: Deep blue flowers on spikes, similar to lavender, bloom from mid- through late summer, sometimes into early fall.

LIKES/DISLIKES: This herb is native to the Mediterranean region and prefers sunny, open areas.

PROPAGATION/MAINTENANCE: Hyssop is easy to grow from seed. Sow seeds indoors in early spring. Germination, at around 80 percent, occurs in about 2 weeks. Transplant outdoors in mid- to late spring. Hyssop grows in clumps and should be spaced 12 inches (30 cm) apart. Provide low to moderate water.

SUN/SOIL: Full sun to partial shade; well-drained, poorer types of soils

COMPANION/COMPLEMENTARY PLANTING: Hyssop likes a community of lavender, rosemary, garlic chives, and catmint.

HARVESTING: Aerial parts, with or without flowers. Use snips or scissors to harvest.

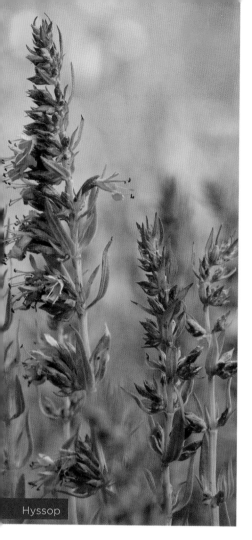

Hyssop

Lady's Mantle

Alchemilla vulgaris

This pretty herb was named in the Middle Ages as a reference to the Virgin Mary. It is beautiful in a shady herb garden, with chartreuse flowers and scalloped leaves that hold the morning dew.

PERSONALITY: Perennial; herbaceous (Zones 5–7)

HEIGHT: 12 to 15 inches (30–38 cm)

BLOOM TRAITS: Clusters of chartreuse flowers from late spring through early summer

LIKES/DISLIKES: Lady's mantle prefers a moist and shady habitat, making it excellent under trees in the garden.

PROPAGATION/MAINTENANCE: Sow seeds in late winter or very early spring in the greenhouse and transplant into the garden in late spring or early summer, when temperatures are not yet too hot. Expect 50 to 60 percent germination, in 3 to 4 weeks. Lady's mantle grows in a clump. Space plants 12 to 15 inches (30–38 cm) apart in full to part shade, with moderate water.

SUN/SOIL: Full to part shade; rich garden soil is preferred, but tolerant of clay or sandy soils that are rich in organic matter

COMPANION/COMPLEMENTARY PLANTING: Breadseed poppy, red-veined sorrel, salad burnet

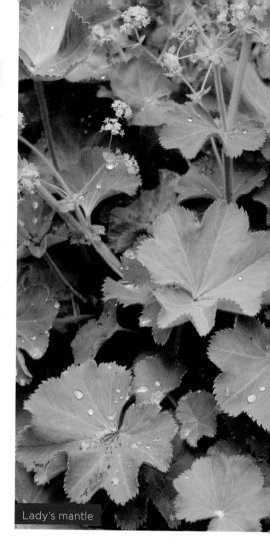

Lady's mantle

MEDICINAL BENEFITS: Hyssop is favored for its minty flavor, as a support for good digestion, and for its mild antimicrobial benefits. It is also used as an expectorant to soothe a cough.

PARTS USED: Aerial parts, with or without flowers, fresh or dried

HOME PHARMACY USES: Infusion, traditional tincture, syrup, elixir, foot soak, honey

EDIBLE FLOWERS: The blue flowers are very pretty for decorating cakes, or add to green and fruit salads for an unusual color.

HARVESTING: Harvest all the aerial parts, in flower or not, using a pair of snips or scissors.

MEDICINAL BENEFITS: Used as a strong astringent topically for the skin and for women's health concerns

PARTS USED: Aerial parts, with or without flowers, fresh or dried

HOME PHARMACY USES: Infusion, traditional tincture, ointment, cream, foot soak, bath herb, infused oil, liniment

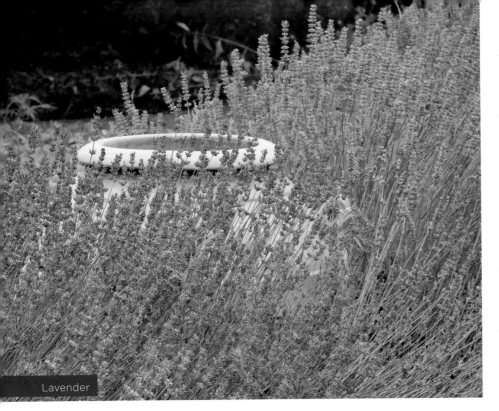
Lavender

Lavender

Lavandula species

Most of us are familiar with the fragrance of lavender, but it is also a fantastic culinary and medicinal plant that has a multitude of applications. The leaves, stems, and flowers are all valuable, making the plant available for harvesting throughout the growing season.

COMMON VARIETIES: French (*L. dentata*), Spanish (*L. stoechas*), and 'Spanish Eyes' (*L. multifida*) are tender perennials (Zones 8–9). 'Provence', 'Hidcote', 'Munstead', and 'Grosso' are hardy perennial (Zones 5–7) varieties of *L. angustifolia* and *L. × intermedia*.

ETHNIC AND OTHER NAMES: *Alhucema* (Spanish)

PERSONALITY: Perennial or tender perennial (depending on species); woody subshrub (Zones 5–8)

HEIGHT: 24 inches (60 cm); varies somewhat depending on the species

BLOOM TRAITS: Varieties of lavender have purple to deep blue flowers, or sometimes pink or even white flowers, and may bloom from early summer to the end of the season.

LIKES/DISLIKES: Lavender prefers dry soil and a sunny, hot environment similar to that of its native Mediterranean region.

PROPAGATION/MAINTENANCE: Seeds should be stratified for 1 to 2 weeks and then sown indoors. Transplant outdoors in mid- to late spring. Germination usually takes 2 to 3 weeks and is about 50 percent. Lavender may be propagated by cuttings, but don't overwater. Liquid or powder rooting hormone helps speed up the rooting process. Warm nighttime temperatures of about 70°F (21°C) and good air circulation will also help cuttings to root more quickly. Lavender grows in clumps and should be spaced 12 to 15 inches (30–38 cm) apart. Water lightly.

SUN/SOIL: Full sun or afternoon shade; well-drained soil is mandatory.

COMPANION/COMPLEMENTARY PLANTING: Grow with echinacea, winter savory, hyssop, and yarrow.

HARVESTING: Harvest leaves and/or flowers with snips at any point during the summer. Cut stems to about 3 inches (7.5 cm) above the ground. If just the flowers are being used in cooking or crafting, harvest carefully with a small pair of scissors: avoid inadvertently cutting into the stem and leaves.

CULINARY USE: Leaves and flowers make an interesting addition to a green salad.

MEDICINAL BENEFITS: Lavender is versatile and recommended for women's and children's health, nervous system conditions, and pain relief. Lavender is very good for skin health, especially for treating burns and acne, as well as moisturizing and toning the skin.

PARTS USED: Aerial parts, fresh or dried

HOME PHARMACY USES: Infusion, traditional tincture, cider vinegar tincture, syrup, elixir, ointment, salve, cream, foot soak, sleep pillow, bath herb, infused oil, honey, butter, liniment, insect repellent

EDIBLE FLOWERS: Put some flowers in vegetable and fruit salads, and incorporate into herb butters and cream cheese spreads. Adding lavender flowers to shortbread cookies will make you famous, and honey infused with lavender flowers is a special treat.

CRAFTING: Lavender has long been a popular ingredient in herbal body care products and aromatherapy applications. Use the flowers and leaves in sachets, sleep pillows, lavender wands, and bath herb blends. They will bring beauty and fragrance to every part of your home.

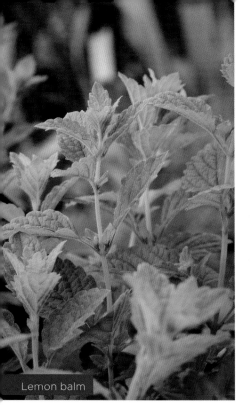

Lemon balm

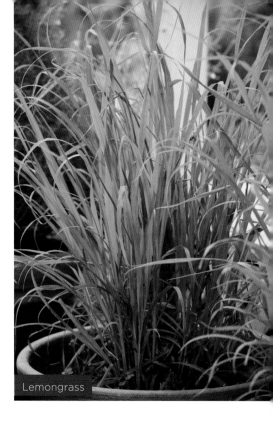

Lemongrass

late spring. Seed germination is 60 to 70 percent and takes about 14 days. Tip cuttings may also be done; dip the stem ends in a liquid or powder rooting hormone before planting. Lemon balm grows in clumps and should be spaced 12 inches (30 cm) apart. This herb reseeds vigorously. Water moderately.

SUN/SOIL: Full sun, partial shade; well-drained soil

COMPANION/COMPLEMENTARY PLANTING: Grow with hollyhock, angelica, and nasturtiums, and in food gardens. Lemon balm is also a great container-grown herb.

HARVESTING: Harvest aerial parts at any time during the growing season. Snips or scissors will work nicely. If you cut only the upper half of the plant, it will quickly regenerate, giving you several harvest cuts over the course of a summer.

Lemon Balm

Melissa officinalis

Lemon balm was the first herb I ever grew. A neighbor gave me a plant as a gift, and I had no idea what an impact it would have on my life. This wonderfully versatile herb has been used for centuries.

ETHNIC AND OTHER NAMES: Melissa, balm, sweet balm, *toronjil* (Spanish)

PERSONALITY: Perennial; herbaceous (Zones 4–9)

HEIGHT: 24 inches (60 cm)

BLOOM TRAITS: Lemon balm has small white flowers that are not especially showy; it blooms on and off throughout the summer months.

LIKES/DISLIKES: Lemon balm is Mediterranean in origin. It prefers a warm climate that is not too wet.

PROPAGATION/MAINTENANCE: Easiest grown from seed that has been stratified at least 1 week. Start indoors, then transplant outside in

CULINARY USE: Lemon balm is delicious added to cream cheese to spread over bagels or pancakes. Freshly chopped leaves can be lightly sprinkled in fruit salad for a lemony flavor. Better yet . . . sprinkle freshly chopped leaves over vanilla ice cream and then drizzle the whole thing with chocolate syrup. Scrumptious.

MEDICINAL BENEFITS: Used for the entire body, lemon balm is beneficial for the digestive tract, children's health, winter illnesses, and to strengthen the immune system. It is recommended for pain relief and nervous system health, and is considered a great stress reliever.

PARTS USED: Aerial parts, fresh or dried. *Note:* The dried plant loses some of its potency after 6 months.

HOME PHARMACY USES: Infusion, traditional tincture, cider vinegar tincture, syrup, elixir, ointment, salve, cream, foot soak, bath herb, infused oil, honey, liniment

Lemongrass

Cymbopogon flexuosus, C. citratus

Lemongrass is a plant of strong economic value in Guatemala. Much of the plant material grown and exported from that country, however, is sprayed heavily with toxic chemicals. Grow your own lemongrass to be sure it is free of unhealthy chemical residues.

ETHNIC AND OTHER NAMES: *Té de limón* (Spanish)

PERSONALITY: Tender perennial; herbaceous (Zones 8–11)

HEIGHT: 3 to 4 feet (0.9–1.2 m)

BLOOM TRAITS: No specific blooms

LIKES/DISLIKES: Lemongrass is a tropical plant native to Sri Lanka and the Seychelles and is used primarily for farming and gardening. It prefers a climate that is moist and hot, but will tolerate warm, dry climates if it is watered regularly.

PROPAGATION/MAINTENANCE: Root divisions work fairly well for West Indian lemongrass (*C. citratus*), which rarely produces viable seed. This species does require a lot of mother plants to yield very many new plantlets, as each mother plant will only divide into a few new plantlets. I have found that East Indian lemongrass (*C. flexuosus*) is best grown from seed. Both varieties do beautifully in our hot greenhouse, providing we keep them well watered. Germination for East Indian lemongrass is about 90 percent; seeds take only a few days to sprout. In temperate climates, transplant outdoors after all frost danger has passed and bring back indoors early in fall before the first frost. Lemongrass is a perennial in tropical climates. It grows in clumps and should be given moderate to large amounts of water. Space plants 12 to 15 inches (30–38 cm) apart.

SUN/SOIL: Full sun, partial shade, shade; prefers a moist, loamy soil

COMPANION/COMPLEMENTARY PLANTING: Lemongrass complements lemon verbena, passionflower, and gotu kola in a garden environment. It is an excellent container plant.

HARVESTING: All of the aerial parts may be harvested from mid- to late summer. The summer heat concentrates the oils and increases the intensity of the flavor.

CULINARY USE: Leafy parts of lemongrass are delicious brewed into tea. The leaves are equally tasty in vegetable soup and in rice.

MEDICINAL BENEFITS: Lemongrass supports a healthy digestive tract, and has some anti-inflammatory benefits.

PARTS USED: Aerial parts, fresh or dried

HOME PHARMACY USES: Infusion, cider vinegar tincture, foot soak, sleep pillow, bath herb, infused oil, honey

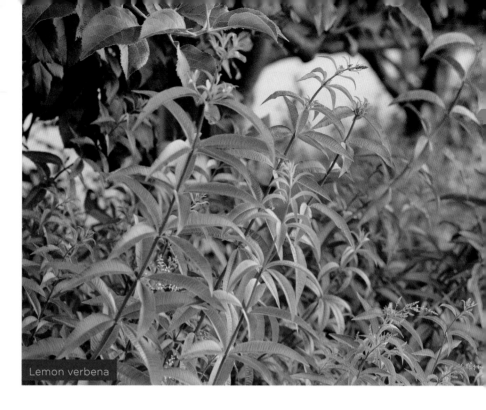

Lemon verbena

Lemon Verbena

Aloysia triphylla

Lemon verbena is very fragrant, strong-tasting, and quite delicious. It is a primary ingredient in herbal tea. Harvest the leaves and dry them carefully to preserve the lemony volatile oils that give this herb its wonderful flavor.

PERSONALITY: Tender perennial; woody (Zones 8–11)

HEIGHT: 3 to 4 feet (0.9–1.2 m)

BLOOM TRAITS: Delicate, fragrant white flowers bloom in mid- to late summer.

LIKES/DISLIKES: A tropical plant that is only a garden guest for subtropical and temperate regions, it is an extensive farm crop in some tropical areas.

PROPAGATION/MAINTENANCE: Take softwood tip cuttings and use liquid or powder rooting hormone. Cuttings require extra heat; we keep night temperatures at 65 to 70°F (18–21°C) and daytime temperatures in the high 80s and 90s (30–37°C). Provide good air circulation, and keep cuttings consistently moist. Rooting percentage varies greatly with sunlight exposure and temperature. Put cuttings under lights for 14 to 20 hours per day while rooting. Transplant outdoors only after weather is warm and well settled in temperate climates. Bring indoors before fall frost. In tropical climates, lemon verbena is grown year-round. It forms clumps; plants should be spaced 12 to 15 inches (30–38 cm) apart. Provide it with moderate to large amounts of water.

SUN/SOIL: Sun, partial shade; prefers rich soil, but will tolerate poor soil if given enough water and fish emulsion fertilizer

COMPANION/COMPLEMENTARY PLANTING: Lemon verbena does very nicely in a container either as a patio plant or indoors in bright light. In mild climates, it is lovely planted in the garden with gotu kola, breadseed poppies, and shiso. It is also a nice inclusion in food gardens, both veggie and fruit.

HARVESTING: Cut aerial parts, with snips, in mid- to late summer. Dry, then strip leaves from stems. Discard stems. Leaves may be handpicked; use immediately after harvest.

CULINARY USE: The leaves are wonderful for sun tea, or add them to a pitcher of fresh water and infuse it gently in the fridge for a refreshing drink on a hot summer day. Lemon verbena leaves and flowers can be infused in honey to make a tasty drizzle over ice cream or custard.

MEDICINAL BENEFITS: Used as a soothing digestive tea and as a calming sleep herb, it is also a common ingredient in herbal insect repellents.

PARTS USED: Leaves and flowers, fresh or dried

HOME PHARMACY USES: Infusion, cider vinegar tincture, elixir, honey, insect repellent

EDIBLE FLOWERS: The flowers are fragrant and very pretty added to a green salad or a fruit salad.

CRAFTING: The fragrance of lemon verbena flowers and leaves is amazing and makes a fantastic ingredient in sachet blends and herbal bath blends.

Licorice

Glycyrrhiza glabra

Licorice is one of nature's sweeteners; you can use it in beverages and oatmeal, or as a garnish.

ETHNIC AND OTHER NAMES: *Réglisse* (French), *Lakritze* (German), *regolizia* (Italian)

PERSONALITY: Tender perennial; herbaceous (Zones 9–11)

HEIGHT: 4 to 5 feet (1.2–1.5 m)

BLOOM TRAITS: Stunning lavender and white flowers bloom in mid- to late summer.

LIKES/DISLIKES: Licorice is a Mediterranean plant by nature and prefers a hot and somewhat arid climate.

PROPAGATION/MAINTENANCE: Seeds must be stratified for several weeks. Just before sowing, scarify them and then soak for 2 hours in warm water. Sow immediately, preferably indoors, and then transplant outside in mid- to late spring. Outdoor sowing is possible, but results are much less predictable. My experience is that seed, once stratified, scarified, and soaked, will germinate at a rate of 70 to 80 percent, whereas untreated seed achieves only a 20 percent success rate. Sprouting normally takes about 2 weeks. Each year licorice will die back in the winter and come up vigorously in late spring. The plant will gradually get larger over time; space 24 inches (60 cm) apart. I usually harvest older licorice and start over with small plants. Water moderately.

SUN/SOIL: Full sun, partial shade; well-drained soil

HARVESTING: Harvest licorice rhizomes in the third year of

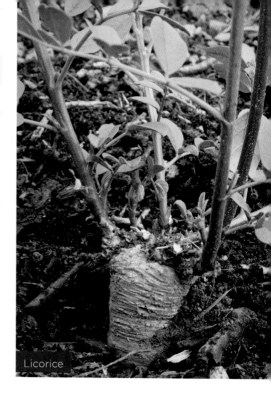
Licorice

growth. Use a needle-nose spade to lift them out of the soil. They are normally quite large, even in our clay soil, and require a fair amount of energy to dig. Harvest in spring or fall.

CULINARY USE: This herb is a wonderful sweetener for any food where a licorice flavor combines with sweet, but use a light hand, as licorice root is often said to be 100 times sweeter than table sugar. Kids often really like oatmeal cereal or lemon balm tea sweetened lightly with licorice.

MEDICINAL BENEFITS: Licorice is a fine tonic herb for winter illnesses and immune system, digestive tract, respiratory tract, and adrenal gland support. It is also excellent for children's health. Some people will be advised to avoid licorice; consult a reliable herbal reference for details.

PARTS USED: Rhizome, fresh or dried

HOME PHARMACY USES: Decoction, traditional tincture, syrup, elixir, honey

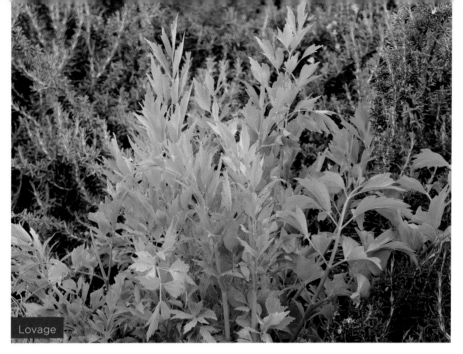

Lovage

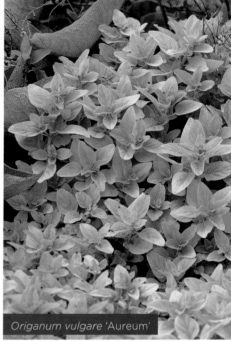

Origanum vulgare 'Aureum'

Lovage

Levisticum officinale

Lovage has been used for cooking and in herbal medicine since Roman times. It is now found in temperate gardens around the world.

ETHNIC AND OTHER NAMES: Garden osha (not true osha, which is *Ligusticum porteri*), *céleri bâtard* (French)

PERSONALITY: Perennial; herbaceous (Zones 5–8)

HEIGHT: 2 to 3 feet (0.6–0.9 m)

BLOOM TRAITS: Umbels of white flowers appear in late spring to early summer.

LIKES/DISLIKES: Native to mountainous regions of southern Europe and common in the Mediterranean area

PROPAGATION/MAINTENANCE: Stratify seeds for 1 to 2 weeks and then sow indoors. Expect near 50 percent germination, which takes about 2 weeks. Transplant this clump-grower outdoors, 24 inches (60 cm) apart, in mid- to late spring. Water moderately.

SUN/SOIL: Sun, shade, partial shade; needs well-drained soil

COMPANION/COMPLEMENTARY PLANTING: Grow lovage with fennel, hyssop, and catmint, or in a food garden.

HARVESTING: Harvest the roots in spring or fall with a needle-nose spade or garden fork. Hand-pick or snip the leaves and stems at any point during the growing season. With a pair of snips or scissors, cut off the seed umbels when fully ripened (late summer or early fall). Gently rub off the seeds between your palms.

CULINARY USE: Lovage is a really good celery substitute in soups, potato salad, stuffing for poultry dishes, and wherever a strong celery flavor is desired. Use fresh leaves and stems or dried seeds.

MEDICINAL BENEFITS: Excellent for treating winter illnesses and respiratory tract concerns

PARTS USED: Roots, leaves, stems, and seeds, used fresh or dried

HOME PHARMACY USES: Infusion, decoction, traditional tincture, cider vinegar tincture, syrup, elixir, foot soak, bath herb, honey

Marjoram
(Sweet, Za'atar, Wild)

Origanum majorana, O. syriaca, O. vulgare

Marjorams are close cousins to oregano, but they are different enough to be thought of separately.

ETHNIC AND OTHER NAMES: *E'zov* (Hebrew for za'atar marjoram), *marjolaine* (French)

PERSONALITY: Tender perennial; herbaceous (Zones 9–10)

HEIGHT: 12 to 24 inches (30–60 cm)

BLOOM TRAITS: Delicate white, occasionally lavender, flowers from mid- to late summer

LIKES/DISLIKES: Marjorams tend to grow in sunny open areas, in sandy or gravelly soils. They do not survive frosts, and must be handled as annuals or windowsill herbs in colder climates.

PROPAGATION/MAINTENANCE: Grow all species of marjoram from seed. Most have high germination rates of nearly 80 to 90 percent, although za'atar marjoram (*O. syriaca*) germinates at around 70

percent. Expect germination in less than 2 weeks. Za'atar marjoram can also be grown from tip cuttings, but this is more difficult, as the cuttings rot easily if overwatered. If you are taking cuttings, use liquid or powder rooting hormone to facilitate the process, and keep the cuttings in a warm location. Transplant marjoram outdoors after all danger of frost is past. Space about 12 inches (30 cm) apart and provide low to moderate water.

SUN/SOIL: Full sun to partial shade; best are well-drained soils with high organic matter

COMPANION/COMPLEMENTARY PLANTING: Marjorams are great combined with garlic chives, sage, rosemary, and chamomile. They thrive in containers both indoors and outdoors during warm months, but do not overwater them in pots.

HARVESTING: Aerial parts, with or without flowers, using snips or scissors

CULINARY USE: Marjorams are often used with meats, especially poultry and sausage. They are also quite good added lightly to potato dishes. Za'atar marjoram is used in Middle Eastern countries to season lentils, potatoes, and stews.

MEDICINAL BENEFITS: Marjoram is supportive of digestion and has antiseptic properties.

PARTS USED: Aerial parts, fresh or dried

HOME PHARMACY USES: Infusion, traditional tincture, skin wash, foot wash, honey

Marsh Mallow

Althaea officinalis

In the late 1800s, a confection called marshmallow was made from the roots of this herb. The roots were cooked with sugar and whipped until they were light and airy. Although the resulting sweet treat was different from the modern-day marshmallow (which is made up mostly of corn syrup), this is where that campfire favorite originated.

ETHNIC AND OTHER NAMES: *Pâte de guimauve* (French)

PERSONALITY: Perennial; herbaceous (Zones 5–8)

HEIGHT: 3 to 4 feet (0.9–1.2 m)

BLOOM TRAITS: Very pale pink flowers bloom up the stalk from mid- to late summer.

LIKES/DISLIKES: Marsh mallow prefers open meadows near streams, lakes, or ponds.

PROPAGATION/MAINTENANCE: Stratify seeds for several weeks. Plant seeds outside as soon as the soil can be worked. They can also be sown indoors and transplanted outside in mid- to late spring. Expect good germination of 70 to 80 percent. Sprouting takes 2 to 3 weeks. Marsh mallow will grow in clumps, and should be spaced 12 inches (30 cm) apart. Water moderately.

SUN/SOIL: Sun, partial shade, shade; prefers a loamy soil, but like many herbs is quite adaptable

HARVESTING: Harvest the roots in spring or fall. They are large and deep, so use a needle-nose spade or a garden fork. Leaves and flowers may be hand-picked at any time during the growing season.

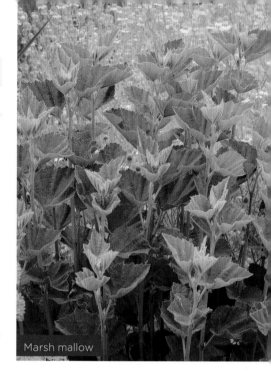

Marsh mallow

CULINARY USE: Cook the roots as you cook carrots — delicious baked with a beef roast or chicken. They can also be peeled and chopped into a vegetable soup. Young leaves can be used, alongside spinach and lettuces, in salads.

MEDICINAL BENEFITS: A soothing herb for the gastrointestinal tract, urinary tract, and throat, marsh mallow is often used for winter illnesses and to relieve skin conditions.

PARTS USED: Roots, leaves, and flowers, fresh or dried

HOME PHARMACY USES: Infusion, decoction, traditional tincture, cider vinegar tincture, syrup, elixir, ointment, salve, cream, infused oil, honey

EDIBLE FLOWERS: The flowers are simple and very sweet, making them the perfect decoration atop frosted tea cakes for a proper English tea party. They are also pretty added into salads.

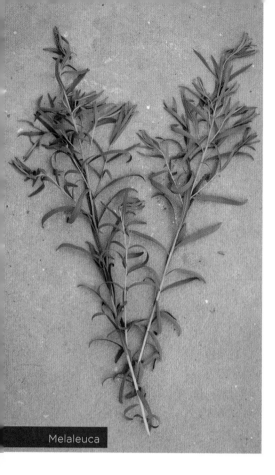

Melaleuca

Melaleuca, Tea Tree

Melaleuca alternifolia

This Australian tree yields tea tree oil, which has become well recognized for its strong antimicrobial and antiseptic properties. It is found in products ranging from toothpaste to household cleaning supplies.

PERSONALITY: Tender perennial; woody (Zones 8–10)

HEIGHT: 10 feet (3 m) or more

BLOOM TRAITS: Feathery white flower spikes

LIKES/DISLIKES: Prefers moist, sunny, open areas that are protected somewhat from windy conditions

PROPAGATION/MAINTENANCE: Sow tiny seeds and press into soil or cover ever so lightly with fine soil. Keep moist and germinate at temperatures of 60 to 70°F (15–21°C). Transplant into the garden in warm-climate regions and space 6 feet (1.8 meters) apart. In cooler climates, grow as a container tree in a pot at least 15 inches (38 cm) in diameter. If container trees get too tall, cut them back to 12 inches (30 cm) above the pot's edge.

SUN/SOIL: Full sun to partial shade; light, well-drained and rich soil

HARVESTING: Softwood (young) leafy branch tips can be harvested with snips or scissors.

MEDICINAL BENEFITS: Highly antimicrobial and antiseptic in nature; use topically for cuts and scrapes or as a mouthwash for bleeding, sensitive gums

PARTS USED: Softwood leafy stems, fresh or dried

HOME PHARMACY USES: Skin wash, mouthwash, liniment, ointment, salve, cream, foot soak

HOUSEHOLD USES: Prepare a traditional tincture of the tender leafy stems. Into a household spray bottle pour ½ ounce (15 mL) tincture to ½ ounce (15 mL) water, and add 10 drops of grapefruit or lavender essential oil per 1 ounce (30 mL) of solution. Use this household cleaner on linoleum floors, countertops, and sinks.

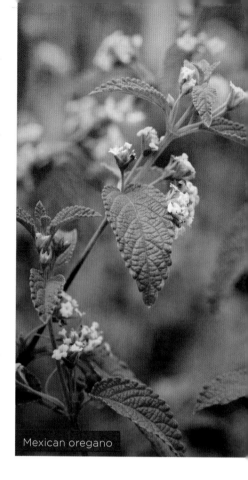

Mexican oregano

Mexican Oregano

Lippia graveolens

Seri Indians in Mexico sustainably wild-harvest Mexican oregano — or xomcahiift, as they call it — by hand, as their ancestors have done for centuries.

PERSONALITY: Perennial; woody (Zones 8–9)

HEIGHT: 3 to 5 feet (0.9–1.5 m)

BLOOM TRAITS: Clusters of white flowers in late summer

LIKES/DISLIKES: Grows in sandy, gravelly soil among rocks. It can survive on 5 inches (12.7 cm) of rain annually in the Sonoran Desert.

PROPAGATION/MAINTENANCE:
Propagate from softwood tip cuttings when the plant is not in flower. Dip the cuttings in liquid or powder rooting hormone and stick into a moist, loose soil medium. Cuttings root more easily if kept on bottom heat of 70°F (21° C). Rooted plants can be grown outdoors in warm, arid climates. Space plants 2 feet (0.6 m) apart and water sparingly. Mexican oregano does well as a container herb on the patio in hot weather and moved indoors in bright light during cold months. Protect from frost.

SUN/SOIL: Full sun; poorer sandy or gravelly soils that drain well

COMPANION/COMPLEMENTARY PLANTING: Grow with agastaches, epazote, white sage, and prickly pear

HARVESTING: Hand-pick leaves from woody branches. Seri Indians describe the motion as a gentle raking of the leaves from the branches with one's fingers, using care not to cause damage to the woody parts of the plant.

CULINARY USE: Leaves, fresh or dried, are added to fish and rice dishes. This is a very strong and delicious oregano, so use a light hand. Finely chopped leaves incorporated into an herb butter are delicious on home-baked breads and noodles.

MEDICINAL BENEFITS: A rich source of antioxidants and anti-inflammatory agents

PARTS USED: Leaves, dried or fresh

HOME PHARMACY USES: Traditional tincture, ointment, salve, cream, bath herb, food soak, liniment

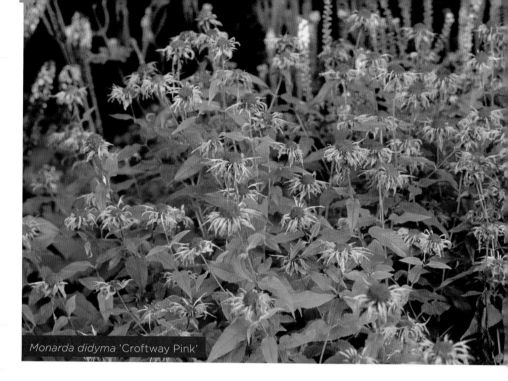

Monarda didyma 'Croftway Pink'

Monarda

Monarda species

Monarda is a tasty, spicy herb. It is wonderful as a culinary seasoning and makes a good substitute for Greek oregano.

ETHNIC AND OTHER NAMES: Bee balm, wild oregano, bergamot, Oswego tea, *oregano de la Sierra* (Spanish)

PERSONALITY: Perennial; herbaceous (Zones 4–9)

HEIGHT: 2 to 3 feet (0.6–0.9 m)

BLOOM TRAITS: Red, lavender, pinkish lavender, yellow, or pink- and purple-spotted flowers bloom early to late summer in most regions.

LIKES/DISLIKES: Monarda prefers sunny meadows and gardens and is often found growing near waterways.

PROPAGATION/MAINTENANCE: Seeds are best stratified for 3 months before sowing. Expect sporadic, 60 to 70 percent germination in 2 to 3 weeks. Tender tip cuttings have a lower success rate. Transplant seedlings or rooted cuttings outdoors in late spring. Root divisions propagate easily. Space 12 inches (30 cm) apart. Plants grow in clumps and require moderate watering.

SUN/SOIL: Full sun, partial shade. *M. fistulosa* var. *menthifolia* and *M. didyma* prefer rich soil and fair moisture; *M. fistulosa* likes dry, well-drained soil; and *M. punctata* prefers loose, sandy, dry soil.

HARVESTING: Harvest aerial parts at any time during the growing season. Use a pair of snips.

CULINARY USE: Coarsely grind the dried aerial parts and use as a wonderful substitute for oregano or marjoram.

MEDICINAL BENEFITS: Excellent for winter illness symptoms, respiratory conditions, and the digestive tract

PARTS USED: Aerial parts, fresh or dried

HOME PHARMACY USES: Infusion, ointment, salve, cream, foot or bath soak, infused oil, liniment, honey, syrup, elixir, traditional and cider vinegar tincture

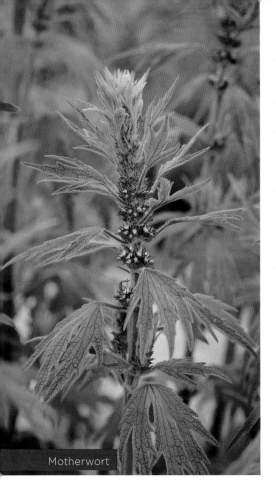

Motherwort

PERSONALITY: Perennial; herbaceous (Zones 4–8)

HEIGHT: 2 to 4 feet (0.6–1.2 m)

BLOOM TRAITS: Motherwort has small whorls of lavender flowers from mid- to late summer.

LIKES/DISLIKES: Commonly found in disturbed areas in temperate climates. It grows abundantly near streams and rivers.

PROPAGATION/MAINTENANCE: Stratify seeds for several weeks. Sow directly outdoors or start indoors and transplant outside in mid- to late spring. Seeds germinate in about 2 weeks at a rate of 75 to 80 percent. This clump-growing herb should be spaced 15 to 20 inches (38–50 cm) apart. Water moderately. Remember to cut back motherwort to 3 inches above the ground just after flowering but before seeds mature, as motherwort self-seeds dramatically.

SUN/SOIL: Full sun, partial shade, shade; no special soil needs

HARVESTING: Harvest the aerial parts from spring through fall. Snips or scissors will work nicely.

MEDICINAL BENEFITS: Motherwort is used for women's ailments, as a heart tonic herb, and for some nervous system and digestive tract conditions.

PARTS USED: Aerial parts, fresh or dried

HOME PHARMACY USES: Infusion, traditional tincture, cider vinegar tincture, elixir, syrup, honey

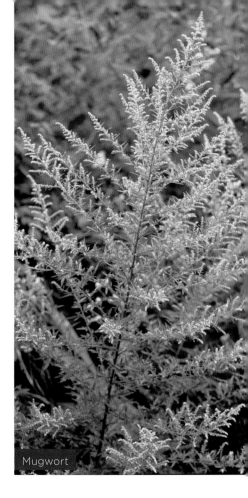

Mugwort

Motherwort

Leonurus cardiaca

Wort is an Old English word meaning "to heal," and when attached to mother we get a picture of how this plant has been used. It was and still is often given to women just after childbirth to facilitate the recovery process. The Latin name comes from the words for "lion" and "heart," appropriate for an herb that is considered a good heart supporter.

ETHNIC AND OTHER NAMES:
Jaboncillo (Spanish)

Mugwort

Artemisia vulgaris

During the Middle Ages, people believed that putting a leaf of mugwort in their shoes would prevent them from becoming weary. The herb was reputed to enable a traveler to walk 40 miles before noon!

ETHNIC AND OTHER NAMES: Cronewort, *altamisa* (Spanish)

PERSONALITY: Perennial; herbaceous (Zones 4–8)

HEIGHT: 4 to 5 feet (1.2–1.5 m)

BLOOM TRAITS: Spikes of whitish green flowers pale in comparison to the stunning purple stems and green leaves with silvery undersides.

LIKES/DISLIKES: Mugwort comes from Mediterranean mountain regions, where it is commonly found growing in disturbed areas.

PROPAGATION/MAINTENANCE: Stratify the seeds for several weeks and then sow indoors. Germination takes about 2 weeks and sprouting is near 70 percent. Without stratification, you can expect closer to 50 percent germination. Transplant outdoors in mid- to early spring. Mugwort stays in a clump but it grows quite large; space plants 15 to 20 inches (38–50 cm) apart. Water lightly to moderately.

SUN/SOIL: Full sun, partial shade; no special soil needs

HARVESTING: Harvest aerial parts with snips or scissors any time during the growing season.

MEDICINAL BENEFITS: Mugwort is primarily used for menopausal symptoms in women and for digestive tract support.

PARTS USED: Aerial parts, fresh or dried

HOME PHARMACY USES: Infusion, traditional tincture, cider vinegar tincture, syrup, elixir, ointment, salve, cream, foot soak, sleep pillow, bath herb, infused oil, honey, liniment

CRAFTING: Mugwort sleep pillows are fun to make and to gift to someone special. Tradition says that sleeping with a mugwort sleep pillow tucked into your pillow slip will most certainly contribute to colorful, vivid dreams. Use dried leaves to make the sleep pillow.

Mullein

Verbascum thapsus

Mullein is a great indicator of soil contamination. If the soil is high in heavy metals or chemical contaminants, mullein's normally straight stalk will often grow twisted and distorted. Do not harvest from such plants; they likely are not safe for use. Occasionally the mullein stalks will be forked but still growing relatively straight. This indicates simply that the stalk was broken off somehow and responded by sending up multiple stalks from that point.

ETHNIC AND OTHER NAMES: *Punchón* (Spanish)

PERSONALITY: Biennial; herbaceous (Zones 3–9)

HEIGHT: 5 to 6 feet (1.5–1.8 m)

BLOOM TRAITS: In the second year, a stalk of individual yellow flowers emerges. Blooming begins at the bottom and continues up to the tip over the course of a couple of weeks in mid- to late summer.

LIKES/DISLIKES: Grows in mountain meadows, open grasslands, and along streams and rivers. Prefers a disturbed area with dry, well-drained soil. Mullein does not grow in tropical regions; it likes a more arid climate.

PROPAGATION/MAINTENANCE: Seeds are easy. Sow seeds directly outdoors in fall or early spring or sow them indoors in early spring to transplant into the garden in mid- to late spring. Germination is normally between 75 to 80 percent. It takes about 2 weeks to sprout. Reseeds vigorously and grows in clumps. Space plants 15 inches (38 cm) apart and water lightly to moderately.

SUN/SOIL: Full sun; well-drained soil

COMPANION/COMPLEMENTARY PLANTING: Grow with mugwort, feverfew, and echinacea

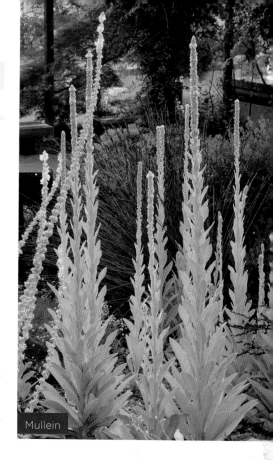
Mullein

HARVESTING: The whole plant is used, but the various parts are harvested at different times. Harvest roots with a needle-nose spade or garden fork in the fall of the first year's growth or in the spring of the second. Hand-pick leaves at any time during the growing season; I prefer late spring and early summer. Hand-pick flowers in full bloom. To harvest the flowering tops, snip off the upper 3 to 6 inches (7–15 cm) of stalk, when it is heavily flowering and full of buds just about to pop. Lay out the plant material for several hours in a shady location to give weevils a chance to exit the plant parts.

MEDICINAL BENEFITS: Roots are specific for the urinary tract; leaves and flowers are used for the respiratory tract, the skin, and the ears.

PARTS USED: Roots, leaves, and flowers, fresh or dried

HOME PHARMACY USES: Infusion, decoction, traditional tincture, cider vinegar tincture, syrup, ointment, salve, cream, infused oil

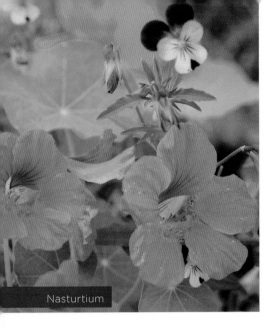

Nasturtium

Nasturtium

Tropaeolum majus

Nasturtiums are usually thought of as pretty annual flowers, but that description does a great disservice to this plant. The flowers, leaves, and seeds of this herb are culinary delights. Make this herb part of your kitchen's bag of tricks and you will not be disappointed.

COMMON VARIETIES: 'Milkmaid', 'Empress of India', 'Ladybird', Jewel series, trailing nasturtium

ETHNIC AND OTHER NAMES: Indian cress

PERSONALITY: Annual

HEIGHT: 12 to 15 inches (30–38 cm)

BLOOM TRAITS: Flowers begin in late spring and continue until a killing frost occurs. Blooms come in shades of yellow, orange, and red, along with bicolor combinations.

LIKES/DISLIKES: Nasturtiums prefer lush, semi-shady places. They grow nicely in dappled shade — under trees, in hanging baskets, in containers as patio plants. They will vine or trail but usually climb if there is something nearby they can use as a trellis.

PROPAGATION/MAINTENANCE: Sow seed directly into the garden or into its permanent container. Nasturtiums will just barely tolerate transplanting if you handle them with great care, and do not disturb the roots. They respond by becoming stunted, if they survive at all. The seeds sprout in about 2 weeks' time with a germination rate of 80 to 90 percent. Space the seeds about 8 inches (20 cm) apart when sowing and put 2 seeds in each spot to hedge your bets against birds and mice. Nasturtiums prefer moderate to heavy watering. If you go heavy on the fertilizer, they will have gorgeous green leaves but no flowers.

SUN/SOIL: Partial shade; adaptable to all soil types that are reasonably well-drained and have good amounts of organic matter. For containers, use a mix of 1 part compost to 3 parts potting soil. Do not incorporate fertilizer for that growing season.

COMPANION/COMPLEMENTARY PLANTING: Grow in community with vegetables, strawberries, spilanthes, parsley, and sunflowers

HARVESTING: Hand-pick younger leaves and flowers, or use scissors to harvest. Seeds should be handpicked.

CULINARY USE: Fresh young leaves are wonderful as a green salad ingredient to impart some spicy zing. They are tasty on sandwiches, or on top of burritos in place of some or all of the lettuce. The seeds can be pickled and used as a nutty-zippy substitute for capers. The pickled seeds are especially good with tuna and hard-cooked eggs, along with a few veggies, for a different take on the usual tuna salad.

EDIBLE FLOWERS: Nasturtium flowers are pretty in vegetable salads of all kinds. They have a peppery, broccoli-type flavor. Try them atop steamed vegetables on a bed of rice or floated in vegetable soup. The flower buds are also tasty.

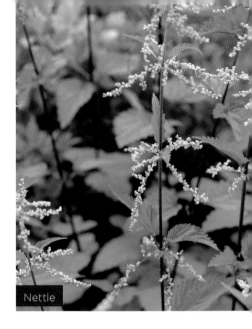

Nettle

Nettle

Urtica dioica

The nettle plant has gotten an undeserved bad reputation because of its sting. The sensation, which feels like a bad sunburn and may be accompanied by small blisters, is caused by formic acid and occurs only when the plant is touched in its fresh state. Cooked or dried nettles do not cause stinging. If you do get stung by nettles, the discomfort will be gone in an hour or so. Wearing protective clothing and gloves is a good idea when working with this herb. It is also wise to plant nettles away from paths and out of the reach of young children.

ETHNIC AND OTHER NAMES: *Ortiga* (Spanish)

PERSONALITY: Perennial; herbaceous (Zones 5–9)

HEIGHT: 2 to 4 feet (0.6–1.2 m)

BLOOM TRAITS: Tiny, cream-colored, pearl-like flowers bloom from early to late summer.

LIKES/DISLIKES: Nettles grow around the world. This species is native to Eurasia and is now naturalized in North America and Europe. It grows in disturbed areas wherever there is good moisture: near streams, rivers, ponds, and lakes.

PROPAGATION/MAINTENANCE: Stratify seeds and sow them directly in the garden, or sow indoors and transplant in late spring. About half of the seeds sown will germinate. Propagation by root divisions is best done in early spring. Wear gloves when working with seedlings or when dividing plants. The plants spread, so space them about 12 inches (30 cm) apart. Provide moderate to heavy amounts of water.

SUN/SOIL: Full sun, partial shade, shade; prefers a soil high in organic matter (4 to 5 percent)

COMPANION/COMPLEMENTARY PLANTING: Plant with sunflowers, grapes, and fennel

HARVESTING: Harvest the aerial parts at any point during the growing season except when flowering. Wear heavy gloves and use snips or scissors. If you are handling fresh leaves, keep those gloves on.

CULINARY USE: Nettles are well recognized as an important vegetable and herb in many parts of the world. Fresh nettles can be made into soup, added to casseroles, or used as a spinach substitute.

MEDICINAL BENEFITS: Nettles are definitely a whole-body tonic, rich in vitamins and minerals, and are a fabulous medicinal food. Valuable for male and female reproductive health, respiratory and urinary tract concerns, immune health, childhood ailments and allergy relief. They are also great for the skin and hair.

PARTS USED: Aerial parts, fresh or dried

HOME PHARMACY USES: Infusion, traditional tincture, cider vinegar tincture, elixir, ointment, cream, salve, foot soak, bath herb, infused oil, honey, liniment

Oats

Avena sativa

The ancient Egyptians were known to cultivate oats, which they used for food and medicine. They knew that harvesting oatseed at the milky stage would provide the highest nutritional and medicinal benefit. This wise culture also regarded oats as an important skin herb.

ETHNIC AND OTHER NAMES: Oatseed, oatstraw, *avena* (Spanish)

PERSONALITY: Annual; herbaceous

HEIGHT: 4 to 5 feet (1.2–1.5 m)

BLOOM TRAITS: This grass sports light green grain spikelets that turn golden upon full maturity. Flowering will occur approximately 1 month after planting, depending on weather.

LIKES/DISLIKES: Like many grasses, oats grow in open, sunny areas. They have been cultivated in nearly every temperate climate around the world.

PROPAGATION/MAINTENANCE: Sow seeds directly outdoors in mid- to late spring. No special treatments are needed. Oats will grow in clumps and should be spaced about 8 inches (20 cm) apart. Water moderately.

SUN/SOIL: Full sun; prefers a soil with good organic matter content (4 to 5 percent is ideal)

COMPANION/COMPLEMENTARY PLANTING: Oats are a grain in the grass family, and often folks don't think about planting them in their gardens. They do very nicely, though, and because they are an annual, they can be turned into the soil as a green manure once you've harvested all you want from them. They also do nicely in large containers. I find that two 15-inch round clay pots are all I really need. Once I have harvested the milky oats or the matured oat grain, I empty the pots into the compost barrel.

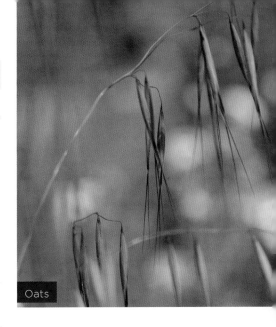

Oats

HARVESTING: To harvest oatseed, pick in the milky stage (when the green grains get plump and spurt out a milky juice when squeezed). Strip the grains from the spikelets by pulling them through your fingertips. Have a bucket or bag ready to catch the oat grains as you move through the patch. If you are harvesting oatstraw, cut and dry the aerial parts (stems, leaves, grains) when the plant is in the milky stage. If you want oats for cooking, allow the grains to come to full maturity and then harvest them.

CULINARY USE: Oats are one of the most nutritious of all foods and, in a word: tasty! Besides being a hearty cereal grain, oats are delicious in muffins and breads. Oat topping on fruit crisps is a great favorite here at the farm.

MEDICINAL BENEFITS: Oats are a whole-body tonic for all ages, but are especially useful for the nervous system, skin, and bone health. Oats are also quite good for male and female reproductive health.

PARTS USED: Milky-stage seeds, grains, and aerial parts, fresh or dried; if used in tinctures, the seeds should be used fresh.

HOME PHARMACY USES: Infusion, traditional tincture, cider vinegar tincture, ointment, salve, cream, bath herb

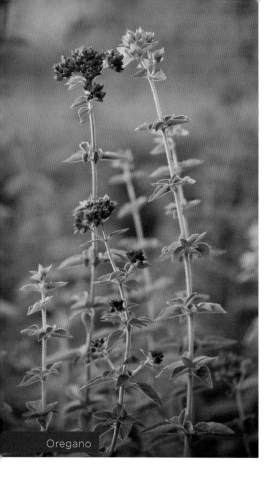
Oregano

Oregano

Origanum species

Oregano is usually thought of as a culinary herb, but it is also highly antiseptic. Consider preparing oregano as a topical remedy for cuts and scrapes. This herb has also been used to relieve nervousness, irritability, insomnia, tension, and anxiety.

COMMON VARIETIES: Italian, Greek, 'Hot & Spicy', variegated

ETHNIC AND OTHER NAMES: *Origan* (French), *Dost* (German), *oregano* (Italian), *orégano* (Spanish)

PERSONALITY: Perennial; herbaceous (Zones 5–9)

HEIGHT: To 24 inches (60 cm)

BLOOM TRAITS: Tiny lavender, white, or pink flowers grace oregano throughout the summer.

LIKES/DISLIKES: Oregano is native to the Mediterranean regions. It enjoys a hot, but not too wet, climate.

PROPAGATION/MAINTENANCE: Stratify seeds for 1 week, then sow them indoors. Germination is near 70 percent; seeds take a week or two to sprout. Transplant outside once spring weather is well settled. Oregano can also be propagated by tip cuttings; liquid rooting hormone will assist in the rooting process. Space plants 12 inches (30 cm) apart to allow for spreading. Water lightly to moderately.

SUN/SOIL: Full sun, partial shade, well-drained soil

HARVESTING: Harvest the aerial parts of oregano at any time during the growing season. Snips or scissors work nicely.

CULINARY USE: Oregano makes a perfect seasoning in spaghetti and sprinkled over pizza. We also like to season buttered popcorn with a blend of oregano, garlic, and thyme.

MEDICINAL BENEFITS: Oregano is recommended during winter illnesses and to support the digestive system. It is also strongly antiseptic for skin concerns.

PARTS USED: Aerial parts, fresh or dried

HOME PHARMACY USES: Infusion, traditional tincture, ointment, salve, foot soak, bath herb, infused oil

Parsley

Petroselinum crispum, P. crispum var. neapolitanum

I plant parsley around the perimeter of the garden to satisfy rabbits and deer. They do not seem to be inclined to venture farther into the garden, and the parsley does not mind the regular "trimming."

COMMON VARIETIES: 'Giant of Italy', Italian, 'Starkes Leafy Curled', 'Triple Curled Forest'

ETHNIC AND OTHER NAMES: *Persil* (French), *Petersilie* (German), *prezzemolo* (Italian), *perejil* (Spanish), *persilja* (Swedish)

PERSONALITY: Biennial; herbaceous (Zones 5–8)

HEIGHT: 12 to 20 inches (30–50 cm)

BLOOM TRAITS: In the second year, parsley will bloom with white flower umbels. Flowering usually occurs from early to midsummer.

LIKES/DISLIKES: Parsley is a Mediterranean plant by nature and will do best in a dry, hot climate.

PROPAGATION/MAINTENANCE: Stratify seeds for at least 1 week. The day before sowing, soak them in water for 12 to 24 hours. Parsley takes a long time to germinate, up to 4 weeks, but by stratifying and soaking the seeds, germination occurs in 2 weeks or less. Germination rate is usually in the neighborhood of 70 percent. Sow seeds indoors and transplant outside in mid- to late spring, or sow directly in the garden in early spring. This clump-growing herb should be spaced 12 inches (30 cm) apart. Water moderately.

SUN/SOIL: Full sun, partial shade; no special soil needs

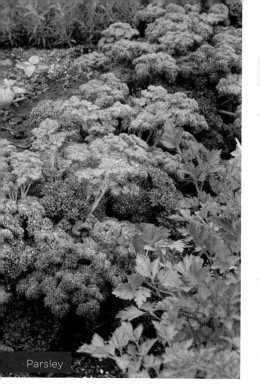

Parsley

Passionflower

Passiflora incarnata, P. edulis

Passionflower vine is a perfect way to add height to the garden. Let the vines climb up a beautiful trellis, building, or fence. Passionflower can also be grown in a large container with a mini-trellis as a houseplant or as a patio plant during the warm months.

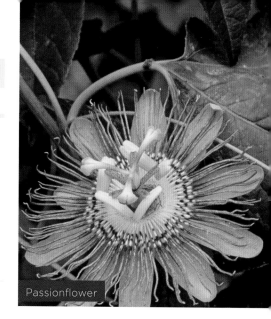

Passionflower

ETHNIC AND OTHER NAMES: Maypop and apricot vine (*P. incarnata*), purple passionfruit and granadilla (*P. edulis*)

PERSONALITY: Perennial; herbaceous (Zones 5–9)

HEIGHT: 8 feet (2.39 m) and much taller

BLOOM TRAITS: Amazing, colorful, and very exotic white and lavender flowers bloom from mid- to late summer.

LIKES/DISLIKES: Passionflower is native to the southeastern United States; it prefers moisture and humidity and will not tolerate a severe winter. It can be treated as a perennial if you mulch at the root zone for extra protection against winters in Zone 5 and colder.

SUN/SOIL: Shade, partial shade; prefers a rich, humusy soil

COMPANION/COMPLEMENTARY PLANTING: Passionflower is pollinated by bats, so plant it where it is accessible to these creatures, such as near bat houses and building eaves.

PROPAGATION/MAINTENANCE: Propagation from seeds is very difficult. The most successful method is to stratify them in moist peat moss in the refrigerator for 1 week, then sow indoors in a very warm greenhouse. Seedlings usually appear in about 3 weeks.

Parsley column

HARVESTING: Gather aerial parts at any point during the growing season. I prefer to use scissors, but snips will also work well. If you plan to use the roots, dig them in the fall of the first year or the spring of the second year. Use a garden fork or needle-nose spade.

CULINARY USE: Although parsley is mainly recognized as a garnish, it deserves more respect. The fresh leaves make a vitamin- and mineral-rich ingredient when added to green salads or cold pasta dishes, or minced into deviled eggs. Parsley is also great in potato salad. Dried parsley is a nice seasoning for soups and sauces.

MEDICINAL BENEFITS: Parsley is a strong antioxidant. It is beneficial to the digestive tract and is often recommended for urinary tract concerns.

PARTS USED: Aerial parts and roots, fresh or dried

HOME PHARMACY USES: Infusion, decoction, traditional tincture, cider vinegar tincture

Passionflower right column

Germination is typically low, between 20 and 40 percent. Plant outdoors only after all danger of frost is past. I grow passionflower from tip cuttings. I use a liquid rooting hormone and keep the cuttings warm and moist until rooting occurs, in about 2 weeks. I have good success growing it this way and keep a mother plant permanently on hand to provide cuttings. Space 24 inches (60 cm) apart and give these spreading, vining plants a trellis at least 8 feet high to climb on. Water moderately to heavily.

HARVESTING: Harvest aerial parts, including any flowers or fruits, at any point during the growing season. Use snips and a big basket (we use 30-gallon plastic tree baskets).

CULINARY USE: The fruits are quite tasty and edible. They resemble a green apricot in both size and outside appearance.

MEDICINAL BENEFITS: Passionflower is a strong sedative and nervine herb.

PARTS USED: Aerial parts, fresh or dried

HOME PHARMACY USES: Infusion, traditional tincture, syrup, elixir, foot soak, bath herb, honey

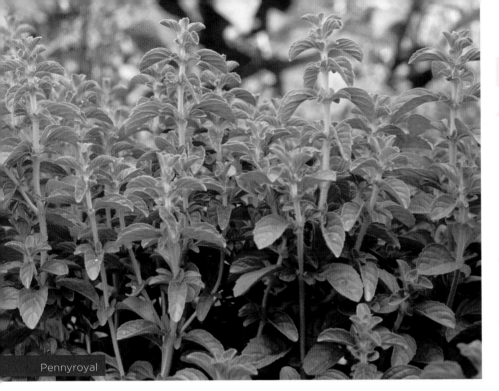
Pennyroyal

Peppermint

Mentha piperita

Few plants are as diverse in their uses as peppermint. Familiar as an ingredient in chewing gum, candy, toothpaste, and even cleaning products, peppermint can be used medicinally to address nearly every body system.

COMMON VARIETIES: Chocolate mint, blue balsam peppermint, Kentucky peppermint, candy mint

ETHNIC AND OTHER NAMES: *Menta peperita* (Italian), *hierbabuena* (Spanish), *Pfefferminze* (German), *menthe poivrée* (French), *pepparmynta* (Swedish)

PERSONALITY: Perennial; herbaceous (Zones 5–9)

HEIGHT: 24 inches (60 cm)

BLOOM TRAITS: Spikes of purple flowers bloom in mid- to late summer.

LIKES/DISLIKES: Often found as a garden escapee in disturbed soil areas near streams and ponds; also common in city alleys

PROPAGATION/MAINTENANCE: Propagate peppermint from root divisions or cuttings. Both methods are easy and foolproof. Do not grow peppermint from seed if you want a good, strong plant; seed crops of peppermint have very little smell or taste to them. This is a vigorous, spreading herb; space plants 12 inches (30 cm) apart. Peppermint requires moderate to heavy watering, but if you grow the herb on the drier side, it will behave itself better in the garden.

SUN/SOIL: Full sun, partial shade, shade; no special soil needs

Pennyroyal

Mentha pulegium

Pennyroyal has an unwarranted reputation for being dangerous. It is true that pregnant women should not use this plant, but many other herbs should also be avoided during pregnancy. Pennyroyal essential oil, however, does have some cautions attached to it and should be used externally only and with extreme care. It is often included in herbal pet products to repel fleas and ticks, but it should not be used on cats.

ETHNIC AND OTHER NAMES: *Poleo chino* (Spanish)

PERSONALITY: Perennial; herbaceous (Zones 7–9)

HEIGHT: 10 to 12 inches (25–30 cm)

BLOOM TRAITS: Sports graceful lavender whorls in mid- to late summer.

LIKES/DISLIKES: Pennyroyal is native to the hot Mediterranean regions.

PROPAGATION/MAINTENANCE: Root divisions and cuttings are easy propagation methods. Sow seed indoors, then transplant outdoors in mid- to late spring. Germination rate is near 65 percent and sprouting occurs in about 2 weeks. Pennyroyal has a spreading nature; space plants 12 inches (30 cm) apart. Water moderately.

SUN/SOIL: Full sun, partial shade, shade; needs well-drained soil

HARVESTING: Aerial parts are harvested at any point during the growing season. Cut with snips or scissors

MEDICINAL BENEFITS: Good for women's health (do not use if pregnant), winter illnesses, and digestive support

PARTS USED: Aerial parts, fresh or dried

HOME PHARMACY USES: Infusion, traditional tincture, syrup, foot soak, bath herb, honey, insect repellent

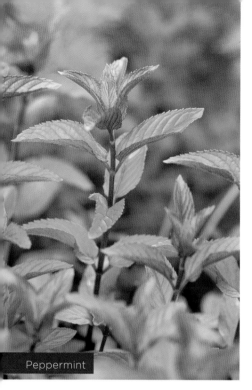

Peppermint

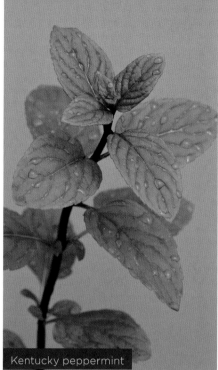

Kentucky peppermint

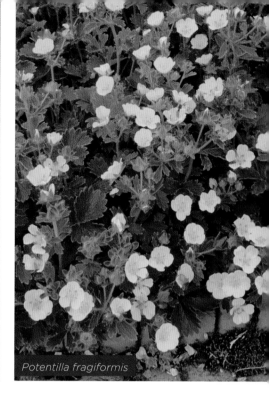

Potentilla fragiformis

COMPANION/COMPLEMENTARY PLANTING: Grow peppermint next to other aggressive plants like yarrow and wormwood to keep each one in its place. Peppermint can be grown in a large pot very successfully, but do not plant it in the same pot with other herbs, as mints are not good neighbors and will choke out everything else in the pot.

HARVESTING: Aerial parts are cut, with snips or scissors, at any point during the growing season. Harvesting just before it flowers will yield a sweeter taste. Flowering peppermint often has a strong, burning, even slightly bitter taste.

CULINARY USE: Finely chop several fresh peppermint leaves and add to a leafy green salad or pasta salad. You can also freeze 6- to 8-inch sprigs of any type of mint to use in cookies. While the mint is still frozen, crumble one or two sprigs of it into chocolate-chip cookie dough and mix well, then bake as usual for wonderfully minty cookies. This method also works for other types of cookies, such as oatmeal and peanut butter.

MEDICINAL BENEFITS: Useful for nearly every part of the body, including the digestive tract, muscular system, respiratory tract, and women's reproductive system. It is also helpful for pain relief, skin concerns, winter illnesses, and children's health.

PARTS USED: Aerial parts, fresh or dried

HOME PHARMACY USES: Infusion, traditional tincture, cider vinegar tincture, syrup, elixir, ointment, salve, cream, foot soak, sleep pillow, bath herb, infused oil, honey, butter, liniment

CRAFTING: Peppermint leaves are a great addition to sachets, bath herbs, sleep pillows, hand creams, and potpourri. I use them to stuff handmade herbal stocking dolls that I stitch during the winter in front of the woodstove. Peppermint — and other herbs — makes the dolls smell delightful and add to their magic.

Potentilla

Potentilla species

Potentilla's flowers make it a cheerful addition to the herb garden. It will grow in most North American climates and is very adaptable to soil and moisture variances.

ETHNIC AND OTHER NAMES: Five-fingers, cinquefoil, tormentil

PERSONALITY: Perennial; herbaceous, woody (Zones 4–8)

HEIGHT: Herbaceous species, 6 to 20 inches (15–50 cm); woody shrubs, 2 to 4 feet (0.6–1.2 m)

BLOOM TRAITS: Flowers appear all summer and are mainly yellow, occasionally apricot or white.

LIKES/DISLIKES: Potentillas are found growing at higher elevations in mountainous areas. They prefer meadows and pastures; bushy varieties are sometimes found along roadsides. This herb is popular in landscapes, often as a hedgerow plant.

PROPAGATION/MAINTENANCE: It is nearly impossible to get viable seed; you must propagate by cuttings or by the more reliable root divisions or crown divisions. Cuttings may require several weeks to root. Once the root structure has developed, plant outdoors. If propagating by division, make sure that every section has some root attached to it, and plant in prepared garden space. Keep well watered until roots have a chance to establish themselves. Occasionally, a species of potentilla will have a spreading nature, but most often it grows in a clump. Space herbaceous species 10 to 15 inches (25–38 cm) apart; space shrub species 2 to 3 feet (0.6–0.9 m) apart. Provide moderate to heavy water.

SUN/SOIL: Full sun, partial shade, shade, depending on species; prefers well-drained, somewhat sandy soil, but is quite adaptable

HARVESTING: Harvest aerial parts at any point during the growing season. Handpick or use snips or scissors.

MEDICINAL BENEFITS: Potentilla is an astringent herb used for skin problems, some gastrointestinal conditions, and gum tissue health.

PARTS USED: Aerial parts, fresh or dried

HOME PHARMACY USES: Infusion, decoction, traditional tincture, cider vinegar tincture, syrup, elixir, ointment, salve, cream, foot soak, bath herb, honey, butter, liniment

EDIBLE FLOWERS: Like all of its cousins in the rose family, potentilla flowers are edible. Use them to beautify fruit and leafy green salads.

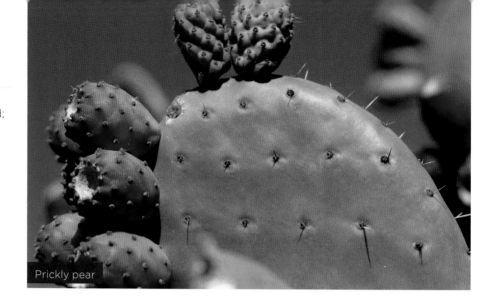
Prickly pear

Prickly Pear

Opuntia species

Prickly pear is an important medicinal food among the cultures of Mexico and the southwestern United States. Adult-onset diabetes is a severe problem in these groups, and adding prickly pear to their diet helps maintain blood-sugar levels.

PERSONALITY: Perennial; succulent (Zones 6–11, depending on species)

HEIGHT: 10 to 15 inches (25–38 cm)

BLOOM TRAITS: Flowers bloom in pinks and yellows, depending on species, from late spring into early summer.

LIKES/DISLIKES: Most prickly pears range from high mountain desert regions into the lower desert. They rely on spring rains to help sustain them through the dry summer.

PROPAGATION/MAINTENANCE: Simulate the desert environment by stratifying prickly pear seeds for 1 to 2 weeks. Just before sowing, soak seeds for 15 minutes in 3 percent hydrogen peroxide. Sow immediately in a loose soil mix and keep temperatures warm. Germination rates (and time) vary greatly, from 10 to 70 percent (and 2 weeks to

4 months). Keep seeds evenly moist and be patient. Transplant outdoors when seedlings are 1 year old and well established. Water thoroughly, then wait a few days before watering again. Do not overwater. Some species spread more aggressively than others. Space plants 12 to 15 inches (30–38 cm) apart. Water lightly when mature.

SUN/SOIL: Full sun; prefers well-drained, sandy soil

COMPANION/COMPLEMENTARY PLANTING: Plant with white sage, California poppy, and catmint

HARVESTING: Wearing gloves, snip off the pads, flowers, and fruits of prickly pear. Singe the spines off the harvested plants, using a campfire flame or even a butane lighter, then prepare the cactus for use.

CULINARY USE: Once the spines have been singed off, cut the pads into strips or cubes and sauté with chopped onions and garlic to taste. Use the fruit to make jelly.

MEDICINAL BENEFITS: Good for balancing blood sugar levels and for gastrointestinal complaints, prickly pear is also useful as a skin herb.

PARTS USED: Aerial parts, fresh

HOME PHARMACY USES: Syrup, medicinal food, ointment, salve, cream, honey

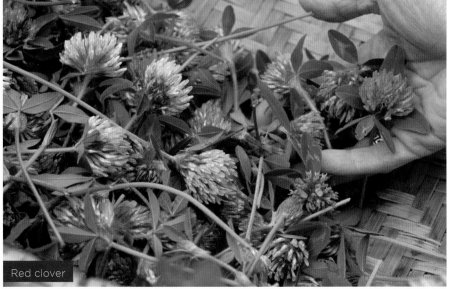

Red clover

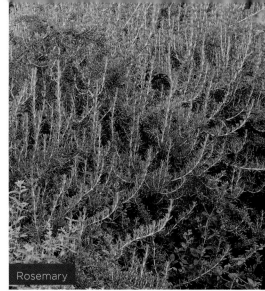

Rosemary

Red Clover

Trifolium pratense

Handle the blossoms gently when harvesting to preserve their color and their nutritional and medicinal benefits. They are very delicate.

ETHNIC AND OTHER NAMES: *Trébol* (Spanish)

PERSONALITY: Perennial; herbaceous (Zones 5–9)

HEIGHT: 12 to 15 inches (30–38 cm)

BLOOM TRAITS: Red clover is found growing in disturbed areas, but it is especially fond of mountain meadows and the banks of rivers and streams. It is often seen along mountain roadsides where runoff gathers.

PROPAGATION/MAINTENANCE: Stratify seeds for several weeks and then sow directly outdoors. Germination will occur in 7 to 10 days at a rate of 75 percent or so. Space these clumping plants 12 inches (30 cm) apart. Water moderately.

SUN/SOIL: Full sun, partial shade; no special soil needs

HARVESTING: Harvest the blossoms only, and pick them carefully by hand. This is time-consuming, but necessary. To dry this herb properly, pick in the early morning while dew is still on the blossoms. Handle them gently; they bruise easily. Lay flowers on a screen in a single layer and let them dry. They will be a deep purplish red when fully dried. Store in a glass jar or paper bag, out of direct light and heat.

CULINARY USE: Add the flowers to the cooking pot when preparing oatmeal, rice, soups, stews, and dried beans. They are a rich source of nutrition.

MEDICINAL BENEFITS: A tonic, red clover is often suggested for women's and children's health concerns, winter illnesses, and immune system support.

PARTS USED: Flowers, fresh or dried

HOME PHARMACY USES: Infusion, traditional tincture, cider vinegar tincture, syrup, elixir, ointment, salve, cream, honey

EDIBLE FLOWERS: Cut fresh blossoms in half and add to a green leafy salad for nutrition and beauty.

Rosemary

Rosmarinus species

Rosemary is a traditional symbol of good health, fidelity, and remembrance. It is one of the best antioxidant herbs and is also excellent for enhancing circulation. Rosemary helps increase the oxygen supply to the brain, thus sharpening concentration and memory.

COMMON VARIETIES OF ROSEMARY: 'Tuscan Blue', 'Madeline Hill', 'Arp', 'Majorcan', 'Spice Islands'

ETHNIC AND OTHER NAMES: *Romero* (Spanish), *romarin* (French), *Rosmarin* (German and Swedish), *ramerino* (Italian)

PERSONALITY: Tender perennial; herbaceous (Zones 8–11). Varieties 'Arp' and 'Madeline Hill' are hardy to −5°F and 7,200 feet elevation.

HEIGHT: 12 to 36 inches (30–90 cm), although it can grow considerably taller

BLOOM TRAITS: Blue flowers bloom profusely when the plants experience cooler nighttime temperatures (not below 38°F; 3°C) to set the buds. Some varieties blossom in shades of pink and white.

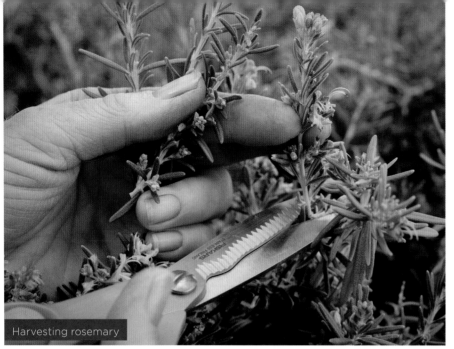
Harvesting rosemary

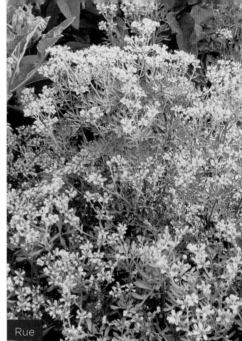
Rue

ROSEMARY, *continued*

LIKES/DISLIKES: Rosemary is from the Mediterranean region. It prefers hot temperatures and dry soil conditions.

PROPAGATION/MAINTENANCE: Propagate rosemary from tip cuttings and use a liquid rooting hormone to encourage better root formation. Warmth and good air circulation are essential. Keep cuttings moist, but not soggy, until rooting structure is strong. Rosemary grows in clumps; space plants 12 to 15 inches (30–38 cm) apart. Water lightly to moderately.

SUN/SOIL: Full sun; well-drained soil

COMPANION/COMPLEMENTARY PLANTING: Grows beautifully in community with lavender, hyssop, santolina, and California poppy. Rosemary is also a popular herb planted in food gardens and can be grown indoors or outdoors in bright light as a container herb.

HARVESTING: Harvest aerial parts, using snips, any time during the growing season. Multiple harvests will be possible if no more than 25 percent of a plant is taken at once.

CULINARY USE: Rosemary is magnificent with poultry dishes, all things potato, and baked into bread. It is strong-flavored and delicious. Add a small amount, then adjust to taste.

MEDICINAL BENEFITS: Rosemary is an outstanding source of antioxidants. It is beneficial to the immune system and for winter illnesses, and is often recommended for the digestive tract, the circulatory system, brain health, the respiratory system, and the skin.

PARTS USED: Aerial parts, fresh or dried

HOME PHARMACY USES: Infusion, traditional tincture, cider vinegar tincture, syrup, elixir, ointment, salve, cream, foot soak, bath herb, infused oil, liniment, honey

EDIBLE FLOWERS: Flowers are tasty sprinkled into salads, used in herb butter or cream cheese spreads, and to decorate cakes. Crystallized rosemary flowers on cakes and sugar cookies are especially beautiful.

Rue

Ruta graveolens

In the Catholic Latin American cultures, rue is considered a sacred herb. It is often referred to as herb-of-grace, and is used in religious rituals. Rue is believed to offer protection for health and well-being.

ETHNIC AND OTHER NAMES: *Ruda* (Spanish)

PERSONALITY: Perennial; herbaceous (Zones 5–9)

HEIGHT: 12 to 15 inches (30–38 cm)

BLOOM TRAITS: Flowers are yellow and bloom in mid- to late summer.

LIKES/DISLIKES: Rue likes to grow in both cool and hot climates. It will tolerate some wet environments as well as arid ones. It is originally native to the Mediterranean regions, where it prefers to grow in disturbed soil.

PROPAGATION/MAINTENANCE: Stratify seeds for 1 week before planting to encourage better germination. Sow seeds indoors and expect about 50 percent germination in 7 to 10 days. Extra-warm temperatures (near 70°F; 21°C) help tremendously. Transplant outside when spring weather is well settled. Rue will grow in clumps; space 10 to 12 inches (25–30 cm) apart. Provide light to moderate amounts of water.

SUN/SOIL: Full sun; no special soil needs

COMPANION/COMPLEMENTARY PLANTING: Rue helps deter pest insects in the garden. Plant it in areas where aphids, whiteflies, and thrips are present.

HARVESTING: Aerial parts are harvested from mid- to late summer. Harvest the upper half of the plant using snips or scissors. Some fair-skinned people may notice skin irritation when handling rue, due to the volatile oils contained in the leaves. Those gardeners would be wise to wear gloves when harvesting and processing rue.

MEDICINAL BENEFITS: Rue is used for women's health concerns and for ear ailments. *Caution:* It should not be used by pregnant women.

PARTS USED: Aerial parts, dried

HOME PHARMACY USES: Infusion, traditional tincture

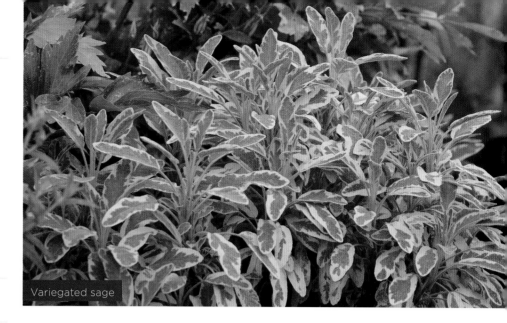
Variegated sage

Sage

Salvia officinalis

Sage is a delicious culinary seasoning and a strong medicinal herb. Caution: *Nursing mothers should forgo this herb: It will pass into the breast milk, and because most infants do not like the taste of sage, they will refuse to nurse.*

COMMON VARIETIES: Tricolor, purple, golden variegated, 'Sage of Bath', 'Woodcote'

ETHNIC AND OTHER NAMES: *Salvia* (Spanish), *sauge* (French), *salvia* (Italian), *Salbei* (German)

PERSONALITY: Perennial; herbaceous (Zones 4–8)

HEIGHT: 24 inches (60 cm)

BLOOM TRAITS: Purple flowers appear in mid- to late summer. 'Sage of Bath' has pink flowers.

LIKES/DISLIKES: Sage is a Mediterranean plant by nature. It thrives in hot or cool, dry environments, often in disturbed soil.

PROPAGATION/MAINTENANCE: Stratify seeds for several weeks, then sow indoors. Expect a germination rate of about 60 percent in 10 to 14 days. Transplant outside, 12 inches (30 cm) apart, in mid- to late spring. This clumping herb requires light to moderate watering.

SUN/SOIL: Full sun; well-drained soil

COMPANION/COMPLEMENTARY PLANTING: Grow with chives and calendula, and in food gardens. Sage is a good container herb.

HARVESTING: Aerial parts are harvested at any point during the growing season, using snips or scissors. Harvest only the upper half of the plant and it will regenerate more quickly, enabling subsequent harvests in the same season.

CULINARY USE: Sage is the traditional seasoning in stuffing for turkey, chicken, and pork dishes. It is quite nice added to grains like couscous and quinoa.

MEDICINAL BENEFITS: Used for winter illnesses, digestive tract and respiratory tract concerns, and throat conditions, sage is also important for skin and hair health, and for women's health.

PARTS USED: Aerial parts, fresh or dried

HOME PHARMACY USES: Infusion, traditional tincture, cider vinegar tincture, syrup, elixir, ointment, salve, cream, foot soak, bath herb, infused oil, honey, liniment

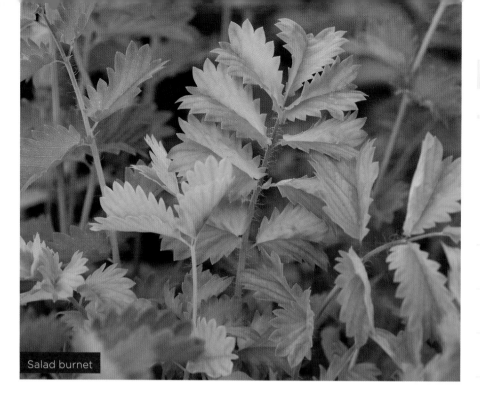

Salad burnet

Salad Burnet

Sanguisorba minor

This herb tastes a lot like a cucumber and can be used in salads as a substitute for that vegetable.

PERSONALITY: Perennial; herbaceous (Zone 5–10)

HEIGHT: 12 to 15 inches (30–38 cm)

BLOOM TRAITS: Pink flowers off and on throughout the summer

LIKES/DISLIKES: Open, grassy pastures and meadows, where soil is moist but well drained

PROPAGATION/MAINTENANCE: Sow seeds in early spring indoors or in mid- to late spring outdoors directly in the garden. Germination is approximately 70 percent and occurs in about 2 weeks. Transplant outdoors in late spring, spacing plants about 12 inches (30 cm) apart. Moderate water is preferred.

SUN/SOIL: Full sun or dappled shade; adaptable to different soil types as long as they are well drained

COMPANION/COMPLEMENTARY PLANTING: Grow with catnip, cutting celery, and dill.

HARVESTING: Aerial parts; snips or scissors work well

CULINARY USE: The leaves have a cucumber-like taste and can be used in any dish where this flavor is desired. Add a few leaves chopped into a tomato-mozzarella salad, cold pasta dishes, soups, and casseroles. A few sprigs in the filling for deviled eggs is quite good. Younger leaves have a less bitter flavor.

Santolina

Santolina species

Santolina is an herb that does not burn very easily, and because of this it is often planted as a hedge to serve as a natural firebreak in landscapes where wildfires are common.

COMMON VARIETIES: 'Napoleon', 'Morning Mist'

ETHNIC AND OTHER NAMES: Lavender cotton (*S. chamaecyparissus*)

PERSONALITY: Perennial; herbaceous (Zones 6–9)

HEIGHT: 12 to 24 inches (30–60 cm)

BLOOM TRAITS: Gray santolina (*S. chamaecyparissus*) has yellow button flowers about the size of a dime. Green santolina (*S. rosmarinifolia*) sports button flowers of yellowish green. 'Napoleon' and 'Morning Mist' santolinas also have yellow button flowers. All varieties bloom in early to midsummer.

LIKES/DISLIKES: A warm weather-lover, santolina grows best in hot, dry climates. It is originally from the Mediterranean region.

PROPAGATION/MAINTENANCE: Tip cuttings are the best way to propagate santolina. Use a liquid rooting hormone to encourage rooting. Keep cuttings evenly moist but not wet. When cuttings have developed a strong root structure, transplant outdoors. Make sure that spring weather is fully settled before planting outside. Space plants 15 inches (38 cm) apart. The plants will grow in clumps and require light watering.

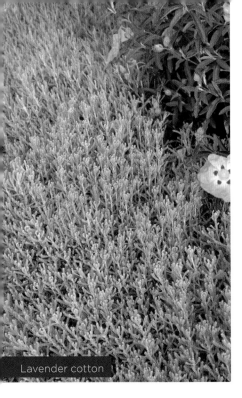

Lavender cotton

SUN/SOIL: Full sun; well-drained soil

COMPANION/COMPLEMENTARY PLANTING: Santolinas repel insects, so plant them next to problematic plants to help prevent infestation. Pair santolina with catmint, California poppy, and rue for a beautiful effect.

HARVESTING: Harvest the aerial parts at any time during the growing season, with scissors or snips.

MEDICINAL BENEFITS: Santolina is an important component of herbal insect repellents.

PARTS USED: Aerial parts, fresh or dried

HOME PHARMACY USES: Insect repellent

Savory, Summer

Satureja hortensis

Summer savory grows as a small, bushy plant. When it blooms, the plant is covered with delicate, pale lavender flowers. This pretty herb seems to twinkle with so many tiny blossoms.

ETHNIC AND OTHER NAMES: *Bohnenkraut* (German)

PERSONALITY: Annual; herbaceous

HEIGHT: 12 to 20 inches (30–50 cm)

BLOOM TRAITS: Flowers are pale lavender to white; blooming occurs throughout the summer.

LIKES/DISLIKES: Summer savory is a Mediterranean plant by nature. It prefers a hot and somewhat dry climate.

PROPAGATION/MAINTENANCE: Sow seed indoors and expect sprouting in about 2 weeks. No special seed treatment is required. Germination averages 60 percent. Transplant outside in late spring. Space this clumping plant 10 to 12 inches (25–30 cm) apart. Water lightly to moderately.

SUN/SOIL: Full sun, partial shade; well-drained soil

HARVESTING: Harvest aerial parts with snips or scissors throughout the summer. I like to harvest my summer savory while it is in flower, but that timing is not crucial.

CULINARY USE: Summer savory is a wonderful seasoning for lamb, potato, and green bean dishes. Or sprinkle lightly into a green salad, but use just a touch.

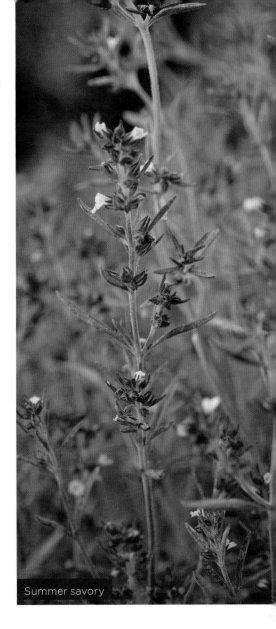

Summer savory

MEDICINAL BENEFITS: Primarily recommended for the digestive, respiratory, and urinary tracts, summer savory is also a good astringent for throat conditions and skin health.

PARTS USED: Aerial parts, fresh or dried

HOME PHARMACY USES: Infusion, traditional tincture, cider vinegar tincture

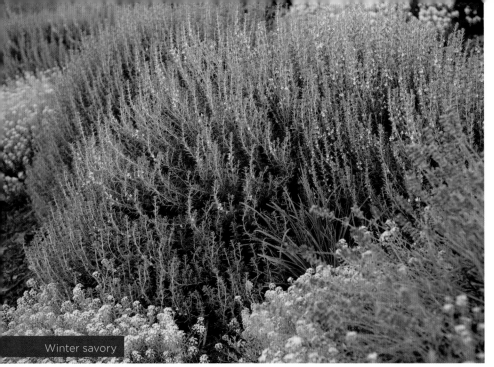

Winter savory

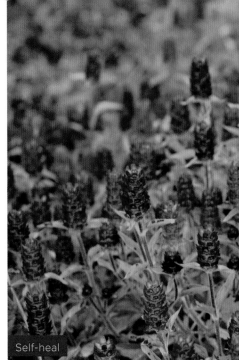

Self-heal

Savory, Winter

Satureja montana

Native to Turkey and North Africa, winter savory is a hardy evergreen herb boasting attractive flowers. It is a flavorful addition to a simmering pot of soup or stew.

ETHNIC AND OTHER NAMES: *Bergbohnenkraut* (German), *sariette vivace* (French)

PERSONALITY: Perennial; woody (Zones 5–8)

HEIGHT: 12 inches (30 cm)

BLOOM TRAITS: Purple, blue, and occasionally white flowers in mid- to late summer

LIKES/DISLIKES: This savory tolerates cold winters, but it also likes sunny, open areas and more arid conditions. It is quite tolerant of hot, sunny summers.

PROPAGATION/MAINTENANCE: Start seed indoors in early spring. Germination is about 80 percent and takes around 2 weeks. Transplant outdoors in mid- to late spring and space plants 12 to 15 inches (30–38 cm) apart. Provide low to moderate water.

SUN/SOIL: Full sun; well-drained soils are a must, but this plant is tolerant of different soil types.

COMPANION/COMPLEMENTARY PLANTING: Grow with hyssop, lavender, thymes, and sage

HARVESTING: Aerial parts, harvested with snips or scissors

CULINARY USE: The leaves are wonderful added to soups and stews, especially those made with lamb. Winter savory is a good seasoning with cabbage, potatoes, and other root vegetables. The dried herb is used to coat the outside of goat cheese.

EDIBLE FLOWERS: The flowers are a tasty addition to herb butter and delicious with vegetables.

Self-Heal

Prunella grandiflora subsp. pyrenaica, P. vulgaris

Self-heal is a beautiful perennial that acts as a well-behaved ground cover. It blooms generously for nearly two months in my garden. I plant it with irises because the foliage contrast is appealing.

PERSONALITY: Perennial; herbaceous (Zones 4–9)

HEIGHT: 8 to 10 inches (20–25 cm)

BLOOM TRAITS: Flowers, varying from pinks and purples to white, bloom in early and midsummer.

LIKES/DISLIKES: In temperate climates, self-heal is a common woodland and forest plant. It is also found in mountain meadows, and is happiest near a stream or a creek. It will grow only in a temperate climate.

PROPAGATION/MAINTENANCE: Stratify seeds for at least 1 month before sowing. Sow indoors and watch for germination within 3 weeks, at a rate of approximately 70 percent. Transplant outdoors

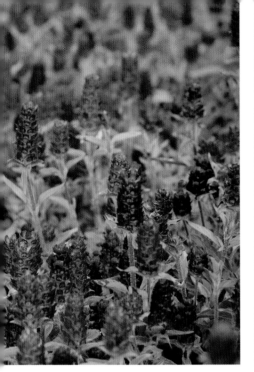

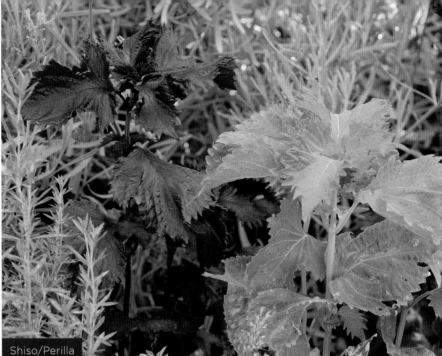

Shiso/Perilla

in mid- to late spring. Space this spreader 10 to 12 inches (25–30 cm) apart and water moderately.

SUN/SOIL: Full sun, partial shade; prefers a humusy soil

COMPANION/COMPLEMENTARY PLANTING: Grow with wood betony, thymes, and violets.

HARVESTING: Harvest the aerial parts of self-heal with snips or scissors while the plant is in flower.

MEDICINAL BENEFITS: Self-heal is used for women's health concerns, the digestive tract, the throat, and skin conditions.

PARTS USED: Flowering aerial parts, fresh

HOME PHARMACY USES: Infusion, traditional tincture, syrup, elixir, ointment, salve, cream, foot soak, bath herb, infused oil, honey

Shiso/Perilla

Perilla frutescens

Due to its spicy flavor and pretty colors, this Asian herb has found great favor when added to salads and Asian dishes.

COMMON VARIETIES: Britton shiso, red shiso

PERSONALITY: Annual

HEIGHT: 12 to 24 inches (30–60 cm)

BLOOM TRAITS: The lavender blooms are quite pretty, but they signal the end of the life cycle for shiso. Once the plant begins to flower, it works toward maturing seed, after which the plant will die.

LIKES/DISLIKES: Shiso grows best in warm to hot climates and partially shaded locations, such as under hardwood trees.

PROPAGATION/MAINTENANCE: Sow seed anytime for indoor container growing, or in mid-spring indoors for later transplanting into the garden once all danger of frost is past. Seeds germinate in 1 to 2 weeks at about 80 percent. Space the plants

10 to 12 inches (25–30 cm) apart and water thoroughly. Keep flowers pinched off in an effort to prevent the plant from trying to go to seed, although at some point it will, and its life cycle will be complete.

SUN/SOIL: Partial to full shade; Moist, loamy soil, high in organic matter. For indoor growing, place shiso in bright but indirect light and prevent warm air (from heat vents) from blowing directly on the plant.

COMPANION/COMPLEMENTARY PLANTING: Grow with gotu kola, lemon verbena, and spilanthes. Shiso also makes an excellent container herb indoors or on the patio in warmer months.

HARVESTING: Harvest leaves, with or without flowers, with a pair of snips or scissors.

CULINARY USE: Add the fresh leaves to Oriental dishes, use as the outer wraps for sushi (Britton shiso preferred), or toss into salads for a cinnamon-curry flavor. Red shiso is highly favored as a natural coloring agent when pickling ume boshi plums, radishes, and ginger. In salads, the leaves provide extra color and flavor.

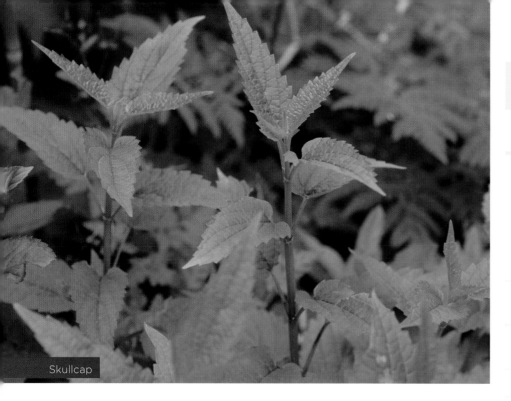
Skullcap

Sorrel, French and Red-Veined

Rumex acetosa, R. sanguineus var. *sanguineus*

Sorrel is a delicious vegetable that also doubles as a medicinal herb. Once a wild-harvested food in Europe and parts of Asia, sorrel is now grown as a garden plant throughout much of the world.

ETHNIC AND OTHER NAMES: Garden sorrel, bloody dock

PERSONALITY: Perennial; herbaceous (Zones 4–9)

HEIGHT: 12 to 24 inches (30–60 cm)

BLOOM TRAITS: Spikes of greenish white flowers form large, spiky plumes, typical of members of the knotweed family (which includes buckwheat).

LIKES/DISLIKES: Prefers open meadowlike areas with plenty of moisture

PROPAGATION/MAINTENANCE: Grow sorrel from seed sown in early spring. It is easy and requires no special treatment. Germination occurs in about 2 weeks at a rate of around 80 percent. Transplant outdoors in mid- to late spring and space 12 to 15 inches (30–38 cm) apart. Needs lots of water ideally, but plants are tolerant of moderate watering if grown in partial shade.

SUN/SOIL: Full sun to partial shade (red-veined sorrel is less tolerant of full sun); moist, loamy soil preferred, but tolerant of other soil types if they are high in organic matter

COMPANION/COMPLEMENTARY PLANTING: Sorrels are equally at home in herb and food gardens. Grow in community with watercress, lovage, and cilantro

Skullcap

Scutellaria lateriflora

Skullcap takes its name from its flowers, which look like small skulls wearing hats. They are rather small flowers, but if you look closely, you are sure to see the resemblance.

ETHNIC AND OTHER NAMES: *Casida* (Spanish)

PERSONALITY: Perennial; herbaceous (Zones 4–8)

HEIGHT: 8 to 24 inches (20–60 cm)

BLOOM TRAITS: Skullcap blooms with light blue flowers from mid- to late summer.

LIKES/DISLIKES: Skullcap prefers to grow where there is a good amount of spring moisture. It will grow near streams and wash areas where water is flowing.

PROPAGATION/MAINTENANCE: Stratify seeds for a minimum of 1 week before sowing. Sow indoors and expect to see sprouting in approximately 2 weeks.

Germination rates are usually pretty good, near 75 to 80 percent. Transplant outside after all danger of frost is past. This herb grows in clumps; space 12 inches (30 cm) apart. Provide a moderate amount of water.

SUN/SOIL: Full sun, partial shade; prefers well-drained, moist soil

COMPANION/COMPLEMENTARY PLANTING: Plant with feverfew, catnip, and valerian for a lovely effect.

HARVESTING: Aerial parts are harvested when the herb is in full flower. I cut skullcap with scissors, but snips will also work. Harvest from about 3 inches above the ground.

MEDICINAL BENEFITS: Skullcap is an excellent nervine and sedative that relieves stress, anxiety, and pain while nourishing the nervous system.

PARTS USED: Flowering aerial parts, fresh

HOME PHARMACY USES: Traditional tincture, liniment

PROPAGATION/MAINTENANCE: Sow untreated seeds indoors in mid- to late spring and transplant outside when frost danger is past. Or, plant seeds directly in the garden soil in late spring. Germination rate is about 80 percent and takes place in 1 to 2 weeks. Plants grow in clumps; space 12 to 15 inches (30–38 cm) apart. Water lightly to moderately.

SUN/SOIL: Full sun; well-drained soil

COMPANION/COMPLEMENTARY PLANTING: Very nice with fennel, angelica, and calendula or in food gardens

HARVESTING: Harvest seed heads, with a pair of strong snips, when fully ripe in late summer or early fall.

CULINARY USE: Sprinkle seeds lightly onto pasta or rice salads for a nutty flavor. The seeds are also delicious with green salads. I also like to include shelled sunflower seeds in my homemade trail mix as a snack for hiking youngsters. We call the trail mix *gorp* and it is always quite popular.

MEDICINAL BENEFITS: Good for the urinary, respiratory, and digestive tracts, and useful for winter illnesses

PARTS USED: Seeds, dried

CRAFTING: To make wild-bird treats, attach a wire to the top of a pinecone (to use as a tree hanger), then coat the cone with unsalted peanut butter. Next, roll the cone in a dish filled with unsalted sunflower seeds and millet; the seeds will stick to the peanut butter. Hang the pinecone treat in a tree near your favorite window and have a great time watching the birds as they feast.

Sweetgrass

Hierochloe odorata

This fragrant herb holds ceremonial importance to indigenous peoples of temperate regions of the Americas. Sweetgrass is used for making ritual braids and aromatic baskets.

PERSONALITY: Perennial grass (Zones 5–9)

HEIGHT: 12 to 15 inches (30–38 cm)

BLOOM TRAITS: As with most grasses, sweetgrass sports yellowish, insignificant flowers in plumes that quickly mature into seed grains. Flowering occurs in mid- to late summer.

LIKES/DISLIKES: Sweetgrass prefers sunny, open, grassy meadows and prairie habitats. It grows in most temperate regions.

PROPAGATION/MAINTENANCE: Grow sweetgrass from seed or root divisions. Seeds germinate readily if sown in late fall or early spring. Keep evenly moist and expect germination in about 2 weeks. Root divisions are equally successful. Dig up a chunk of the grass and divide the root zone into pieces about 1 inch (2.5 cm) long. Transplant root pieces into evenly moist soil, using 12-inch (30 cm) spacing. Use care not to overwater, as small pieces take time to build up a more extensive root system. Once established, water moderately.

SUN/SOIL: Full sun preferred, but will tolerate partial shade; adaptable to all well-drained soil types

COMPANION/COMPLEMENTARY PLANTING: Sweetgrass spreads, so plant it in the garden near other equally aggressive plants like yarrow and mints. To prevent spreading from becoming problematic, grow sweetgrass in a large container (15-inch or [38 cm] diameter).

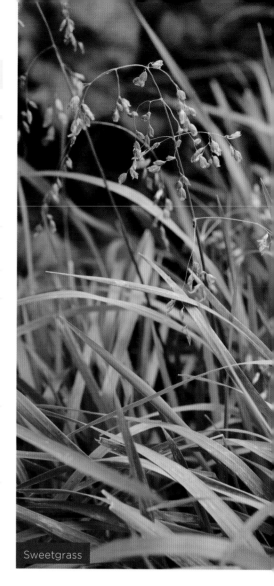

Sweetgrass

HARVESTING: Cut aerial parts using snips or scissors. Let grass stems wilt slightly before using.

CRAFTING: Sweetgrass can be braided, using slightly wilted fresh grass, into tight braids that are used ceremonially. They also create an aromatic smoke when burned in a chiminea or outside fire pit. The grass can be woven into beautiful and fragrant small baskets to hold special treasures.

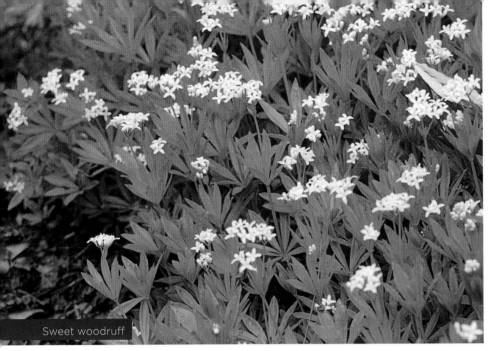

Sweet woodruff

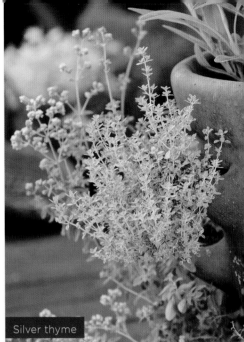

Silver thyme

Sweet Woodruff

Galium odoratum

Historically, sweet woodruff was added to May wine and drunk on May Day (May 1). It was said to "make a man merry" and it still makes for an especially refreshing drink.

PERSONALITY: Perennial; herbaceous (Zones 4–8)

HEIGHT: 8 to 12 inches (20–25 cm)

BLOOM TRAITS: Delicate, lightly fragrant white flowers in late spring and early summer

LIKES/DISLIKES: Sweet woodruff is a woodland plant by nature. It prefers shade, humusy soil, and lots of moisture. When grown in too much sunlight, the foliage becomes pale and yellowish rather than its normal deep green.

PROPAGATION/MAINTENANCE: Sow seeds as fresh as possible, and keep them in the shade to germinate. Germination rates vary from 40 to 70 percent, depending on the freshness of the seed. I find tip cuttings to be a more successful way to propagate this herb. Dip cuttings in liquid or powder rooting hormone and stick them into moist soil. Place cuttings in a shady location to root. Once a strong root structure is established, transplant outdoors and space 10 to 12 inches (25–30 cm) apart. Water heavily for ideal growing.

SUN/SOIL: Shade; rich loamy soil is preferred, but adaptable to other soil types if kept in a moist, shady area

COMPANION/COMPLEMENTARY PLANTING: Grow with watercress, lady's mantle, and heartsease.

HARVESTING: Leaves and/or flowers are cut with snips or scissors and dried in shallow baskets or on screens. Fragrance intensifies as the herb dries.

MEDICINAL BENEFITS: Use topically as a first-aid herb for cuts and scrapes.

PARTS USED: Aerial parts, fresh or dried

HOME PHARMACY USES: Skin wash, ointment, salve, cream, bath herb, foot soak

CRAFTING: The dried aerial parts are excellent for a fresh-smelling potpourri. Sew sweet woodruff into sachets to protect clothing and linens from insect damage.

Thyme

Thymus species

During the Middle Ages in Europe, thyme enjoyed important symbolic value. It was believed to protect people from harm, and soldiers bathed in thyme water to heighten their bravery.

COMMON VARIETIES OF THYME: Lemon thyme (*T. citriodorus*), silver-variegated thyme (*T. citriodorus var. aureus*), Spanish wood thyme (*T. mastichina*), Doone Valley thyme (*T. citriodorus* 'Doone Valley Lemon'), creeping thyme (*T. serpyllum*), woolly thyme (*T. pseudolanuginosus*)

ETHNIC AND OTHER NAMES: *Tomillo* (Spanish)

PERSONALITY: Perennial; herbaceous (Zones 5–9)

HEIGHT: 12 to 15 inches (30–38 cm)

BLOOM TRAITS: Flowers vary and may be purple, pink, or white. Blooming occurs on and off throughout the summer.

LIKES/DISLIKES: Native to the Mediterranean regions of Europe, thyme prefers a hot, dry climate and soils that are not too rich.

PROPAGATION/MAINTENANCE: Seed can be sown indoors for transplanting outside in late spring. Germination rates are 60 to 70 percent; sprouting takes place in about 1 week. Thyme can also be grown from cuttings, dipped in liquid rooting hormone for enhanced rooting, and from root divisions. Regardless of the method you choose, you should have good success. Space this spreading herb 10 to 12 inches (25–30 cm) apart. It requires light to moderate water.

SUN/SOIL: Full sun, partial shade; well-drained and somewhat dry soil

COMPANION/COMPLEMENTARY PLANTING: Grow in community with hyssop, garlic chives, and rosemary.

HARVESTING: Harvest the aerial parts with snips or scissors at any point during the summer.

CULINARY USE: Thyme is fantastic to season vegetable and grain dishes, and is superb with sweet corn and potatoes or in home-baked bread.

MEDICINAL BENEFITS: Thyme is beneficial for winter illnesses and immune system support. It is often recommended for digestive and respiratory concerns, sore muscles, throat conditions, nervous system support, and skin health. It is strongly antibacterial and antiseptic. The lemon varieties of thyme are highly valued in preparing "tummy" formulas for children, as they taste delicious and sweet and will quickly calm an upset stomach.

PARTS USED: Aerial parts, fresh or dried

HOME PHARMACY USES: Infusion, traditional tincture, cider vinegar tincture, syrup, elixir, ointment, salve, cream, foot soak, bath herb, infused oil, honey, butter, liniment

EDIBLE FLOWERS: Add just the flowers or leaves and flowers to pasta and potato salad for wonderful color along with great flavor.

Turmeric

Curcuma longa

Turmeric is a delicious spice, native to the tropics of India, often used in curries. It is a powerful dye for paper and fabrics, and a useful medicinal.

ETHNIC AND OTHER NAMES: *Curcuma* (French), *gurkmeja* (Swedish), *Kurkuma* or *Gelbwurz* (German)

PERSONALITY: Tender perennial; herbaceous (Zones 10–11)

HEIGHT: 12 to 24 inches (30–60 cm)

BLOOM TRAITS: Turmeric seldom blooms in cultivation.

LIKES/DISLIKES: Turmeric is a tropical plant that like its cousin ginger grows in the understory of tropical forests. It prefers a shady, moist habitat.

PROPAGATION/MAINTENANCE: Turmeric is propagated by root divisions. Divide a fresh root of turmeric into pieces, with each piece containing at least one eye (similar to a potato eye, this is where the root will sprout). Plant the root pieces sideways, as you would an iris, and not too deep, only about 2 inches. Keep the pot in a warm place and the soil evenly moist, and be patient. Turmeric takes several weeks to sprout. Turmeric will spread, although not aggressively, so space plants 15 to 24 inches (38–60 cm) apart. If growing in a container, which is how I grow mine here in Colorado, plant in a pot that is 15 to 24 inches (38–60 cm) in diameter and about 8 inches (20 cm) deep. Provide plenty of water to keep soil moist but not soggy.

SUN/SOIL: Shade; soil should be rich in organic matter and not too heavy, so loamy or sandy soil is good. When growing in a container, provide a loose potting soil mix.

COMPANION/COMPLEMENTARY PLANTING: Turmeric is a container herb for most of us, unless you

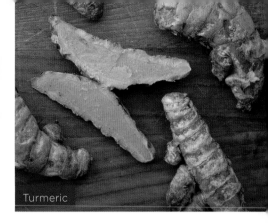
Turmeric

live in a tropical climate. It does very nicely on a shady patio or under trees that provide dappled shade. It is a nice addition to food gardens, and if you are an indoor herb gardener, turmeric will be great to include in your collection. It is best planted in its own pot, but ginger, Vietnamese coriander, and watercress can be good neighbors.

HARVESTING: Turmeric is best harvested in midwinter. Cut back the leaves and unearth the roots, removing all the soil. If your turmeric is container-grown, this process is quite easy. If your turmeric is growing in the garden, use a needle-nose spade or garden fork to lift out the roots. Harvest the roots you want to use and then replant the rest.

CULINARY USE: Turmeric is a key ingredient in curry seasoning blends, and you can also use it as an herbal food coloring for soups and rice dishes. It is sometimes used as a coloring agent in cheese.

MEDICINAL BENEFITS: The root is considered an excellent anti-inflammatory herb and is often recommended for chronic health challenges.

PARTS USED: Roots, dried or fresh

HOME PHARMACY USES: Infusion, traditional tincture, cider vinegar tincture, salve, ointment, cream

CRAFTING: The root yields a bright yellow-orange dye that is used to tint fabrics and paper. It is sometimes used as an ingredient for cosmetics in Southeast Asia.

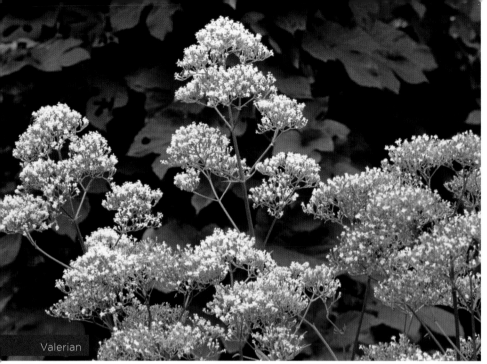

Valerian

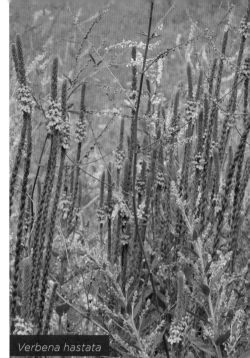

Verbena hastata

Valerian

Valeriana officinalis

Valerian root is recognized for its very strong, unpleasant fragrance. Interestingly, in spring beautifully scented flowers bloom on this pungent plant. It is an excellent medicinal herb that is widely valued.

ETHNIC AND OTHER NAMES: *Valeriana* (Spanish)

PERSONALITY: Perennial; herbaceous (Zones 4–7)

HEIGHT: 3 to 4 feet (0.9–1.2 m)

BLOOM TRAITS: Valerian flowers are intensely fragrant and white with just the palest touch of pink. They bloom in late spring and early summer.

LIKES/DISLIKES: A woodland plant by nature, valerian prefers to grow near streams, lakes, and ponds. It thrives in conditions from sun to shade providing it grows in moist soil.

PROPAGATION/MAINTENANCE: Seeds germinate well at 60 to 70 percent with no special treatment.

Sprouting takes place in 7 to 14 days. Transplant outdoors in late spring. Seed may also be sown directly into the garden in early spring. Space plants 12 to 15 inches (30–38 cm) apart; they will grow in clumps. Moderate to heavy watering is necessary.

SUN/SOIL: Full sun, partial shade (preferred), shade; likes a humusy soil

HARVESTING: The roots are harvested in the fall of the first year or the spring of the second. Valerian is a perennial plant, but the roots follow the behavior of biennial roots and begin to deteriorate in quality by the fall of the second year. For easiest harvest, use a garden fork or needle-nose spade, and dig on a day when the soil is consistently moist but not overly wet.

MEDICINAL BENEFITS: Valerian is used as a strong sedative and pain reliever.

PARTS USED: Roots, fresh or dried

HOME PHARMACY USES: Decoction, traditional tincture

Vervain

Verbena species

When vervain flowers, the blooms begin at the bottom of the green spikelet and circle their way toward the top. Gradually, over a period of several weeks, this herb finishes growing its delicate lavender flowers at the tip of the spikelet. They remind me of fairy-garden flowers.

ETHNIC AND OTHER NAMES: Herb-of-grace, verbena, *dormilón* (Spanish)

PERSONALITY: Perennial; herbaceous (Zones 3–7)

HEIGHT: 3 to 5 feet (0.9–1.5 m)

BLOOM TRAITS: Blue to purple flower spikes that stretch from spike base to tip bloom from mid- to late summer.

LIKES/DISLIKES: Blue vervain most often grows in open, grassy prairies, although it also enjoys moist locations. Its purple flowers are easily visible from some distance as it grows among native grasses and other wildflowers. Vervain is native to the Mediterranean mountains and grows best in disturbed soil.

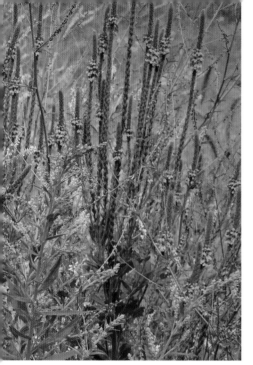

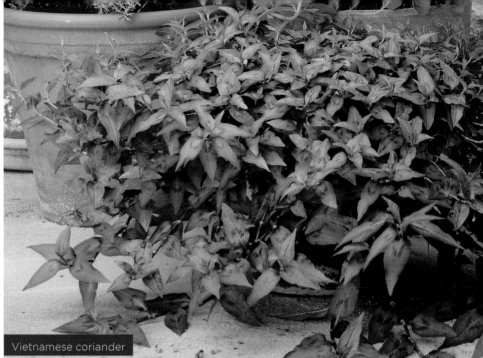

Vietnamese coriander

PROPAGATION/MAINTENANCE: Stratify the seeds for at least 2 weeks and then sow indoors. Transplant by mid- to late spring. Space 12 inches (30 cm) apart; a clump of vervain may easily grow 4 to 6 stalks on 1 plant. Water moderately.

SUN/SOIL: Sun, partial shade; well-drained soil that is reasonably high in organic matter

HARVESTING: It is preferable to harvest the aerial parts while the plant is blooming. I harvest the upper half of the plant at this time with snips or scissors.

MEDICINAL BENEFITS: Blue vervain and vervain both relieve a variety of cold and flu symptoms, such as achy muscles, respiratory congestion, and digestive tract discomfort. They are good stress-relief herbs, and are excellent for use with children.

PARTS USED: Flowering aerial parts, fresh or dried

HOME PHARMACY USES: Infusion, traditional tincture, cider vinegar tincture, syrup, elixir, ointment, salve, cream, foot soak, bath herb, honey

Vietnamese Coriander

Polygonum odorata

Vietnamese coriander can be grown in nontropical gardens as an annual ground cover. For a lovely houseplant, grow it indoors in containers or in a hanging basket, with its bicolored leaves cascading.

ETHNIC AND OTHER NAMES: *Rau ram* (Vietnamese), *daun kesom* (Malaysian), Vietnamese mint

PERSONALITY: Tender perennial; herbaceous (Zones 10–11)

HEIGHT: 8 to 10 inches (20–25 cm)

BLOOM TRAITS: In tropical climates, blossoms are reddish pink; in temperate climates, it is unlikely to bloom.

LIKES/DISLIKES: Vietnamese coriander grows near waterways in tropical, partially shaded areas. It sprawls like a ground cover and prefers a humid climate.

PROPAGATION/MAINTENANCE: Grow from cuttings or root divisions. Stems easily root wherever they come in contact with moist soil. No rooting hormone is needed. You can also dig up a chunk of the plant, trim back the tops to soil level, and separate the root mass into small pieces 1 to 2 inches (3–5 cm) in length. Plant root pieces in moist soil and expect rooting in just a couple of days. Transplant rooted plants into the garden with a spacing of 15 to 24 inches (38–60 cm). The plant will be perennial in tropical areas, but it is annual in temperate climates. It is also easy to grow in containers. Provide a lot of water.

SUN/SOIL: Full to partial shade; moist, sandy, or loamy soil high in organic matter

HARVESTING: Harvest the aerial parts, using snips or scissors.

CULINARY USE: Add Vietnamese coriander to salads for a flavor that's reminiscent of cilantro, but spicy and peppery. In Asia, it is traditionally used with pork, chicken, and fish dishes. It is also added to soups and stir-fries with a light hand. This herb has a strong flavor that people either love or hate.

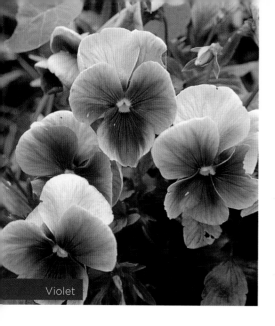

Violet

Violet

Viola species

Violets are a wonderful, old-fashioned addition to any herb garden. When they bloom, in spring and early summer, the air is filled with their lovely fragrance — amazing for such tiny flowers.

COMMON VARIETIES: Sweet violet, Labrador purple violet, wood violet

PERSONALITY: Perennial; herbaceous (Zones 2–11, depending on species)

HEIGHT: 4 to 8 inches (10–20 cm)

BLOOM TRAITS: Most of us are familiar with the purple flowers, but violets also come in yellow, pink, and white. They usually bloom in spring.

LIKES/DISLIKES: Many violets are woodland plants that prefer a shady and moist growing environment. Some species, however, grow in a variety of habitats.

PROPAGATION/MAINTENANCE: Stratify seed for a minimum of 3 months, then sow indoors in early spring. Seed prefers dark conditions to germinate, which occurs

sporadically over several weeks; expect between 30 and 40 percent overall germination. Transplant outdoors in mid- to late spring. These clumping plants reseed vigorously. Space violets 6 to 8 inches (15–20 cm) apart and water moderately to heavily.

SUN/SOIL: Full sun, partial shade, shade (depending on species); prefers a soil high in organic matter (4 to 5 percent)

COMPANION/COMPLEMENTARY PLANTING: Grow with self-heal, skullcap, and sweet woodruff.

HARVESTING: Hand-pick leaves at any time during the growing season. Pick the flowers in spring, but leave some for seed production.

CULINARY USE: Add leaves to salads or use as a lettuce substitute on sandwiches.

MEDICINAL BENEFITS: Often used for heart health, digestive tract and respiratory concerns, skin conditions, and throat ailments, violets are also helpful for women's and children's health, stress relief, and nervous system support.

PARTS USED: Leaves and flowers, fresh or dried

HOME PHARMACY USES: Infusion, traditional tincture, cider vinegar tincture, syrup, elixir, ointment, salve, cream, foot soak, bath herb, infused oil, liniment, honey

EDIBLE FLOWERS: Violet flowers can grace many dishes from fruit and leafy salads to cakes, herb butters and cream cheese spreads, jellies, and herbal flower honey. Float the flowers in beverages like limeade for a festive look. Freeze violet flowers in an ice-cube tray, then plunk a cube into iced tea.

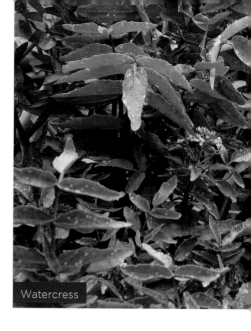

Watercress

Watercress

Nasturtium officinale

Watercress has been enjoyed as a salad herb since ancient times. It is crisp and flavorful, and full of nutrients besides.

PERSONALITY: Perennial; aquatic plant (Zones 5–10)

HEIGHT: 10 to 12 inches (25–30 cm)

BLOOM TRAITS: Delicate white flowers in spring and occasionally early summer. Blooms while temperatures are still moderate.

LIKES/DISLIKES: This herb would choose a home with its feet almost floating in a gently moving stream. It does want to be planted in actual earth, not free-floating; choose a shady spot. Never plant watercress at the edge of still water.

PROPAGATION/MAINTENANCE: Watercress is easily grown from seed sown in early spring or before the intense heat of summer arrives. Sow directly in the garden or transplant outdoors in early spring a week or so before the last frost is expected. Germination occurs in 1 to 2 weeks at around an 80 percent

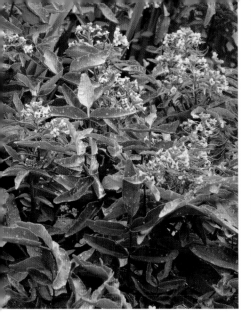

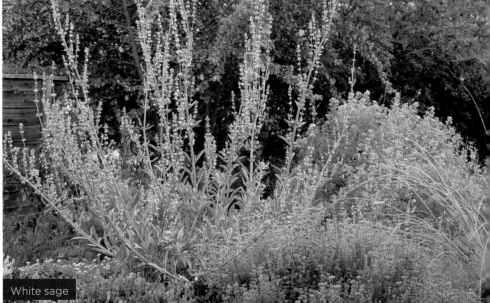

White sage

success rate. Site plants in a shady part of the garden, where the soil stays moist, or along the water's edge of a free-moving streamside. Watercress does spread a bit, but not in a troublesome way. Space plants 12 to 15 inches (30–38 cm) apart and water heavily.

SUN/SOIL: Full or partially dappled shade; moist, rich, loamy soil

COMPANION/COMPLEMENTARY PLANTING: Grow in community with gotu kola, lemon verbena, and angelica.

HARVESTING: Harvest aerial parts, with or without flowers, using snips or scissors.

CULINARY USE: Watercress is a fantastic salad herb. Mix with lettuces, a bit of dill weed, and some edible flowers for a delicious and nutritious lunch or dinner salad. You can also use the greens to top a sandwich or pita pocket wrap.

White Sage

Salvia apiana

White sage is used to make ceremonial smudge sticks used in Native American traditions. It has been greatly overharvested from the wild and is now nearly extinct in some regions. White sage is now on the United Plant Savers at-risk list, and we are hopeful that this plant will find its way into organic cultivation very soon. It is easy to grow in the garden or as a container herb.

ETHNIC AND OTHER NAMES: *Salvia blanca* (Spanish)

PERSONALITY: Tender perennial; herbaceous (Zones 8–11)

HEIGHT: 12 to 24 inches (30–60 cm)

BLOOM TRAITS: Pale blue flowers bloom in late summer.

LIKES/DISLIKES: White sage is native to southern California and northern Baja California. It prefers a sunny area and has good tolerance for hot, dry, windy conditions.

PROPAGATION/MAINTENANCE: Stratify seeds for 1 week and then sow indoors. Provide a warm nighttime temperature of 70°F (21°C) and daytime temperatures between 80 and 90°F (27–32°C). Germination is usually near 40 percent, and seeds take 2 to 3 weeks to sprout. Keep them evenly moist, but once seedlings are up, do not overwater. Transplant outdoors in late spring. They will grow in clumps; space plants 12 inches (30 cm) apart.

SUN/SOIL: Full sun; well-drained soil

HARVESTING: Harvest aerial parts with snips or scissors in late summer.

MEDICINAL BENEFITS: Useful for women's health concerns, digestive tract conditions, and throat and skin health; white sage is often recommended for winter illnesses and respiratory ailments.

PARTS USED: Aerial parts, fresh or dried

HOME PHARMACY USES: Traditional tincture, insect repellent

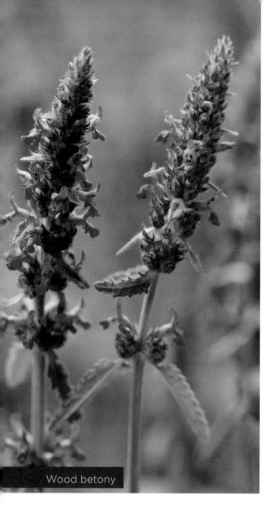

Wood betony

HEIGHT: 12 inches (30 cm)

BLOOM TRAITS: Purple, and very occasionally pink or white, blooms from midsummer on

LIKES/DISLIKES: Wood betony is a woodland plant that prefers a moist and shady growing habitat.

PROPAGATION/MAINTENANCE: Wood betony seeds should be stratified for several weeks before starting them indoors. Transplant them outdoors 10 to 12 inches (25–30 cm) apart in mid- to late spring. Each year a clump will gradually become larger, but this plant is not a rapid spreader. Its water needs are moderate to high.

SUN/SOIL: Shade, partial shade; rich garden soil is best but also grows in clay soil

HARVESTING: The aerial parts are harvested at any time during the growing season. I harvest wood betony when it is in flower, but this is not mandatory. Use scissors or snips.

MEDICINAL BENEFITS: A fantastic pain-relieving herb, wood betony is also often used to address stress and disrupted sleep patterns.

PARTS USED: Aerial parts, fresh or dried

HOME PHARMACY USES: Infusion, traditional tincture, syrup, ointment, salve, cream, foot soak, bath herb, liniment

Wood Betony

Stachys officinalis

Wood betony prefers a woodland setting. It is sometimes confused with another North American plant, Pedicularis canadensis, which is also sometimes called wood betony. However, the true wood betony is a European herb, a glorious member of the mint family. It is much easier to grow than Pedicularis and is very beautiful in the garden.

PERSONALITY: Perennial; herbaceous (Zones 5–8)

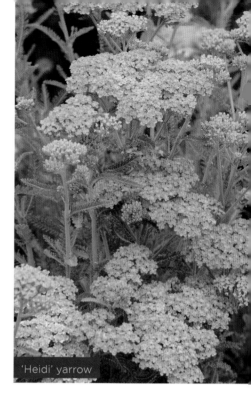

'Heidi' yarrow

Yarrow

Achillea millefolium, A. millefolium var. rosea, A. filipendulina

Native American peoples call the yarrow plant chipmunk tail because the leaf looks just like the tail of those small creatures. The lacy texture adds charm to a garden. Although some varieties of yarrow have yellow flowers, do not use them internally. Use only the white flowers of the species Achillea millefolium and the pink flowers of Achillea millefolium var. rosea.

COMMON VARIETIES OF YARROW: Traditional (white), 'Cerise Queen' (red), 'Cloth of Gold' (yellow), Colorado mix, 'Heidi'

ETHNIC OR OTHER NAMES: *Milenrama, plumajillo* (Spanish)

PERSONALITY: Perennial; herbaceous (Zones 3–9)

HEIGHT: 2 to 3 feet (0.6–0.9 meter)

BLOOM TRAITS: White, shades of pink and red, or yellow flowers appear in mid- to late summer.

LIKES/DISLIKES: Yarrow can be found in open, grassy areas such as mountain meadows and prairies. It prefers disturbed soil and grows only in temperate climates.

PROPAGATION/MAINTENANCE: Stratify seeds for a month before sowing. Sow indoors and transplant outside in mid- to late spring, or sow directly outdoors in early spring. Germination is around 70 percent; sprouting occurs in 7 to 14 days. Root divisions are another easy way to propagate yarrow. Take divisions in spring or fall for ideal results. Yarrow will spread, and needs to be spaced 12 inches (30 cm) apart. Provide plants low to moderate amounts of water.

SUN/SOIL: Full sun or partial shade; prefers well-drained soil

HARVESTING: Harvest the aerial parts in mid- to late summer, preferably while the plant is in full flower. Snips or scissors work well.

MEDICINAL BENEFITS: Yarrow is used for women's and children's health concerns, winter illnesses and respiratory conditions, the throat and the skin, and gastrointestinal health. It is also considered beneficial for circulation and muscle aches.

PARTS USED: Flowering aerial parts, fresh or dried

HOME PHARMACY USES: Infusion, traditional tincture, cider vinegar tincture, syrup, elixir, ointment, salve, cream, foot soak, bath herb, infused oil, honey, liniment

EDIBLE FLOWERS: Yarrow flower umbels can be separated into individual flowers and added to cookie batter for a confetti effect.

CRAFTING: All types of yarrow are beautiful dried. Used in wreath-making, herbal swags, and dried bouquets. Dried flower stalks are nice too.

Yerba Mansa

Anemopsis californica

Yerba mansa is often substituted for goldenseal, an at-risk herb. There is concern about yerba mansa being overharvested from wild populations, and cultivation is strongly encouraged. It can be tricky to grow from seed, so consider starting with a young nursery-grown plant to establish a patch in your garden.

ETHNIC AND OTHER NAMES: Lizard tail

PERSONALITY: Perennial; herbaceous (Zones 5–10)

HEIGHT: 12 inches (30 cm)

BLOOM TRAITS: Conical flowers with white petals bloom in late spring to early summer.

LIKES/DISLIKES: This is a desert plant that is native to the southwestern parts of North America. It prefers hot climates and chooses to grow near a water source, like ponds, streams, and lakes.

PROPAGATION/MAINTENANCE: Seeds can be tricky to germinate. Sow indoors in a very warm greenhouse. Seeds require daytime temperatures of 90 to 104°F (32–40°C) for 1 to 2 weeks and constant nighttime temperatures between 60 and 70°F (15–21°C). Keep seeds well watered before and after sprouting. Sprouting takes place in 4 to 6 weeks, at a germination rate of 70 to 80 percent. Transplant outside, 12 inches (30 cm) apart, in early summer when temperatures are consistently warm. Yerba mansa spreads by runners, similar to strawberries, and requires moderate to heavy watering.

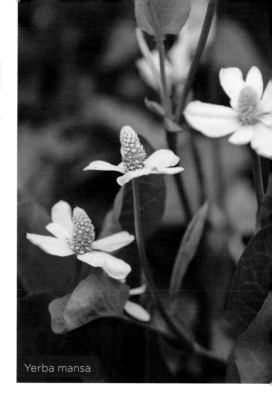

Yerba mansa

SUN/SOIL: Full sun, partial shade; prefers a moist, alkaline soil that is reasonably high in organic matter

HARVESTING: If it has been a very hot growing season with abundant water, harvest the roots or whole plants in the fall of the first year. Harvest anytime after the plant is 2 years old. I let the plants go to seed before harvesting them. Use a garden fork to lift the plants from the soil. Replant any runners that were attached to harvested plants.

MEDICINAL BENEFITS: Used for acute stages of winter illnesses and respiratory conditions, and for lymphatic support

PARTS USED: Whole plant and roots, fresh or dried

HOME PHARMACY USES: Decoction, traditional tincture, syrup, elixir, ointment, salve, foot soak, infused oil, liniment

Yucca

Yucca species

Yucca can be used in an amazing number of ways. The root is the medicinal part, but the leaves are made into fabric, mats, baskets, and twine. The flowers are delicious.

ETHNIC AND OTHER NAMES: Soapweed, *amole* (Spanish)

PERSONALITY: Perennial; herbaceous (Zones 5–10)

HEIGHT: 15 inches (38 cm) and taller

BLOOM TRAITS: Large, beautiful, cream-colored blooms appear in late spring and through the summer.

LIKES/DISLIKES: Most yuccas grow in arid regions, but they will also thrive in moist areas. They prefer wide-open, sunny places where the soil is well drained. They are common in disturbed areas.

PROPAGATION/MAINTENANCE: Stratify seed for 3 months in the freezer or for 2 weeks in moist sand in the refrigerator. Sow seed indoors and supply extra heat for optimum germination and growth. Germination percentages are usually good for treated seed, often in the neighborhood of 60 to 70 percent. Germination time is sporadic and can take up to 4 weeks, so be patient. Transplant outside, 15 inches (38 cm) apart, in late spring or early summer. Yucca grows in clumps and requires light watering.

SUN/SOIL: Full sun; well-drained soil

COMPANION/COMPLEMENTARY PLANTING: Plant in community with coyote mint, prickly pear, agastaches, and vervains.

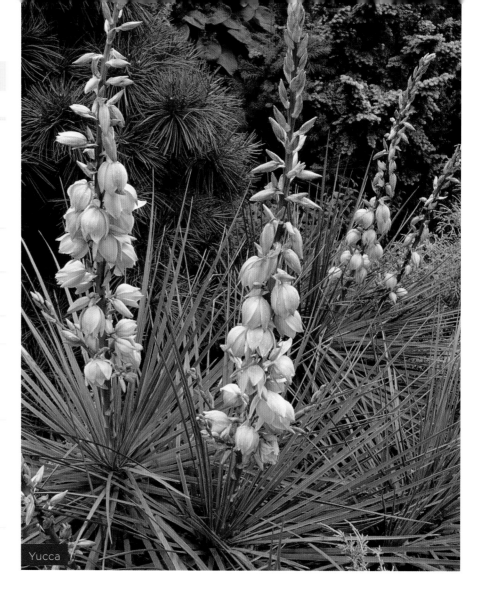

Yucca

HARVESTING: Harvest yucca roots in the fall of the second year's growth. Use a garden fork or needle-nose spade — or both — to dig roots. Leaves may be harvested in the late spring or throughout the summer using a sharp pair of snips. Wear gloves when working with these plants; they tend to poke the skin. Hand-pick flowers in spring.

MEDICINAL BENEFITS: The root is beneficial for joint conditions.

PARTS USED: Roots, leaves, and flowers, fresh or dried

HOME PHARMACY USES: Decoction, traditional tincture, cider vinegar tincture, syrup, ointment, salve, cream, foot soak, bath herb, infused oil, liniment

EDIBLE FLOWERS: Yucca flowers are tasty and beautiful in salads, especially in combination with squash blossoms.

CRAFTING: The fibers in yucca leaves are very strong, sturdy enough to weave into mats and baskets.

PLANT NAME CROSS-REFERENCE

COMMON NAME	LATIN BOTANICAL NAME	ETHNIC AND OTHER NAMES
Agastache	*Agastache rupestris, A. cana*	Sunset hyssop, double bubblegum mint
Angelica	*Angelica archangelica*	
Anise hyssop	*Agastache foeniculum*	
Astragalus, Chinese	*Astragalus membranaceus*	*Huang qi* (Chinese)
Basil	*Ocimum* species	*Albacar* (Spanish), *tulsi* (Indian for Holy Basil), *basilic* (French), *Basilikum* (German), *basilico* (Italian)
Borage	*Borago officinalis*	*Borraja* (Spanish)
Breadseed poppy	*Papaver somniferum*	Mawseed, opium poppy, white poppy
Calendula	*Calendula officinalis*	French pot marigold, pot marigold
California poppy	*Eschscholzia californica*	
Catmint	*Nepeta × faassenii*	
Catnip	*Nepeta cataria*	*Nebada* (Spanish)
Cayenne	*Capsicum* species	*Poivre de Cayenne* (French), *pepe di caienna* or *peperone* (Italian), *pimiento* or *chile* (Spanish), *Cayennepfeffer* (German), *kajennpeppar* (Swedish)
Chamomile	*Matricaria recutita, Chamaemelum nobile*	*Manzanilla* (Spanish)
Chasteberry	*Vitex agnus-castus*	Vitex, *palo santo* (Spanish)
Chives	*Allium schoenoprasum*	*Ciboulette* (French), *cipollina* (Italian), *cebolleta* (Spanish)
Cilantro, Coriander	*Coriandrum sativum*	*Coriandre* (French), *coriandolo* (Italian), *Koriander* (German)
Clary sage	*Salvia sclarea*	
Comfrey	*Symphytum × uplandicum*	
Costmary	*Tanacetum balsamita*	Balsamita, *menthe-coq, grande balsamite* (French)
Coyote mint	*Monardella odoratissima*	
Cutting celery	*Apium graveolens*	
Dill	*Anethum graveolens*	
Echinacea	*Echinacea* species	Purple coneflower
Epazote	*Chenopodium ambrosioides*	Mexican tea, *pazote* (Spanish)
Eucalyptus	*Eucalyptus* species	Blue gum tree
Fennel	*Foeniculum vulgare, F. vulgare* 'Rubrum'	*Fenouil* (French), *hinojo* (Spanish), *Fenchel* (German), *finocchio* (Italian)
Feverfew	*Tanacetum parthenium*	*Altamisa mexicana* (Spanish)
Garlic	*Allium sativum*	*Ajo* (Spanish), *Knoblauch* (German), *aglio* (Italian), *ail* (French)
Garlic chives	*Allium tuberosum*	Chinese chives, *jiu-zi* (Chinese)
Ginger	*Zingiber officinale*	*Ajenjibre* (Mexican Spanish), *jengibre* (Spanish), *gingembre* (French), *Ingwer* (German), *zenzero* (Italian), *ingefära* (Swedish)
Goldenrod	*Solidago* species	
Goldenseal	*Hydrastis canadensis*	

COMMON NAME	LATIN BOTANICAL NAME	ETHNIC AND OTHER NAMES
Gotu kola	*Centella asiatica*	
Heartsease	*Viola tricolor, V. cornuta*	Johnny-jump-up, wild pansy
Hollyhock	*Alcea* species	
Hops	*Humulus lupulus*	*Hopfen* (German), *luppolo* (Italian), *houblon* (French), *lúpulo* (Spanish)
Horehound	*Marrubium vulgare*	*Marrubio* (Spanish)
Horseradish	*Armoracia rusticana*	*Raifort* (French), *Meerrettich* or *Kren* (German), *rafano* (Italian), *rabano picante* (Spanish), *pepparrot* (Swedish)
Hyssop	*Hyssopus officinalis*	
Lady's mantle	*Alchemilla vulgaris*	
Lavender	*Lavandula* species	*Alhucema* (Spanish)
Lemon balm	*Melissa officinalis*	Melissa, balm, sweet balm, *toronjil* (Spanish)
Lemongrass, East Indian, West Indian	*Cymbopogon flexuosus, C. citratus*	*Té de limón* (Spanish)
Lemon verbena	*Aloysia triphylla*	
Licorice	*Glycyrrhiza glabra*	*Réglisse* (French), *Lakritze* (German), *regolizia* (Italian)
Lovage	*Levisticum officinale*	Garden osha (although it is not true osha, which is *Ligusticum porteri*), *céleri bâtard* (French)
Marjoram (sweet, za'atar, wild)	*Origanum majorana, O.syriaca, O. vulgare*	*E'zov* (Hebrew for za'atar marjoram), *marjolaine* (French)
Marsh mallow	*Althaea officinalis*	*Pâte de guimauve* (French)
Melaleuca, Tea tree	*Melaleuca alternifolia*	
Mexican oregano	*Lippia graveolens*	*Xomcachiift* (Seri Indian)
Monarda	*Monarda* species	Bee balm, wild oregano, bergamot, Oswego tea, *oregano de la Sierra* (Spanish)
Motherwort	*Leonurus cardiaca*	*Jaboncillo* (Spanish)
Mugwort	*Artemisia vulgaris*	Cronewort, *altamisa* (Spanish)
Mullein	*Verbascum thapsus*	*Punchón* (Spanish)
Nasturtium	*Tropaeolum majus*	Indian cress
Nettles	*Urtica dioica*	*Ortiga* (Spanish)
Oats	*Avena sativa*	Oatseed, oatstraw, *avena* (Spanish)
Oregano	*Origanum* species	*Origan* (French), *Dost* (German), *oregano* (Italian), *orégano* (Spanish)
Parsley	*Petroselinum crispum* var. *neapolitanum*	*Persil* (French), *Petersilie* (German), *prezzemolo* (Italian), *perejil* (Spanish), *persilja* (Swedish)
Passionflower	*Passiflora incarnata, P. edulis*	Maypop, apricot vine (*P. incarnata*), purple passion fruit, granadilla (*P. edulis*)
Pennyroyal	*Mentha pulegium*	*Poleo chino* (Spanish)
Peppermint	*Mentha piperita*	*Menta peperita* (Italian), *hierbabuena* (Spanish), *Pfefferminze* (German), *menthe poivrée* (French), *pepparmynta* (Swedish)
Potentilla	*Potentilla* species	Five-fingers, cinquefoil, tormentil

Vegetable Slow-Cooker Soup,
    Hearty, 164
Verbena species. *See* vervain
vervain (*Verbena* species), 234–35,
    234–35
Vietnamese coriander (*Polygonum
    odoratum*), 72, *72*, 235, *235*
vinegar tinctures, 140
Viola species. *See* heartsease;
    violet
violet (*Viola* species), 236, *236*
    culinary uses for, 159, *159, 162,
        167*
    Flower Power Salad, 159
    harvesting, 120, *120*
    seed pod of, 122, *122*
viruses, 98
Vitex agnus-castus. See
    chasteberry

W

Water, Refreshing Mint-and-Fruit-
    Infused, 167
water chestnut substitute, 168, *168*
watercress (*Nasturtium officinale*),
    236–37, *236–37*
weed control, 88–90
    pulling weeds, 89
    tips, 89
    tools for, *89,* 89–90
    what a "weed" is, 88–89
weeds, cooking with. *See* cooking
    with garden weeds
wet climates, sharp sand for, 59, *59*

whiteflies, 107, *107*
white sage (*Salvia apiana*), 237, *237.
    See also* clary sage; sage
whole-grain oats, 166
Whole Grains Poultry Seasoning,
    153
whole plants, harvesting, 115, 118,
    118
wild garden, 34, *34, 35*
wildlife, 84, 99. *See also* animal
    pests; bats; birds
wildlife herb gardens, 46
wild marjoram. *See* marjoram
wild plants, saving, 12
wild roots, 115
windowsill gardens, 55
wood betony (*Stachys officinalis*),
    238, *238*
woodland/forest ecosystem herb
    garden, 32
wooly lamb's ears, 52

Y

yarrow (*Achillea* species), 23, *238,*
    238–39
yerba mansa (*Anemopsis califor-
    nica*), 68, 239, *239*
yucca (*Yucca* species), 240, *240*

Z

Za'atar marjoram. *See* marjoram
Zingiber officinale. See ginger
zone map, USDA, 244, *244*

Other Storey Titles You Will Enjoy

***The Herbal Home Remedy Book,* by Joyce A. Wardwell.**
A wealth of herbal healing wisdom, with advice on how to collect and store herbs, make remedies, and stock a home herbal medicine chest.
176 pages. Paper. ISBN 978-1-58017-016-1.

***Herbal Remedy Gardens,* by Dorie Byers.**
More than 35 illustrated plans for easy-to-maintain container and backyard herbal gardens.
224 pages. Paper. ISBN 978-1-58017-095-6.

***Herbal Tea Gardens,* by Marietta Marshall Marcin.**
A tea lover's gardening bible, complete growing instructions and recipes for blending and brewing.
192 pages. Paper. ISBN 978-1-58017-106-9.

***Making Herbal Dream Pillows,* by Jim Long.**
Step-by-step instructions and lavish, full-color illustrations that show how to create herbal dream blends and pillows.
64 pages. Hardcover with jacket. ISBN 978-1-58017-075-8.

***Organic Body Care Recipes,* by Stephanie Tourles.**
Homemade, herbal formulas for glowing skin, hair, and nails, plus a vibrant self.
384 pages. Paper. ISBN 978-1-58017-676-7.

Rosemary Gladstar's Herbal Recipes for Vibrant Health.
A practical compendium of herbal lore and know-how for wellness, longevity, and boundless energy.
408 pages. Paper. ISBN 978-1-60342-078-5.

These and other books from Storey Publishing are available
wherever quality books are sold or by calling 1-800-441-5700.
Visit us at *www.storey.com.*